PHOTODERMATOLOGY

PHOTODERMATOLOGY

Edited by
J.L.M. Hawk

Department of Photobiology
St John's Institute of Dermatology
St Thomas' Hospital
London
UK

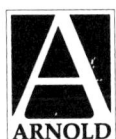

A member of the Hodder Headline Group
LONDON ● SYDNEY ● AUCKLAND
Co-published in the United States of America by
Oxford University Press Inc., New York

First published in Great Britain in 1999 by
Arnold, a member of the Hodder Headline Group,
338 Euston Road, London NW1 3BH

http://www.arnoldpublishers.com

Co-published in the United States of America by
Oxford University Press Inc.,
198 Madison Avenue, New York, NY10016
Oxford is a registered trademark of Oxford University Press

Whilst the advice and information in this book are believed to be true and
accurate at the date of going to press, neither the author[s] nor the publisher
can accept any legal responsibility or liability for any errors or omissions
that may be made. In particular (but without limiting the generality of the
preceding disclaimer) every effort has been made to check drug dosages;
however, it is still possible that errors have been missed. Furthermore,
dosage schedules are constantly being revised and new side-effects
recognized. For these reasons the reader is strongly urged to consult the
drug companies' printed instructions before administering any of the drugs
recommended in this book.

British Library Cataloguing in Publication Data
A catalogue record for this book is available from the British Library

Library of Congress Cataloging-in-Publication Data
A catalog record for this book is available from the Library of Congress

ISBN 0 340 74094 9

1 2 3 4 5 6 7 8 9 10

Typeset in 10/12 Palatino by The Florence Group, Stoodleigh, Devon
Printed and bound by The Bath Press, Bath, Avon

What do you think about this book? Or any other Arnold title?
Please send your comments to feedback.arnold@hodder.co.uk

CONTENTS

CONTRIBUTORS

KENNETH A. ARNDT
Dermatologist-in-Chief
Department of Dermatology,
Professor of Dermatology
Harvard Medical School
Beth Israel Deaconess Medical Center,
330 Brookline Avenue, Boston,
MA 02215, USA

PAUL. R. BERGSTRESSER
Department of Dermatology,
UT Southwestern Medical Center,
Dallas, Texas, USA

BRIAN L. DIFFEY
Professor of Photobiology,
Regional Medical Physics Department,
Newcastle General Hospital,
Newcastle NE4 6BE, UK

JEFFREY S. DOVER
Department of Dermatology,
New England Deaconess Hospital,
110 Francis Street,
Boston MA0215, USA

GEORGE H. ELDER
Department of Medical Biochemistry,
University of Wales College of Medicine,
Heath Park, Cardiff CF4 4XN,
Wales, UK

PETER M. FARR
Consultant Dermatologist,
Royal Victoria Infirmary,
Newcastle on Tyne, UK

JAMES FERGUSON
Consultant Dermatologist,
Photobiology Unit,
Ninewells Hospital and Medical School,
Dundee DD1 9SY, Scotland, UK

BARBARA E. GILCHREST
Professor and Chair of Dermatology,
Department of Dermatology,
Boston University School of Medicine,
Boston MA 02118, USA

JOHN L.M. HAWK
Department of Photobiology,
St John's Institute of Dermatology,
St Thomas' Hospital,
London SE1 7EH, UK

ROBERT M. HERD
Department of Dermatology,
East Campus,
Beth Israel Deaconess Medical Center,
330 Brookline Avenue, Boston,
MA 02215, USA

RACHEL E. HERSCHENFELD
Department of Dermatology,
Boston University School of Medicine,
Boston MA 02118, USA

ERHARD HÖLZLE
Professor of Dermatology,
Department of Dermatology,
City Hospital Oldenburg,
Dr-Eden-Str. 10, 28133 Oldenburg,
   Germany

BARBARA HONIG
Instructor, Department of Dermatology,
Johns Hopkins University School of
   Medicine,
Metropolitan Medical associates, P.A.,
Russell Morgan Building, Third Floor,
   5601 Loch Raven Boulevard,
   Baltimore MA 21239, USA

HERBERT HÖNIGSMANN
Division of Special and Environmental
   Dermatology,
University of Vienna Medical School,
Vienna, Austria

ALAN R. LEHMANN
MRC Cell Mutation Unit,
University of Sussex,
Falmer,
Brighton BN1 9RR, UK

NICHOLAS J. LOWE
UCLA School of Medicine,
Skin Research Foundation of
   California,
2001 Santa Monica Boulevard 490W,
Santa Monica,
CA 90404, USA

JANE M. McGREGOR
Department of Photobiology,
St John's Institute of Dermatology,
St Thomas' Hospital,
London SE1 7EH, UK

HÉLÈNE DU P. MENAGÉ
Department of Photobiology,
St John's Institute of Dermatology,
St Thomas' Hospital,
London SE1 7EH, UK

WARWICK L. MORISON
Department of Dermatology
Johns Hopkins University
Baltimore MD 21287, USA

GILLIAN M. MURPHY
Photobiology Unit,
Department of Dermatology,
Beaumont and Mater Misericordiae Hospitals,
Dublin, Ireland

PAUL G. NORRIS
Department of Dermatology,
Addenbrooke's Hospital,
Cambridge CB2 2QQ, UK

BERNHARD ORTEL
Wellman Laboratories of Photomedicine,
50 Blossom Street, MGH, Boston,
MA 02114, USA

GARY L. STEVENS
Department of Dermatology,
UT Southwestern Medical Center,
Dallas, Texas, USA

CHARLES R. TAYLOR
Wellman Laboratories of Photomedicine,
50 Blossom Street, MGH, Boston,
MA 02114, USA

LAURA E. TOWNE
Refer to co-authors Warwick L. Morison and
   Barbara Honig

FREDERICK URBACH
Temple Medical Practices,
220 Commerce Drive,
Fort Washington, PA 19034, USA

IAN R. WHITE
St John's Institute of Dermatology,
St Thomas' Hospital,
London SE1 9RT, UK

ANTONY R. YOUNG
Department of Photobiology,
St John's Institute of Dermatology,
St Thomas' Hospital,
London SE1 9RT, UK

FOREWORD

Thomas B. Fitzpatrick and
Klaus Wolff

This book is a celebration of the alliance of photobiology and photomedicine. In the 1960s, a large database in photochemistry and photobiology had been developed, although the light sources used by photobiologists for these studies emitted largely, if not exclusively, ultraviolet (UV) C (100–280 nm) radiation, which has no application to human disease. However, also in the early 1960s, there was the beginning of scientific enquiry into the human photosensitivity disorders with the development of a monochromatic irradiation source by Professor Ian Magnus of London, teacher and mentor of Dr John Hawk, editor of this book, and one of the pioneers of the introduction of scientific method into medical photobiology.

Thus, there has existed, until relatively recently, a large gap between the photobiologist-photochemists and the physician-scientists in the development of photobiology. However, this hiatus has rapidly narrowed in the past two decades, with a new subspecialty, photomedicine, now becoming the unifying conceptualization to bring together these two diverse groups of scientists, working at all the different levels of organization between the molecule and the patient.

The International Conference on Photosensitization and Photoprotection held in Tokyo in 1972 can be considered the first major international meeting of scientists and physicians working in photobiology, and the monograph *Sunlight and Man*, based on the proceedings of that meeting – a 'line in the sand' at that time – was the first major publication to put photomedicine on to the map of scientific disciplines. Many have since followed, but the present book created by John Hawk is certainly the most comprehensive and up-to-date, state-of-the-art publication in the subject and has been made possible with the help of a new generation of highly competent scientific photobiological authors.

The rapprochement of basic science and clinical investigation crystallized in this book came about in part as a result of the widespread increase in popularity of phototherapy coincident with the introduction in 1974 of carefully controlled psoralen photochemotherapy (PUVA) into the treatment of cutaneous disease. However, it should not be forgotten that serendipitous photomedicine historically dates back to the beginning of civilization, when skin treatment by exposure to sunlight, or heliotherapy, was found to improve certain cutaneous disease states, which was enhanced in the case of depigmenting disorders by the associated use of certain extracts of plants and seeds. With a long history in India and Egypt, this latter technique of PUVA was first employed in the Western world in 1918 when Axmann painted oil of bergamot on to similar depigmented spots, but it was not until 1948 that El Mofty first reported on his wide experience with the use of psoralens in the treatment of vitiligo and one of us (TBF), with Aaron Lerner, introduced this modality into the United States.

Other forms of photochemotherapy were also investigated in the early years, photodynamic tumour therapy having been attempted as early as 1905 when Jesionek and Tappeiner injected eosin into basal cell carcinomas subsequently exposed to UV radiation, while Goeckermann combined topical tar with phototherapy in the treatment of psoriasis, although this combination was later shown to have only additive therapeutic effects and not to represent true photochemotherapy. UV radiation has also been used under more or less defined conditions as an adjunctive therapy for a whole variety of skin conditions, but it was only after the introduction of PUVA as a systemic treatment, and the appreciation of its dramatic effectiveness in psoriasis, that an enthusiastic and rapid expansion of interest in photobiology initiated a new era in therapeutic photomedicine.

The gradual development of new light sources and the ability to better define disease action spectra also steadily led to the discovery of new or the better definition of already known UV(or visible light)-induced diseases such as erythropoietic protoporphyria (by Magnus), photoallergic contact dermatitis, polymorphic light eruption, drug photosensitivity and solar urticaria, to name just a few. Most importantly, however, the combination of photobiology, molecular biology, immunology and clinical medicine through the collaboration of photophysicists, molecular biologists, photochemists and physicians, especially dermatologists, has brought a new understanding of the mechanisms of photocarcinogenesis and the DNA repair-deficient photodermatoses, in particular, as well as of the various other photosensitivity states, and has also opened up whole new fields of basic and clinical research, such as photoimmunology and photoageing. Thus, the modulation by UV radiation of cytokine networks and the crosstalk between resident and migrating immune cells are presently a major focus for basic research that will very probably lead to

a new understanding of the mechanisms of light-induced diseases and to new approaches to their treatment.

However, let us return to the discipline of therapeutic photomedicine, which has been a burgeoning field for only the past two decades. The 'jumpstart' for this was the introduction of carefully supervised PUVA in 1974 when the first controlled clinical trials of the efficacy of this therapy were undertaken in Boston and later Vienna, following the development of a newly developed high intensity source of UVA (315–400 nm) radiation. These large clinical trials in the USA and Europe rapidly established PUVA as a most effective treatment for psoriasis, but until this remarkable success based on the newly available UVA sources, the lighting industries in the USA and Europe had not been interested in the development of UV equipment for medical applications. However, there are now a number of lighting product groups around the world supplying sophisticated units able to deliver a whole range of UV spectral outputs and intensities: broad-band UVB lamps (280–340 nm), narrow-band UVB lamps (312 nm) and various UVA lamps (320–400 nm) for the effective control of a multitude of skin diseases, including in particular the malignant cutaneous T cell lymphoma (mycosis fungoides); thus, PUVA alone or in combination with oral retinoids is now being used in the treatment of over 23 diseases.

However, what about the photomedicine of the future? There will no doubt be new irradiation units for use alone or in combination with new chemicals for a whole host of different forms of photochemotherapy. Thus, targeted drug delivery will very likely employ either the selective tissue affinity of photosensitizers, as in photodynamic tumour therapy or selective carcinoma cell photolysis, or carriers of specific absorbing molecules, or chromophores, which may be monoclonal antibodies, liposomes, hormones or other dedicated molecules. The principle will therefore be the attachment of a photosensitizing molecule to a special carrier, which will then home to specific molecules on target cells and, following light activation, specifically destroy these targets. In fact, the effectiveness of this principle has already been shown in the treatment of rhabdomyosarcomas in mice (with monoclonal antibody haematoporphyrin derivative conjugates) and in the destruction of leukaemia cells *in vitro* (with similar or antibody-chlorine E6 conjugates); such approaches are therefore likely soon to become applicable in a clinical setting. In addition, liposomes with incorporated phototoxic molecules can be covalently attached to monoclonal antibodies and employed in the *in vitro* purging of malignant or other selected cells from bone marrow aspirates or the peripheral blood. Further, the refinement of *ex vivo* PUVA treatment systems such as photopheresis, along with a better definition of their mechanisms, will eventually allow them to be employed with a higher degree of specific targeting in a whole range of cutaneous and extracutaneous disease states, which will thereby continue to broaden their applications in the clinical medicine of the future. However, the most exciting potentials for drug targeting will be at the molecular level. Thus, antisense oligonucleotides coupled to photoactivable drugs because of the specificity of DNA base pairing will be guided to susceptible sites within specific genes, opening up the possibility of activating a chromophore by UVA irradiation once an oligonucleotide is in place and thereby inactivating a gene or its transcripts. A considerable amount of sophisticated research is still required before this concept can be effectively translated into clinical medicine, but it now seems reasonable to assume that this will be feasible in the future.

These likely therapeutic advances, along with the present explosion of knowledge in molecular immunology, make the future of photomedicine ever more exciting. When the mechanisms controlling cytokine networks and how they are perturbed or modulated by UV radiation or visible light are clarified and once it has been determined how such perturbations or modulations can be pharmacologically counteracted or corrected, not only may we arrive at the paradoxical state in the development of phototherapy where light may no longer be needed but we may also have succeeded in unravelling the mysteries of causation of the many clinical photobiological events affecting either all exposed normal subjects or else the many with photosensitivity disorders and we may then be able to treat these many conditions finally and fully. This excellent book shows most comprehensively just how far we have come along the path towards these goals in so short a time and for this we have to thank John Hawk and his exceptionally competent band of authors. Photobiologists, of all disciplines, now read on!

PREFACE

It is extraordinary that the matter comprising the sun and all living organisms on this earth once probably formed part of the same vast celestial dust cloud, which on the one hand condensed into an extremely massive central object emitting largely damaging radiation by virtue of its mass and associated gravitational forces, and on the other into planets from one of which emerged, by perhaps random evolutionary events, the human organism which is now highly susceptible to the effects of that radiation. This battle between such vastly different end products from the same putative original matter has been waged ever since both were formed, and an uneasy truce now rules, perhaps with man temporarily moving ahead, as his mental capacities have increased sufficiently to outwit his otherwise heavily favoured competitor. It is this contest and the associated offensive events and defensive strategies which are now the subject of this book.

Thus the sun has continued to pour out unending streams of potentially harmful particles of energy, and the human organism has continuously adapted to survive this onslaught from primeval times, at least as long as needed to enable its successful reproduction and survival; however, in the very recent modern era of increasing competence in human health management, we have also at last begun to use our cerebral capabilities to ensure that the damage done to our skins is minimised for as long as we live. To enable this, we have carefully studied the photophysics and photochemistry of solar radiation and its behaviour in space, the atmosphere and our skins, and have also investigated the responses of the human organism and in particular the skin to this attack; as a result, we have now been able to hone strategies to improve our cutaneous survival and well-being, along with also developing preventive and therapeutic medications, and therapeutic surgical techniques, to minimise, neutralise or reverse the damage which does still occur.

This constant war is one that inevitably involves us all upon this earth, each being exposed to sunlight's almost universally damaging effects, and up to about a quarter also suffer abnormal, pathological effects for genetic, iatrogenic or perhaps chance-associated reasons. However, since such events are so important to so many of us, it is now entirely appropriate that the very latest information on these matters should be presented in its latest precise detail in a readable, easily comprehensible style for the ultimate benefit of all who are subject to the sun's rays. It is for this reason therefore that I have taken the opportunity to call together a host of the world's leading experts in the field of photobiology, asking them to produce a state of the art text which summarises in great detail most that is known at the present time about photodermatology, a knowledge that is very considerable. All the senior authors are renowned experts in their fields, and it is with great pleasure that I am able to present to you a collation of their admirable work. Please take advantage, and enjoy the privilege, of it. I have thoroughly enjoyed the editing, and I know you will now thoroughly enjoy the result. Thank you very much indeed to all my authors! Reader, proceed!

John Hawk
Editor

THE HISTORY OF HUMAN PHOTOBIOLOGY

Jane M. McGregor

Human photobiology, or photomedicine, may be defined as the application of the physical and biological principles of photochemistry, photophysics and photobiology to the diagnosis, treatment and understanding of human disease; photodermatology, on the other hand, relates in these matters purely to the skin. That these disciplines derive from such diverse origins, perhaps more than any other medical specialty, is both their strength and their weakness. In his introductory remarks to a major photobiological conference in 1969, Harold Blum stated that:

> The phenomena we have to consider [in photomedicine] are basically photochemical reactions, using the term in a broad sense; but we are forced to study them in a system and under conditions that no self-respecting photochemist would choose if he could help himself. The optics of the system are likewise such as the physicist would not be likely to elect for research; and the physiological properties perhaps even more complicated and uncertain than those with which most biologists are accustomed to deal. So all of us – photochemists, physicists, and biologists of various types and degrees – may be called upon to share our knowledge of different aspects of a difficult problem, which no one of us is likely to resolve entirely by himself. This calls for a good deal of mutual understanding and tolerance, for any one of us is likely to find himself naïve in certain areas no matter how well informed in others.

It is, however, to the philosophers and physicians of the ancient civilizations that we should attribute the earliest history of photomedicine. For example, the Greek sun god, Apollo, was also the spiritual god of healing, providing the first documentation of an association between sunlight and health. Apollo's mortal messenger on earth was Aesculapius, a mythical physician whose healing powers became so famous that his immortal grandfather, Zeus, was said to have become jealous and killed him with a thunderbolt. In 525BC, Herodotus observed that the strength of a man's skull was related to sunlight exposure, predating the formal discovery of the role of sunlight in vitamin D metabolism by over 2000 years. At about the same time, the Egyptians were using psoralens, derived from plant extracts, in combination with sunlight to 'cure' vitiligo, some 2000 years before the advent of modern photochemotherapy.

The more recent evolution of photomedicine, on the other hand, owes a debt to physicists, chemists, biologists and physicians alike. Discoveries made in the century between 1818 and 1912, for example, established the 'Laws

Photodermatology. Edited by J.L.M. Hawk. Published in 1998 by Chapman & Hall, London. ISBN 0 412 72460 X.

of Photochemistry', laws which remain fundamental to our current understanding of the immediate reactions of biological systems to radiation. Increasingly, however, photomedicine is now concerned with the structural, inflammatory and immunological changes which take place in human tissues long after exposure to radiation. These reactions, which are clearly many steps beyond the primary photochemical reaction described by Einstein in 1912, are likely to play important roles in ageing and carcinogenesis as well as in the development of photosensitive eruptions in susceptible individuals. Further, with modern technology, the genetic basis of some of the inheritable photodermatoses and skin cancer-prone syndromes has now been discovered.

Details of the step-by-step advances in the understanding of human photobiology are outlined below.

A CHRONOLOGICAL HISTORY OF PHOTOMEDICINE

2750BC   Aton Ra, from whom the word 'radiation' derives, is worshipped in Egypt as a sun god.

c. 800BC   Worship of Helios, the Greek sun god responsible for the word **heliotherapy**. Apollo, later also a Greek sun god and a god of healing, and his mortal messenger, Aesculapius, the mythical physician, hold sway.

525BC   Herodotus related the strength of the skull to sunlight exposure, predating the more precise explanation of the role of sunlight in vitamin D metabolism by some 2400 years.

1666AD   Isaac Newton '. . . procured me a triangular glass prism, to try therewith the celebrated Phaenomena of colours'.

c. 1798   Robert Willan described what was probably the first reported case of polymorphic light eruption, referred to as 'eczema solaris'.

1800   Sir William Herschel demonstrated the existence of radiation beyond the red end of the visible spectrum, now known as infrared radiation.

1801   Johann Ritter discovered the ultraviolet region of the solar spectrum.

1818   Grotthus formulated the First Law of Photochemistry – that only absorbed radiation is effective in producing a photochemical change.

c. 1820   Humphrey Davy developed the first artificial source of radiation by creating an electrical discharge in air between charcoal electrodes.

1839   Draper verified, through experiment, the validity of the First Law of Photochemistry, now also referred to as the Draper–Grotthus Law.

1842   Description of the Second Law of Photochemistry, or the Bunsen–Roscoe Reciprocity Law, that if the product of radiation intensity and exposure time is constant, the photochemical effect remains the same.

1850   Publication of the Lambert–Beer Law, that the fraction of incident radiation absorbed by a substance in solution is independent of the radiation intensity but increases proportionally with increasing concentrations of the substance.

1852   E.H. Jackson of London patented the first mercury lamp incorporating carbon electrodes.

1859   Charcot proposed that skin erythema might be produced by exposure to the rays of an electric arc.

1862   Bazin first described hydroa vacciniforme.

1877   Downes and Blunt described the antibacterial effect of sunlight on living systems.

1892   Ward demonstrated that the most efficient antibacterial action is produced by the ultraviolet region of the solar spectrum.

1893   Niels Finsen (1860–1904) of Copenhagen, widely regarded as the father of modern phototherapy, described the biological importance of the ultraviolet component of sunlight in his first article *On the Influence of Light on the Skin*. In a series of subsequent articles, written between 1893 and 1896, he then demonstrated the central role of the ultraviolet radiation component of the solar spectrum in producing sunburn erythema.

   He is perhaps most famous for his development of the Finsen lamp, essentially a carbon arc source, which he developed for the artificial production of radiation to treat human disease, most notably lupus vulgaris. In 1903, he was awarded the Nobel Prize in recognition of his contribution to medicine.

1894   Unna first described the relationship between sunlight exposure and skin cancer.

1900   J. Prime described the first clinical study of chemical photosensitivity.

1901   Max Planck formulated the law of quantum physics which states that radiation is emitted in discrete bundles, or quanta, of energy, known in photobiology as **photons**.

1904   Merklen described the first case of solar urticaria.

1908–1912 Stark (1908) and Einstein (1912) postulated the Stark–Einstein Law of Photochemical Equivalence, that each quantum of radiation absorbed activates just one molecule in the primary step of a photochemical process. The number of molecules of reactant consumed or product formed per quantum of radiation absorbed is then known as the **quantum yield**.

1921   Hausser and Vahle published action spectra for the induction of erythema and melanogenesis in human skin. They were the first to employ an irradiation monochromator for such studies, using an artificial mercury lamp source in conjunction with a double quartz prism monochromator.

1924   The Sunlight League was formed in London, in recognition of the importance of sunlight in preventing rickets and its then recently discovered antibacterial properties. Its stated aims included '. . . teaching the nation that sunlight is Nature's universal disinfectant, as well as a stimulant and tonic'.

1929   Gates published an action spectrum for the bactericidal effect of ultraviolet radiation, confirming the previous work of Bie and Bang, two of Finsen's co-workers who had proposed that wavelengths shorter than 300 nanometres (nm) especially around 250 nm, were most effective at killing bacteria.

c. 1930   In recognition of the wide inter-subject variation in photosensitivity and the fact that the biological effects of ultraviolet radiation vary with changes in its wavelength, the Council of Physical Therapy of the American Medical Association introduced the concept of the **erythemal unit**, defined as the radiant exposure at 296.7 nm necessary to produce just perceptible erythema on untanned Caucasian skin (approximately $150 \, \text{J/m}^2$).

1932   At the Second International Congress on Light, held in Copenhagen, it was recommended that the ultraviolet spectrum (UV) should be divided into three spectral regions:

UVA   400–315 nm
UVB   315–280 nm
UVC   < 280 nm

The lower limit of the UVC region is now taken to be 100 nm by the International Commission on Illumination (CIE) and the Health and Safety Executive (HSE) and National Radiation Protection Board (NRPB) in the United Kingdom, but is defined as 200 nm by the National Institute for Occupational Safety and Health (NIOSH) in the United States. In addition, later workers have used less precise definitions of 400–320 nm for UVA and 320–290 nm for UVB.

1933   First edition of the handbook *Actinotherapy Techniques*, produced by the Sollux Publishing Company, detailing the benefits of ultraviolet therapy in a variety of human disorders.

1945   Harold Blum published his studies on the ultraviolet dose–response relationship for the development of skin tumours in mice, demonstrating that wavelengths shorter than 320 nm are most effective.

Major advances after this date are dealt with in the remainder of this book.

HUMAN EXPOSURE TO ULTRAVIOLET RADIATION

Brian L. Diffey

The sun is responsible for the development and continued existence of life on earth. We are warmed by its infrared rays and see with eyes that respond to the visible part of its spectrum. More importantly, visible light is essential for photosynthesis, the process whereby plants, necessary for our nutrition, derive their energy. Besides serving as the ultimate source of his food and energy, sunlight also acts on man to alter his chemical composition, control his rate of maturation and drive his biological rhythms. However, the ultraviolet (UV) component, which comprises only approximately 5% of terrestrial solar radiation, is largely responsible for the deleterious effects associated with sun exposure.

Before the beginning of this century, the sun was our only source of exposure to such radiation but with the advent of artificial sources, the opportunity for additional exposure has increased. Such exposure may be elective (e.g. sunbathing, cosmetic tanning with sunbeds or medical therapy) or adventitious, often as a consequence of occupation (e.g. electric arc welders).

NATURE AND SOURCES OF ULTRAVIOLET RADIATION

Ultraviolet radiation covers only a small part of the electromagnetic spectrum. It consists of

Photodermatology. Edited by J.L.M. Hawk. Published in 1998 by Chapman & Hall, London. ISBN 0 412 72460 X.

energy emitted during transition of a molecular electron from an excited, higher to a less energetic, lower molecular orbital. Each emission is a discrete, oscillating electromagnetic pulse of energy, E (joules, J) and wavelength, λ (nanometres, nm, 10^{-9} m), travelling through space at velocity, c (3×10^8 m/s), such that $E = hc/\lambda$, where $h = 6.63 \times 10^{-34}$ J/s (Planck's constant). Thus a photon of 3000 nm UV radiation has energy 6.63×10^{-19} J, where 1 J accelerates 1 kg over 1 m in 1 s to a velocity of 1 m/s in a frictionless environment. Multiple molecular emissions create a radiation wavefront diverging from its source with gradually diminishing intensity per unit area, the total energy of the wavefront being the sum of its photon energies. Such energy incident on a surface is the radiant exposure, exposure dose or fluence (J/m^2, previously mJ/cm^2) and the rate of incidence, the irradiance, dose rate or intensity (W/m^2, previous mW/cm^2), where 1 W = 1 watt = 1 J/s.

Other regions of the electromagnetic spectrum include radiowaves, microwaves, infrared radiation (heat), visible light, X-rays and gamma radiation, the feature that characterizes any particular region of the spectrum being its wavelength, with UV radiation spanning the region from 400 to 100 nm. Even in the UV portion of the spectrum, however, the biological effects of the radiation vary enormously with wavelength and for this reason that spectrum is further subdivided into three regions:

UVA   400–315 nm
UVB   315–280 nm
UVC   280–200 nm

UVA radiation is further subdivided into UVAI (400–340 nm) and UVAII (340–315 nm). These subdivisions are, however, arbitrary and differ somewhat depending on the scientific discipline involved. Environmental photobiologists normally define the wavelength regions as UVA 400–320 nm; UVB 320–290 nm; and UVC 290–200 nm and choose the division between UVB and UVC as 290 nm, since UV radiation at shorter wavelengths is unlikely to be present in terrestrial sunlight, except at high altitudes. The choice of 320 nm as the division between UVB and UVA, on the other hand, is perhaps more arbitrary, since although radiation at wavelengths shorter than 320 nm is generally more photobiologically active than at longer wavelengths, advances in molecular photobiology indicate that a subdivision at 330–340 nm may be more appropriate (Peak and Peak, 1986).

Ultraviolet radiation is produced either by heating a body to an incandescent temperature, as is the case with solar UV, or by the passage of an electric current through a gas, usually vaporized mercury, the mercury atoms becoming excited by their collisions with electrons flowing between the lamp's electrodes. The excited electrons then return to specific fixed electronic states in the mercury atom and thereby release some of the energy they have absorbed in the form of optical, that is, UV, visible and infrared, radiation.

The spectrum of the radiation thus emitted consists of a limited number of discrete wavelengths (so-called **spectral lines**) corresponding to the electron transitions characteristic of the mercury atom, the relative intensities of the different wavelengths in the spectrum depending upon the pressure of the mercury vapour. Lamps containing mercury vapour at about atmospheric pressure (medium-pressure mercury arc lamps) emit radiation at several different wavelengths in the UVC, UVB, UVA, visible and short infrared regions, while the addition to them of traces of metal halides, such as lead iodide or iron iodide, enhances both the power and composition of this spectrum, particularly in the UVA and visible regions.

A final common way of producing UV radiation is by fluorescent lamps or tubes, which are low-pressure mercury vapour lamps with phosphor coatings applied to the inside of the glass (sometimes referred to as the **envelope**). At low mercury vapour pressures, a predominant spectral line emitted at wavelength 253.7 nm radiation is efficiently absorbed by the phosphor; this then results in the fluorescent re-emission of a wavelength range determined by the chemical nature of the phosphor material. Phosphors are available which produce their fluorescence radiation mainly in the visible (for artificial lighting purposes), the UVA or the UVB regions.

SOLAR ULTRAVIOLET RADIATION

The spectrum of extraterrestrial solar radiation approximates to that of a black body of about 5800 K. Its irradiance outside the atmosphere but at the earth's mean distance from the sun is termed the **solar constant** and is 1.37 kW/m². Of this, about 9% is in the UV region ($\lambda < 400$ nm). The solar output is not, however, constant but varies with an apparent 27-day solar rotation and an 11-year cycle of sunspot activity. This variability affects mostly those wavelengths which are absorbed in the atmosphere ($\lambda < 290$ nm) and the effect on terrestrial UVB (290–320 nm) and UVA (320–400 nm) is minimal. Because of the elliptical solar orbit the sun–earth distance varies by about 3.4% from a minimum at the perihelion (about 3 January) to a maximum at the aphelion (about 5 July). This causes a variation in intensity of about 7% and results in slightly higher UV levels in Southern hemisphere summers than in the Northern hemisphere (Madronich, 1993).

SOLAR ELEVATION

Both the quality (spectrum) and quantity (intensity) of terrestrial radiation vary with the elevation of the sun above the horizon or **solar altitude.** (The complementary angle between the sun and the local vertical is termed the **solar zenith angle**.) The solar altitude depends on the time of day, day of year and geographical location (latitude and longitude). UV intensity changes with this altitude because as the solar zenith angle increases, the number of UV rays emitted by the sun into a given solid angle is distributed over a larger area on the earth's surface. If we neglect absorption in the atmosphere, the intensity at a solar zenith of $\theta°$ is simply equal to the intensity with the sun directly overhead (solar zenith of $0°$) multiplied by the cosine of θ. However, we cannot neglect the attenuation of UV radiation by the atmosphere, particularly ozone (see below for detail), since this also serves to absorb UV in a wavelength-dependent manner and hence change its spectrum relative to that of extraterrestrial sunlight. As a result, as the sun sinks, the UV path length through the atmosphere increases and the UV intensity reaching the earth's surface steadily decreases, particularly at wavelengths shorter than 320 nm. At noon on a summer's day, however, UVB comprises approximately 5% of the terrestrial UV and UVA the remaining 95%. However, since UVB is much more effective than UVA at causing biological damage, it contributes about 80% of the harmful effects we associate with sun exposure at that time, while UVA contributes only the remaining 20%.

ATMOSPHERIC ATTENUATION

The quality and quantity of solar UV are modified by its passage through the atmosphere. The principal events in the stratosphere (~10–50 km above sea level (asl)) are UV absorption by ozone and scattering by molecules such as nitrogen and oxygen. In the troposphere (0–~10km asl), however, absorption by pollutants such as ozone, nitrogen dioxide and sulphur dioxide and scattering by particulates (e.g. soot) and clouds are the main attenuating processes.

CLOUDS

Since pure water is a very weak absorber of UV radiation, clouds, which are composed of either liquid or ice droplets, attenuate primarily by scattering. Cloud droplets have radii from about 1 to 30 μm, considerably larger than UV wavelengths, and thus attenuate UVB and UVA to much the same extent. Clouds thereby reduce UV intensity, although not to the same extent as infrared (heat) intensity, and the risk of skin overexposure is therefore increased because the warning sensation of heat is diminished. Roughly speaking, the ambient annual UV radiation intensity as a result of cloud effects is about two thirds that estimated for clear skies at temperate latitudes, rising to about 75% for the tropics (Frederick and Alberts, 1992).

SURFACE REFLECTION

Reflection of solar UV radiation from most ground surfaces is normally less than 10%. The main exceptions are gypsum sand which reflects about 15–30% and snow which can reflect up to 90%. Contrary to popular belief, calm water reflects only about 5% of incident UV radiation, although up to 20% is reflected in choppy conditions. Since UV rays pass easily into water, however, swimming at the surface of either the sea or open-air pools offers little protection against sunburn.

PERSONAL EXPOSURE TO SOLAR ULTRAVIOLET RADIATION

The solar UV radiation to which an individual is exposed depends upon:

- the intensity of ambient solar ultraviolet radiation

- the fraction of ambient exposure received at an anatomical site
- personal behaviour and time spent outdoors.

The UV dose absorbed by the skin may be further modified by the use of photoprotective agents such as hats, clothing and sunscreens.

Estimates of personal UV exposure can be obtained in two ways: by direct measurement with UV sensitive film badges (Diffey, 1989a) or by independent determination of the three variables above, by measurement, modelling or a combination of both. The results obtained from a number of such studies in Northern Europe (Challoner *et al.*, 1976; Knuschke and Barth, 1996; Larkö and Diffey, 1983; Leach *et al.*, 1978; Schothorst *et al.*, 1985; Slaper, 1987; Webb, 1985) indicate that indoor workers in Northern Europe receive an annual exposure of around 200 **standard erythema doses (SED)***, mainly from weekend and vacation exposure and principally to the hands, forearms and face. This value is approximately 5% of the total ambient radiation available.

Outdoor workers at the same latitudes receive about 2–3 times these exposure doses (Larkö and Diffey, 1983; Webb, 1985), whilst film badge studies (Gies *et al.*, 1995) on three groups of outdoor workers on the Sunshine Coast in Queensland (27°S) suggest that annual exposures there are considerably higher – certainly in excess of 1000 SED per year.

Children have a greater opportunity for outdoor exposure and receive an annual dose in the UK of around 300 SED. For indoor workers, however, the annual exposure associated with occupation (travelling to and from work, going outside at lunchtime) is about 40 SED, while about 100 SED is contributed by weekend exposure and a further 60 SED by vacational exposure. In the case of children, 'occupational' exposure (at playtime and lunchtime) may be about 60 SED, recreational about 180 SED (because children are at school for only about 190 days per year) and vacation with parents about 60 SED. It must be stressed, however, that there will be large variations within a given population group according to individual propensities for outdoor activities.

SUN EXPOSURE OF CHILDREN AND ADOLESCENTS

Different investigators have examined the sun protection behaviour of children (Bennetts *et al.*, 1991; Grob *et al.*, 1993) and adolescents (Cockburn *et al.*, 1989; Fritschi *et al.*, 1992; Grob *et al.*, 1993; Pratt and Borland, 1994), recorded episodes of sunburn in children (Jarrett *et al.*, 1993; Melia and Bulman, 1995), evaluated the success of primary prevention campaigns aimed specifically at children (Boldeman *et al.*, 1991) and adolescents (Hughes *et al.*, 1993; Mermelstein and Riesenberg, 1992) and measured the UV exposure of children taking part in outdoor sporting activities (Melville *et al.*, 1991; Rosenthal *et al.*, 1990).

The variability of exposure within apparently 'homogeneous' groups has been demonstrated in a recent large-scale study of the outdoor UV exposure of 180 children and adolescents (Diffey *et al.*, 1996). The study examined the outdoor exposure of children and adolescents over a three-month summer period in North-East (55°N), South-Central (51°N), and South-West (50°N) England using polysulphone film badges (Fig. 2.1) and exposure diaries recording time spent outdoors. On average, personal exposure was equal to approximately one quarter of the maximum potential dose that could have been received outside, namely 5–6% of the ambient UV radiation.

---

* 1 SED is equivalent to an erythemal weighted exposure dose of 100 J/m²; a minimal erythema on unexposed skin in subjects with skin types I–IV would be expected to require an exposure of between 1.5 and 6 SED. In order to avoid confusion between the minimal erythema dose (MED) and the SED, a numerical value of 100 J/m² was deliberately chosen for the SED to prevent its interpretation as the MED for any particular skin type.

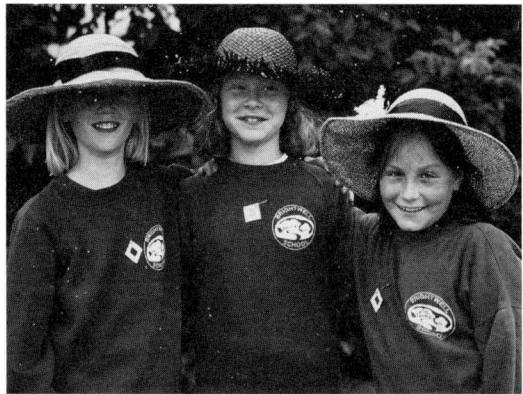

Figure 2.1 Polysulphone film badges worn by children (courtesy of National Radiological Protection Board, UK).

The strongest finding to emerge from this analysis was the observation that during weekdays and weekends, primary school children received about twice the UV exposure of pupils in secondary schools. This difference could not be accounted for entirely by any differences in time spent outdoors which, during weekdays at least, was largely similar for both school levels. Instead, it was probably more a reflection of the behaviour outdoors, with primary school children tending to play more in open spaces. At weekends, in addition, the younger children spent more time outdoors and consequently again received higher doses. That malignant melanoma may have its origins predominantly in sun exposure in childhood cannot be refuted from these data. However, although melanoma is almost twice as common in English females as males (Parkin *et al.*, 1992), the findings of this study do not suggest that it is because girls receive higher exposures than boys.

There was little evidence for geographical variation in exposure during weekdays, when school children are constrained in the time they can spend outdoors. At weekends, however, young people in Durham (55°N) received lower doses and spent less time outdoors than those further South (50–51°N),

a difference not explained solely by differences in ambient UV but suggesting rather that other factors such as culture or climate (e.g. temperature) may be involved and that population exposure cannot therefore be assumed to be a constant fraction of ambient exposure.

The epidemiological evidence linking non-melanoma skin cancer to solar UV radiation is largely indirect and based, among other things, on the relationship between tumour incidence and ambient solar UV levels (Kricker *et al.*, 1994). The results from this study, however, suggest that members of a young population who are reasonably homogeneous ethnically may have significantly different melanoma risks because of differences in their behaviour, resulting in a wide range of personal UV exposures. Indeed, over the 13-week period of the study there were many children who consistently received greater or lesser exposures than their peers.

Whilst this study provided objective data on the magnitude and range of solar UV doses received by English children and adolescents over a three-month period, the results may not necessarily be appropriate to children in other countries, where culture and solar environment are substantially different.

ANATOMICAL DISTRIBUTION OF SUNLIGHT

Film dosimeters enable evaluation of the anatomical distribution of sunlight. Table 2.1 compares the mean percentage of ambient UV radiation received relative to the vertex for a variety of anatomical sites, as measured on rotating manikins and on living subjects pursuing outdoor activities such as tennis, sailing, swimming, walking, golf and gardening. The shoulder area generally receives the highest relative exposure for all activities (approximately two thirds of the vertex), with greater variability between other sites reflecting differences in posture for different activities.

Table 2.1 Sunlight exposure (relative to 100% on vertex) for rotating manikins and living subjects engaged in tennis, golf, gardening or walking

| Site | Manikin | | Living subjects | |
	Diffey et al., 1977	Gies et al., 1992	Holman et al., 1983	Herlihy et al., 1994
Cheek	31	24	15	13
Hand	50	–	24	29
Shoulder	75	94	66	43
Back	43	36	58	40
Chest	68	50	44	23
Thigh	33	–	16	25
Calf	–	–	–	27

FACIAL EXPOSURE TO SOLAR
ULTRAVIOLET RADIATION

The face is particularly prone to solar damage because of its significantly greater exposure as compared with other anatomical sites, which are mostly covered when outside. In fact, a number of workers have used UV-sensitive film badges to measure the solar UV exposure of the face relative to the total ambient exposure in both human subjects (Holman *et al.*, 1983; Melville *et al.*, 1991; Rosenthal *et al.*, 1990, 1991) and manikins (Airey *et al.*, 1995; Diffey and Cheeseman, 1992; Diffey *et al.*, 1977, 1979; Gies *et al.*, 1988). There is considerable variation in these data, however, reflecting factors such as positioning of the film badges at different sites on the face, the behaviour of the individuals, solar altitude and the influence of shade, but representative values at different sites on the face are given in Table 2.2.

Table 2.2 Solar ultraviolet exposure on head taken from number of studies on living subjects and manikins

Site	Relative exposure
Vertex	100
Forehead	20–65
Nose	20–65
Cheek	15–40
Chin	20–35
Back of neck	20–35

The variability in these relative exposures is partly explained by the posture or angle at which the head is held and in a study of the effect of head tilt on relative exposure over the face, Airey *et al.* (1995) showed that exposure of the nose relative to the horizontal dropped from 59% to 11% as the head tilted from 0° to 60° to the normal.

THE EFFECT OF HATS ON FACIAL
EXPOSURE

Because the face is the body region mostly frequently exposed to sunlight, the protection provided by various styles of hat at different sites on the head has been measured by means of model headforms and polysulphone film badges (Diffey and Cheeseman, 1992), the recorded UV exposure being expressed as a fraction of that on an uncovered head during the same period of exposure. The reciprocal of these fractions can be thought of as the **sun protection factor** (SPF) and these results are summarized in Table 2.3. A hat with a wide brim of at least 7 cm not only protects the top of the head but provides excellent shade for the face and neck (Wong *et al.*, 1996), sites at which skin cancers commonly occur.

INFLUENCE OF CLOTHING ON EXPOSURE

Most types of textiles, both natural and man-made, provide good protection against UV radiation, fabrics often having SPFs of 20 or

Table 2.3 Summary of sun protection factors at various sites on head and neck provided by different types of hat (Diffey and Cheesman, 1992)

| Style of hat | *Typical sun protection factor (SPF)* | | | |
	Forehead	Nose	Cheek	Back of neck
Small brim (< 2 cm)	15	1.5	1	1
Medium brim (2–7 cm)	> 20	3	2	2
Large brim (> 7 cm)	> 20	7	3	5
Peaked cap	> 20	5	1.5	1

more, and studies on their spectral transmissions show that many materials absorb more or less uniformly over the whole solar UV spectrum. In other words, most clothing, in common with other forms of shade such as trees, canopies and beach umbrellas, provides a largely quantitative rather than qualitative change in cutaneous UV exposure. The Australian Radiation Laboratory has now tested several thousand samples of such clothing by a variety of laboratory methods (Gies *et al.*, 1994) and found that a number of factors affect the UV protection they offer against solar UV radiation, including in particular their weave, colour, weight, stretch and wetness.

For public information purposes, the concept of an **ultraviolet protection factor (UPF)** has now been introduced in Australia for clothing, analogous to the SPF used for sunscreens, and swing-tags showing these values have been designed for use on all garments, the reverse of the tag carrying a health-related message about the dangers of overexposure to the sun.

DATA LOGGING OF UV EXPOSURE

The relationship between melanoma incidence and sun exposure has given rise to the concept of intermittent exposure as a possible risk factor but the use of integrating dosimeters, such as the polysulphone film badge, does not permit an assessment of short-term exposure (i.e. a few hours or less). However, following the development of miniature electro-optical UVB sensors, it has now become possible to construct small lapel badges incorporating such a sensor electrically coupled to a portable data logger carried in a trouser pocket or worn on a belt. By this means, it is therefore possible to record UVB exposure on a second-by-second basis, which permits a much clearer understanding of human behaviour in sunlight (Diffey and Saunders, 1995). The results from these studies have demonstrated that behaviour outdoors can be a more dominant factor in determining personal exposure than ambient UV intensity and that shade from trees plays a very important role in reducing exposure.

VARIABILITY OF HUMAN EXPOSURE

The daily ambient erythemal UV intensity measured in Durham (55°N) by the author (Fig. 2.2) shows a clear sky summer to winter ratio of about 40:1, with superimposed day-to-day variations as a result of cloud cover. However, population UV exposure will be subject to even greater variation because of differences in individual behaviour. Whilst estimates of personal exposure are best obtained by direct measurement with UV-sensitive film badges (see above), in general these studies have been limited to monitoring the exposure of a few tens of people over periods ranging from a few hours to a few weeks. In order to determine the variability of exposure of different members of a population in detail, however, direct measurement, demanding high compliance over an

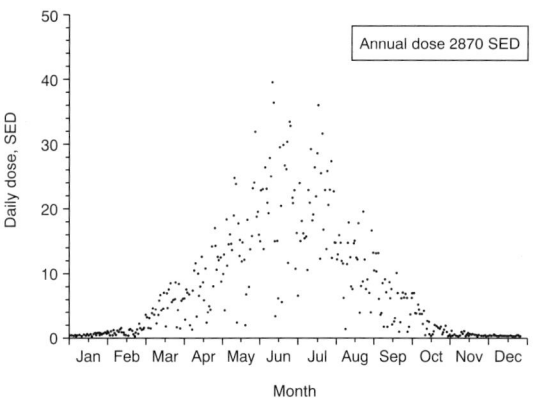

Annual dose 2870 SED

Figure 2.2 Ambient erythemal radiation measured during 1994 in Durham (55°N).

extended period of time by a large number of people, would be required.

An alternative, more feasible idea is to model the variables which affect personal exposure. Within this approach, reported studies (Diffey, 1992; Rosenthal *et al.*, 1991) have taken a typical individual (e.g. outdoor worker) and estimated how long he spends outdoors in hourly intervals throughout the day for different months of the year. This method has been shown to give results in good agreement with the average obtained from personal dosimetry studies for similar exposure scenarios, but it does not yield information about the variability in exposure between members of the same population, such as, for example, the population of British adult indoor workers. Furthermore, it is possible that taking an average person may be representative of nobody at all if the modes

for a given measurement are grouped on either side of the mean (Martin and Bateson, 1993).

Another method has therefore been reported (Diffey, 1996b) where climatological data of erythemal UV intensity throughout the year (taking into account cloud cover) are combined with the perceived behaviour of English adults who work indoors, thus arriving at estimates of the variability of UV exposure to the face. One hundred and twenty adults were asked to imagine that there are 100 people who work indoors in places such as factories, offices, shops and hospitals. Using their judgement, they then estimated how many of the 100 people would spend less than 30 minutes outside on a typical weekday (Monday to Friday) in winter and how many between 30 minutes and one hour, one and two hours, two and four hours, four and six hours and more than six hours. Outside in this context meant being in the open air; travelling in a car or being in a shop counted as being inside. Estimates were made also for a typical summer weekday (Monday to Friday), a typical winter weekend day (either a Saturday or a Sunday), a typical summer weekend day (Saturday or Sunday) and a typical summer holiday to somewhere sunny. The average percentage of people estimated in this way to spend different time periods outdoors for each of these scenarios by the 120 subjects is summarized in Table 2.4.

By combining these average estimates with the day-to-day variability in ambient erythemal UV, it is possible to calculate personal erythemal exposure (assuming 25% of ambient

Table 2.4 Average percentage of British indoor workers who spend different time periods outdoors on a given day (from Diffey, 1996a)

	< 0.5 h	*0.5–1 h*	*1–2 h*	*2–4 h*	*4–6 h*	*> 6 h*
Winter weekday	36	35	18	8	3	0
Summer weekday	11	18	27	25	13	6
Winter weekend	16	23	26	20	11	4
Summer weekend	4	8	17	24	27	20
Summer holiday	0	2	5	14	29	50

whenever outside) for different periods of the year. This approach clearly shows that there are large seasonal variations in personal erythemal exposure which are due not only to seasonal UV changes but, just as importantly, to seasonal variations in behaviour (see Table 2.4). Not surprisingly, holiday exposure accounts for the largest daily UV doses, so whilst there is only a 40-fold difference in clear sky daily erythemal UV from mid-winter to mid-summer at latitudes of 50–55°N, there is something like a 1000-fold variation in daily personal dose throughout the year with a dose to the face of between only 0.02 and 2 SED on about two thirds of the days in a year. Thus, if the daily erythemal personal doses are ranked (Fig. 2.3), we can see that 50% of the annual personal exposure of approximately 200 SED is received on just 33 days per year and that the cumulative exposure for eight months of the year contributes only about 10% to the annual erythemal dose.

BEHAVIOUR IN THE SUN

Whilst climatological factors may influence the levels of UV radiation at the earth's surface, it is the behaviour of people outside which has the greatest impact on personal exposure. Consequently efforts are being made in a number of countries to understand people's behaviour in the sun with a view to

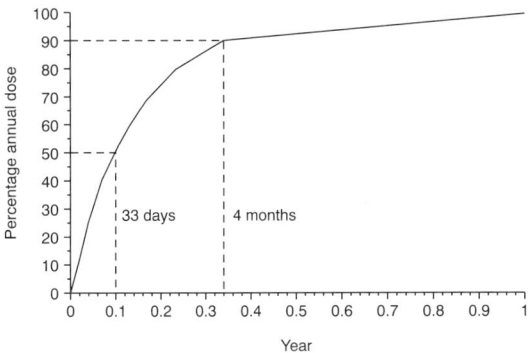

Figure 2.3 Ranked daily solar erythemal doses in indoor workers.

the development of strategies to encourage limitation of their exposure to acceptable values (Morris and Elwood, 1995).

A study conducted on a random sample of 200 adolescents (13–14 years) and 150 three-year-old children in the South of France showed that 42% of sun-sensitive children (based on phenotype characteristics) were not identified as such by their parents and that 60% of similar adolescents thought themselves resistant to the sun (Grob *et al.*, 1993). Sunscreens were used by 48% of the adolescents and 85% of the young children but only about two thirds of these applied the sunscreens adequately. Episodes of sunburn were therefore common despite the fact that most of the adolescents and the mothers of the young children knew that sun exposure in childhood was associated with an increased risk of skin cancer.

The knowledge, attitudes and behaviour of a group of 296 American college students regarding intentional sun exposure were examined by Vail-Smith and Felts (1993). Findings were that frequent sunbathers were more likely to be women and less likely to use a sunscreen than students who sunbathed infrequently, while frequent sunbathers were also more likely to believe that a tan was a sign of health and good looks. In fact, 43% of the female respondents and 61% of the males rarely, if ever, used sunscreens. In common with the French study, therefore, knowledge about the deleterious effects of sun exposure was generally high, but misconceptions about intentional sun exposure were held as well, notably the notion of a safe tan. Both studies highlighted the need for effective educational efforts to dispel myths about sun exposure whilst stressing instead its hazards, particularly in childhood and adolescence.

A further study which questioned Australian adolescents (15–20 years) at the beach on their attitudes towards tanning and beliefs about skin cancer yielded broadly similar findings, the majority not taking adequate sun protection measures (Pratt and Borland, 1994).

Although the males and females were generally similar in their behaviour, sun protection and attitudes, they differed somewhat in the way they protected themselves and in their preferences for a tan, most females going to the beach deliberately to acquire a tan, whilst the males tended to acquire theirs as a result of activities other than direct sunbathing.

Whilst the benefits of health promotion campaigns are widely accepted, it is nonetheless encouraging to see evidence of their effectiveness. Thus, a study carried out by researchers from the Anti-Cancer Council of Victoria in Australia aimed to determine trends in exposure to sunlight, in the context of a melanoma prevention programme, by monitoring the prevalence of sunburn and sun-related attitudes and behaviour (Hill *et al.*, 1993). Telephone interviews took place during three consecutive summers on Monday evenings to collect data concerning interviewee sunburn and behaviour over the previous weekend. As a result, it was found that the proportion of people sunburnt dropped from 11% to 7% over the three years, whilst hat wearing (19% to 29%) and sunscreen use (12% to 21%) increased.

COSMETIC TANNING

The continuing social desirability of a tanned skin is apparent, many people still associating a bronzed body with good health despite widespread media coverage of the detrimental effects of obtaining it. This desire for a tanned skin, coupled with the advent of high-intensity sources of UVA radiation allowing whole-body exposure, led to the growth of the suntan industry from the late 1970s. However, work carried out in the 1980s has shown that UVA exposure in laboratory animals can cause skin cancer (Van Weelden *et al.*, 1988) and it thus seems reasonable to assume that the same may apply to humans in the absence of evidence to the contrary. This realization has led the Photobiology Task Force of the American Academy of

Dermatology (Bickers *et al.*, 1985), the British Photodermatology Group (Diffey *et al.*, 1990) and the International Non-Ionizing Radiation Committee of the International Radiation Protection Association (IRPA, 1991) to recommend that cosmetic tanning with UVA radiation should be discouraged. Yet, despite this advice, the cosmetic tanning industry is a $1 billion-a-year business in the United States and the use of high-intensity UVA tanning devices continues to grow, with an estimated one million Americans visiting tanning salons on any given day (Spencer and Amonette, 1995).

TANNING LAMPS

Before the mid-1970s, the only way of achieving a tan from an artificial source was to use a sunlamp at home. This was invariably an unfiltered medium- or high-pressure mercury arc lamp which emitted a broad spectrum of radiation from UVC through to visible and infrared. These units often incorporated one or more infrared heaters as well and were commonly called sunlamps or health lamps. Because of their high UVC and UVB emission, however, exposure times were short, typically a few minutes, and the lamps were inefficient in tanning; it was also not uncommon for overexposure to occur, resulting in acute eye damage or skin erythema and blistering, while a further disadvantage was that the area of irradiation was limited to a single region such as the face and whole-body tanning was therefore tedious. By later incorporation of several mercury arc lamps into a solarium, however, whole-body exposure was eventually achieved. A preferable method of whole-body irradiation, on the other hand, was by means of fluorescent lamps and in 1981, the American Cancer Society (American Cancer Society, 1981) reported that UVB fluorescent sunlamps were more common in tanning salons in the USA than in Europe. However, this type of unit never appeared in the UK since development of UVA fluorescent lamps in the late 1970s and early 1980s enabled the induction of a tan with UVA radiation.

The tanning industry was quick to seize on this perceived benefit of UVA and as a consequence, UVA lamps with minimal UVB content were promoted. These devices consist of a bed or canopy incorporating between six and 30 fluorescent lamps of either 150 or 180 cm in length. The earliest incorporated a barium silicate phosphor, typified by the Philips TL-09, Wotan L100/79 and Wolff Solarium lamps, their emission spectrum comprising a fluorescence continuum from about 315 to 400 nm, together with the characteristic lines of the mercury spectrum down to 297 nm (Diffey and McKinlay, 1983). The UVA irradiance (Bruyneel-Rapp *et al.*, 1988) at the skin surface was between 50 and 150 W/m², approximately 0.7% of the total UV emission being UVB. In the mid-1980s, however, another such lamp (Philips TL-10R) incorporating a strontium borate phosphor was introduced especially for cosmetic tanning, its principal features being a reflector intrinsic to the lamp envelope and a fluorescence emission spectrum extending from about 340 to 400 nm, peaking at 370 nm, and resulting in a UVB content of only 0.05%; the skin surface irradiance from a sunbed or sun canopy incorporating such lamps is typically around 250 W/m². On the other hand, the most common UVA fluorescent lamps used in sunbeds today are the Cleo range manufactured by Philips Lighting, namely the Cleo R-UVA, Cleo Effect, Cleo Performance and Cleo Professional, whose UVB outputs as a percentage of total UV output are again relatively high at 0.7%, 1.0%, 0.7% and 1.4%, respectively. Finally, a UVA fluorescent lamp for sunbeds with an even higher UVB output (3% of the total UV) is the so-called fast-tan tube, the type of lamp typified by the Bellarium S from the German company Kosmedico, who supply a whole range of tanning lamps.

An alternative to these fluorescent lamps for cosmetic tanning is a variety of optically filtered, high-pressure mercury lamps doped with metal halide additives, whose spectral emission lies entirely within the UVA waveband and which provide very high irradiances at the skin surface of more than 1000 W/m² (Mutzhas, 1986).

CONSUMER USE OF ULTRAVIOLET TANNING DEVICES

Telephone surveys carried out in The Netherlands (Bruggers *et al.*, 1987) and the United Kingdom (Consumer Association, 1987) in the mid-1980s showed that 7–9% of the adult population in each country had used a sunbed in the previous 1–2 years. A more recent survey in the UK (McLaughlan, 1989), with a sample size of 5800, gave a slightly higher figure, 10% of the population having used a sunbed during the previous year (1988) and 19% at some time in the past. The most recent UK survey, commissioned by the Department of Health in 1994 (Bulman, 1995), again found that 9% of respondents had used sunbeds, with 24% aged between 16 and 24 having used a sunbed during 1994. In these and other surveys in the United Kingdom (Diffey, 1986) and the USA (Dougherty *et al.*, 1988; Lillquist *et al.*, 1994), women accounted for 60–85% of users, about half overall being young women between 16 and 30. The commonest reason given for the use of tanning equipment was the acquisition of a pre-holiday tan (Consumer Association, 1987; Lillquist *et al.*, 1994; McLaughlan, 1989); other reasons, however, included perceived health benefits such as reduction of stress, improved relaxation, protection of the skin before going on holiday, retention of a holiday tan and the treatment of skin diseases such as psoriasis and acne (Diffey, 1986: Dougherty *et al.*, 1988).

In the Dutch survey mentioned above (Bruggers *et al.*, 1987), about half the interviewees used tanning equipment at home and the other half facilities at commercial premises such as tanning salons, hairdressers, sports clubs and swimming pools. Very similar results were found in the 1994 UK survey (Bulman, 1995), with twice as many people who used sunbeds at home owning rather than hiring them. The mean number of tanning sessions per year in the Dutch study was 23, while in the UK, half an hour was the most popular length for a session (Diffey, 1986).

Finally, a very recent UK survey of just over 6000 British adults carried out in 1996 by The Sunbed Association has now yielded the following demographic data about modern UK sunbed users:

		% population
Male		5
Female		9
Age	16–34	13
	35–54	6
	55 +	1
Social class	ABC1	8
	C2DE	6
Region	North	10
	Midlands	6
	South	5

Further findings to emerge from this survey include the following:

Why people use sunbeds	%
Look better	58
Feel healthier	34
Pre-holiday tan	28
Other	14
Where people use sunbeds	**%**
Home (owned)	43
Salon	28
Local authority	19
Home (hired)	16
Sunbed sessions in past	
12 months	**%**
1–10	54
11–20	25
21–50	14
> 50	7

THERAPEUTIC EXPOSURE TO ULTRAVIOLET RADIATION

Treatment of skin disease by exposure to UV radiation is termed **phototherapy** and is often used in combination with agents applied topically (for example, dithranol plus UVB phototherapy for psoriasis). When such UV treatment is combined with a photosensitizing agent (for example, oral or topical psoralen plus UVA exposure), the term **photochemotherapy** is used instead (see Chapter 16).

OCCUPATIONAL EXPOSURE TO ULTRAVIOLET RADIATION

SOLAR EXPOSURE

Occupation is the prime determinant of adventitious exposure to sunlight, exposed groups including farmers, construction workers, fishermen, gardeners, oil-field workers, road workers, police officers, sailors and ski instructors. A representative value for the annual, occupational, natural UV exposure of outdoor workers in mid-latitudes (~ 50°N) is around 400 SED, while a corresponding value of 40 SED applies to indoor workers, where occupational exposure occurs only during travel to and from work and weekday lunchtimes.

There are other groups, on the other hand, such as the housebound elderly, some Asian immigrants to the UK and submariners, who receive almost no natural UV exposure and are therefore at possible risk of vitamin D deficiency.

EXPOSURE FROM ARTIFICIAL SOURCES

Artificial sources of UV radiation are used in many different applications in the working environment. In some cases, the source is well contained within an enclosure and under normal circumstances presents no risk of exposure to personnel. In other applications, however, it is inevitable that users will be exposed to some radiation, normally reflected or scattered from adjacent surfaces. Under these conditions, it is clearly important that exposure be kept below the maximum permissible limits for occupational exposure published by national regulatory authorities, either by means of administrative and engineering controls or by the use of protective clothing, eyewear and faceshields.

INDUSTRIAL PHOTOPROCESSES

Many industrial processes, such as the curing of lacquers and inks, involve a photochemical component. The large-scale nature of these processes often necessitates the use of high-power (several kilowatt) UV-emitting lamps such as high-pressure metal halide sources (Phillips, 1983). Although these high-power lamps emit high levels of UV, they are housed in interlocked assemblies to prevent inadvertent irradiation of personnel under normal use.

STERILIZATION AND DISINFECTION

The bactericidal effects of sunlight were first noted by Downes and Blunt in 1877 and this property of UV radiation has since been regularly exploited. Wavelengths in the range 260–265 nm are most effective for this purpose, corresponding to an absorption maximum in the DNA absorption spectrum. For this reason, low-pressure mercury discharge tubes are often used, this source emitting more than 90% of its output in the adjacent 253.7 nm line. Such lamps are often referred to as germicidal, bactericidal or simply UVC lamps.

UVC is used to disinfect sewage effluents, drinking water, water for the cosmetics industry and bathing pools and sometimes inside microbiological safety cabinets to inactivate airborne and surface micro-organisms, the combination of UVC radiation and the ozone produced in air by such radiation having a very powerful oxidizing action capable of reducing the organic content of air and water to extremely low levels. UVC

radiation is particularly injurious to the eyes, but the housing of UVC lamps behind normal glass or plastic provides complete protection for users.

WELDING

Welding equipment falls into two broad categories – gas welding and electric arc welding. Only the latter produces significant levels of UV radiation, the quality and quantity of which depend primarily on the arc current, the shielding gas and the metals being welded.

Welders are most certainly the largest single occupational group exposed to artificial UV radiation, it having been estimated that there may be as many as half a million welders in the USA alone. UV irradiances around electric arc welding equipment are high (Cox, 1987) and it is therefore not surprising that most welders at some time or other experience **welder's flash** (photokeratitis) and sunburn erythema, a survey of electric arc welders in Denmark (Eriksen, 1987) having shown that 65% of those questioned had experienced the latter, although no indication of the frequency was reported.

Measurements of the UV exposure from arc welding by means of polysulphone film have been reported (Barth *et al.*, 1990; Shehade *et al.*, 1987; Tenkate and Collins, 1997). Not surprisingly, outer clothing surface exposures exceed occupational exposure limits to the unprotected eye and skin by several thousand-fold, while in some cases the levels on the inner surface of welders' helmets are such that additional eye protection should be worn (Tenkate and Collins, 1997). Further, even ambient UV levels in the non-welding areas of factories where welding equipment is used can sometimes exceed occupational exposure limits.

PHOTOTHERAPY

Many of the lamps used to treat skin diseases are unenclosed and emit high UV levels, presenting a marked exposure hazard to staff (Diffey and Langley, 1986). At one metre from an Alpine sunlamp (hot quartz lamp), for example, the recommended eight-hour occupational exposure limit in the UK can be exceeded in less than two minutes.

The results of other studies of occupational exposure to staff in hospital phototherapy departments (Larkö and Diffey, 1986; Diffey, 1989b) also show that the annual UV exposure of staff can be estimated from the number of occasions each year on which they experience at least minimal erythema, being approximately 30, 200 and 400 SED for erythema frequencies of once per year, once per month and once per week, respectively.

OPERATING THEATRES

UVC lamps have been used since the 1930s to decrease the levels of airborne bacteria in operating theatres, although the technique is not widely used, filtered air units generally being preferred, presumably to protect the eyes and skin of staff and patients.

RESEARCH LABORATORIES

Sources of UV radiation, including for example lasers, are used by many scientists engaged in experimental aspects of photobiology and photochemistry. In such applications, the primary, direct effect of UV irradiation on the biological or chemical species may be of interest to the researcher or else the secondary, indirect effect, as in fluorescence and absorption techniques. Many such sources are associated with UV hazards (Bowker, 1987).

ULTRAVIOLET PHOTOGRAPHY

There are two distinct forms of UV photography: reflected or transmitted UV photography and UV fluorescence photography. In both applications the effective radiation lies within the UVA waveband.

INSECT TRAPS

Many flying insects are attracted to UVA radiation, particularly at wavelengths around 350 nm, a phenomenon which is the principle of electronic insect traps. In these devices, a UVA fluorescent lamp is mounted in a unit containing a high-voltage grid; the insect, attracted by the UVA lamps, is electrocuted in the air gap between the grid and an earthed metal screen. Such units are common where food is prepared and sold to the public but under normal use, the UV exposure of staff and public is too low to present any hazard.

SUNBED SALONS AND SHOPS

The continuing popularity of UVA sunbeds and sun canopies for cosmetic tanning has resulted in a large number of tanning salons and sunbed shops which may have 20 or more UVA tanning appliances all switched on at once, thus exposing members of the public and, more seriously, staff to continuing high levels of UVA radiation.

DISCOTHEQUES

UVA blacklight lamps are sometimes used in discotheques to induce fluorescence of the clothing of dancers. Whilst such UVA levels are normally low, presenting no eye or skin hazard, UVC lamps have on occasion been installed inadvertently, thus leading to severe photokeratitis.

OFFICES

Signature verification is commonly performed by exposing a signature, written previously with colourless ink, to UVA radiation under which it fluoresces. The lamps used are of very low power and exposure times are short, thus resulting in no occupational hazard for normal conditions of use.

GENERAL LIGHTING

Fluorescent lamps for general lighting in offices and factories emit small quantities of both UVA and UVB. For typical levels of illuminance of around 500 lux from bare fluorescent lamps in the UK, measurements have indicated UVA and UVB irradiances of about 30 mW/m^2 and 3 mW/m^2, respectively (McKinlay and Whillock, 1987). Such levels, however, give rise to annual exposures of no more than 10 SED for indoor workers, doses which can be further appreciably reduced by the use of plastic diffusers. Another study of the personal UV doses of workers engaged in inspecting the paintwork of new cars under bright fluorescent lamps indicated a similar level of exposure (Diffey *et al.*, 1986). However, spectroradiometric measurements of the UV levels from such fluorescent lamps in the USA (Cole *et al.*, 1985) suggested much higher annual doses, at least for persons occupationally exposed for 200 h/year, typical estimates being about 40 SED per year for illuminance levels of 500 lux.

Desktop lamps incorporating tungsten halogen bulbs may also emit significant UV levels, thereby resulting in exposures to the hands and arms of users well above the recommended occupational amounts (McKinlay *et al.*, 1989).

OZONE DEPLETION AND SKIN CANCER

In 1974 Molina and Rowland, who, with Paul Crutzen, were awarded the 1995 Nobel Prize for Chemistry, predicted that manmade chlorine compounds released at ground level would diffuse into the upper atmosphere and gradually destroy its ozone (Molina and Rowland, 1974). However, it took another ten years for scientists from the British Antarctic Survey (Farman *et al.*, 1985) actually to demonstrate an unexpected annual decrease in springtime ozone over the Antarctic continent, the so-called **ozone hole**. As a result, there has been increasing public concern about what is really occurring, fuelled particularly by media speculation of a possible skin cancer epidemic, in that ozone plays a significant part in attenuating solar UV.

Skin cancer is in fact the most common human cancer and its incidence is increasing in many countries. It is well recognized that chronic exposure to sunlight is a causal factor in its development, particularly of non-melanoma skin cancer (NMSC), and therefore concern has been widely expressed that the apparent depletion of stratospheric ozone may lead to a consequent rise in skin cancer incidence (MacKie and Rycroft, 1988; Russell Jones, 1987; UNEP, 1989, 1991).

TRENDS IN ATMOSPHERIC OZONE AND AMBIENT ULTRAVIOLET RADIATION

Significant global decreases in total ozone have been occurring since the late 1970s, the rate of loss in the Northern hemisphere of mid-latitudes (30–50°N) in winter and early spring now being 6–7% per decade. The more important loss in summer months, however, when UV levels are much higher and people exposed more frequently, is less at about 2–3% per decade (Frederick, 1993).

Calculations for the Northern hemisphere, based on measured ozone trends for 1979–1989, suggest that, all other factors being constant, terrestrial erythemally effective UV (which lies mainly within the UVB waveband) should have increased by nearly 1% at 15°N, and by between 4.0% and 4.7% at 35°N and poleward, during this decade (Frederick, 1993). Paradoxically, these predicted increases have not generally been confirmed by ground-based UV monitoring programmes (Diffey, 1996b) and reasons offered to account for the discrepancy include the limited installation period of most UV-monitoring networks, the accuracy of instrument calibration and long-term stability of monitoring equipment, the year-to-year fluctuations in cloud cover (Frederick and Erlick, 1991) and an increase in pollutant ozone and aerosols in the lower atmosphere (Bruhl and Crutzen, 1989). Nevertheless, despite the record low concentrations of total ozone in the Northern winters of 1992 and 1993 (Bojkov *et al.*, 1993), further measurements in the Austrian Alps have again shown no significant increase of cumulative erythemal exposure as compared with a reference series of measurements obtained between 1981 and 1988 (Blumthaler and Ambach, 1994).

In the Southern hemisphere, on the other hand, an apparent definite influence of Antarctic ozone depletion on ambient UVB in Melbourne (latitude 38°S) has been noted by Roy and Gies (1992), continuous monitoring having shown that the levels in February 1991 were 37% and 27% higher than for the same month in 1990 and 1989, respectively. In fact, February 1991 had the lowest ozone values ever recorded for this period, but cloud cover was also very low as compared with recent years and these two important factors rein-force each other and illustrate the difficulty of separating the effects of ozone depletion from those of climate on the ambient UVB. Thus, while there is unequivocal evidence of strato-spheric ozone depletion, we cannot as yet be sure whether this depletion is accompanied by consequent increases in terrestrial UV radi-ation. This does not, however, mean that no definite trend exists, but simply that the 95% confidence interval for such trends is likely to encompass zero.

RISK OF SKIN CANCER

Estimates of skin cancer risk associated with exposure to UV demand a knowledge of UV–cancer dose–response relationships and of the relative effectiveness of the different wavelengths of the source in causing the cancer. Such data, however, remain unknown for malignant melanoma and it is thus unwise to make predictions about the consequences of ozone depletion on the incidence of that cancer, although some information is available for NMSC, thus enabling some quantitative

estimates concerning that condition to be made.

A 1% decrease in ozone has been predicted as likely to lead to a 1.2–1.4% increase in carcinogenic-effective UV radiation (Health Council of The Netherlands, 1994), while for every 1% increase in carcinogenic-effective UVB radiation, it is estimated in turn (Health Council of The Netherlands, 1994) that there will be an approximate 2.5% increase in squamous cell carcinoma (SCC) incidence and a 1.5% increase in basal cell carcinoma (BCC). Combining these figures, we then arrive at overall amplification factors, which can be summarized as:

1% decrease in ozone concentration
$$\rightarrow 1.4 \times 2.5 = 3.5\% \text{ SCC increase}$$
$$\rightarrow 1.4 \times 1.5 = 2.1\% \text{ BCC increase}$$

This approach can also be used to estimate the consequences of a sustained 10% strato-spheric ozone depletion in the UK. The most recent figures for skin cancer incidence in the UK are based on 1989 data from the Office of Population Census and Surveys for England and Wales, the Information and Statistics Division of the NHS Directorate of Information Services for Scotland and the Northern Ireland Cancer Registry and yield a combined figure of just over 40 000 cases of skin cancer annually. Of these, about 30 000 are BCC, 6000 SCC and 4000 malignant melanoma. However, because of under-recording of NMSC (BCC and SCC) in the UK and their rising incidence, the true number of such cancers each year is probably closer to double these figures. Thus, for a sustained 10% ozone depletion, with no alteration in individual exposure habit, we might expect increases of 21% and 35% in the incidences of BCC and SCC, respectively, giving an addi-tional 12 000 cases of BCC and 4000 cases of SCC each year.

This approach may very possibly be applic-able to future generations but not to British people alive today. However, by combining UV climatological data for the United

Kingdom with models of human behaviour (Diffey, 1992), it is possible to estimate future cumulative UVB exposure to the face (the most common site for NMSC) of today's population. Thus, for British adults alive today, ozone depletion continuing indefinitely at current rates is predicted to result in a relatively small additional lifetime risk (< 5%) of NMSC, assuming no changes in climate, time spent outdoors, behaviour or clothing habits, but a significantly higher 10–16% for today's children. Nevertheless, if the production and use of substances which deplete ozone are reduced as expected under the current provisions of the Montreal Protocol (UNEP, 1987), the actual lifetime skin cancer risk is likely to be lower than these estimates. It is thus to be hoped that public awareness about the adverse health effects of sun exposure will achieve these reductions, which could then lead to a decrease, rather than the anticipated increase, in skin cancer incidence.

REFERENCES

Airey, D.K., Wong, J.C.F. and Fleming, R.A. (1995) A comparison of human- and headform based measurements of solar ultraviolet B dose. *Photodermatology, Photoimmunology and Photomedicine*, 11, 155–8.

American Cancer Society (1981) Are tanning centers safe? *Cancer News*, **Spring/Summer**, 19.

Barth, C., Knuschke, P. and Barth, J. (1990) UV-Strahlenbelastung in der Umgebung von Schweissarbeitsplätzen. *Zeitschrift für Gesamte Hygiene* 36, 654–5.

Bennetts, K., Borland, R. and Swerissen, H. (1991) Sun protection behaviour of children and their parents at the beach. *Psychology and Health* 5, 279–87.

Bickers, D.R., Epstein, J.H., Fitzpatrick, T.B., Harber, L.C. and Pathak, M. (1985) Risks and benefits from high-intensity ultraviolet A sources used for cosmetic purposes. *Journal of the American Academy of Dermatology* 12, 380–1.

Blumthaler, M and Ambach, W. (1994) Health and climate change. *Lancet* 343, 303.

Bojkov, R.D., Zerefos, C.S., Balis, D.S., Ziomas, I.C. and Bais, A.F. (1993). *Geophysics Research Letters*, 13, 1351–4.

Boldeman, C., Jansson, B. and Holm, L-E. (1991) Primary prevention of malignant melanoma in a Swedish urban pre-school sector. *Journal of Cancer Education* 6, 247–53.

Bowker, K.W. (1987) Hazards associated with sources of ultra-violet radiation used in a research environment, in *Human Exposure to Ultraviolet Radiation: Risk and Regulations* (eds W.F. Passchier and B.F.M. Bosnjakovic), Elsevier, Amsterdam, pp. 371–5.

Bruggers, J.H.A., deJong, W.E., Bosnjakovic, B.F.M. and Passchier, W.F. (1987) Use of artificial tanning equipment in the Netherlands, in *Human Exposure to Ultraviolet Radiation: Risk and Regulations*, (eds W.F. Passchier and B.F.M. Bosnjakovic), Elsevier, Amsterdam, pp. 235–9.

Bruhl, C. and Crutzen, P.J. .(1989) On the disproportionate role of tropospheric ozone as a filter against solar UV-B radiation. *Geophysics Research Letters* 16, 703–6.

Bruyneel-Rapp, F., Dorsey, S.B. and Guin, J.D. (1988) The tanning salon: an area survey of equipment, procedures, and practices. *Journal of the American Academy of Dermatology* 18, 1030–8.

Bulman, A. (1995) People are overusing sunbeds. *British Medical Journal*, 310, 1327.

Challoner, A.V.J., Corless, D., Davis, A. *et al.* (1976) Personnel monitoring of exposure to ultraviolet radiation. *Clinical and Experimental Dermatology*, 1, 175–9.

Cockburn, J., Hennrikus, D., Scott, R and Sanson-Fisher, R (1989) Adolescent use of sun-protection measures. *Medical Journal of Australia*, 151, 136–40.

Cole, C., Forbes, P.D., Davies, R.E. *et al.* (1985) Effect of indoor lighting on normal skin. *Annals of the New York Academy of Science*, 453, 305–16.

Consumer Association (1987) The truth about tanning. *Which?*, Consumer Association, London, p. 214.

Cox, C.W.J. (1987) Ultraviolet irradiance levels in welding processes, in *Human Exposure to Ultraviolet Radiation: Risk and Regulations*, (eds. W.F. Passchier and B.F.M. Bosnjakovic), Elsevier, Amsterdam, pp. 383–6.

Diffey, B.L. (1986) Use of UVA sunbeds for cosmetic tanning. *British Journal of Dermatology*, 115, 67–76.

Diffey, B.L. (1989a) Ultraviolet radiation dosimetry with polysulphone film, in *Radiation Measurement in Photobiology*, (ed. B.L. Diffey), Academic Press, London, pp. 135–9.

Diffey, B.L. (1989b) Ultraviolet radiation and skin cancer: are physiotherapists at risk? *Physiotherapy*, 75, 615–16.

Diffey, B.L. (1992) Stratospheric ozone depletion and the risk of non-melanoma skin cancer in a British population. *Physics in Medicine and Biology*, **37**, 2237–79.

Diffey, B.L. (1996a) Population exposure to solar UVA radiation. *European Journal of Dermatology*, **6**, 221–2.

Diffey, B.L. (ed.) (1996b) *Measurement and Trends of Terrestrial UVB Radiation in Europe*, Organizzazione Editoriale Medico Farmaceutica, Milan.

Diffey, B.L. and Cheeseman, J (1992) Sun protection with hats. *British Journal of Dermatology*, **127**, 10–12.

Diffey, B.L. and Langley, F.C. (1986) *Evaluation of Ultraviolet Radiation Hazards in Hospitals*, Institute of Physical Sciences in Medicine, London.

Diffey, B.L. and McKinlay, A.F. (1983) The UVB content of 'UVA fluorescent lamps' and its erythemal effectiveness in human skin. *Physics in Medicine and Biology*, **28**, 351–8.

Diffey, B.L. and Saunders P.J. (1995) Behaviour outdoors and its effect on personal ultraviolet exposure rate measured using a portable datalogging dosimeter. *Photochemistry and Photobiology*, **61**, 615–18.

Diffey, B.L., Kerwin, M and Davis, A. (1977) The anatomical distribution of sunlight. *British Journal of Dermatology*, **97**, 407–10.

Diffey, B.L., Tate, T.J. and Davis, A. (1979) Solar dosimetry of the face: the relationship of natural ultraviolet radiation exposure to basal cell carcinoma localisation. *Physics in Medicine and Biology*, **24**, 931–9.

Diffey, B.L., Larkö, O., Meding, B. *et al.* (1986) Personal monitoring of exposure to ultraviolet radiation in the car manufacturing industry. *Annals of Occupational Hygiene*, **30**, 163–70.

Diffey, B.L., Farr, P.M., Ferguson, J. *et al.* (1990) Tanning with ultraviolet A sunbeds. *British Medical Journal*, **301**, 773–4.

Diffey, B.L., Gibson, C.J., Haylock, R and McKinlay, A.F. (1996) Outdoor ultraviolet exposure of children and adolescents. *British Journal of Dermatology*, **134**, 1030–4.

Dougherty, M.A., McDermott, R.J. and Hawkins, M.J. (1988) A profile of users of commercial tanning salons. *Health Values*, **12**, 21–6.

Eriksen, P. (1987) Occupational applications of ultraviolet radiation: risk evaluation and protection techniques, in *Human Exposure to Ultraviolet Radiation: Risk and Regulations*, (eds W.F. Passchier and B.F.M. Bosnjakovic), Elsevier, Amsterdam, pp. 317–30.

Farman, J.C., Gardiner, B.G. and Shanklin, J.D. (1985) Large losses of total ozone in Antarctica reveal season CIOxNOx interaction. *Nature*, **315**, 207–10.

Frederick, J.E. (1993) Ultraviolet sunlight reaching the Earth's surface: a review of recent research. *Photochemistry and Photobiology*, **57**, 175–8.

Frederick, J.E. and Alberts, A.D. (1992) The natural UV-A radiation environment in *Biological responses to Ultraviolet A Radiation*, (ed. F. Urbach), Valdenmar Publishing Company, Overland Park, KS, pp. 7–18.

Frederick, J.E. and Erlick, C. (1991) Trends and interannual variations in erythema sunlight, 1978–1993 *Photochemistry and Photobiology*, **62**, 476–84.

Fritschi, L., Green, A. and Solomon, P.J. (1992) Sun exposure to Australian adolescents. *Journal of the American Academy of Dermatology*, **27**, 25–8.

Gies, H.P., Roy, C.R. and Elliott, G. (1988) *The Anatomical Distribution of Solar UVR with Emphasis on the Eye. Proceedings of the Seventh International Congress of the International Radiation Protection Association.* Pergamon Press, Sydney, pp. 341–4.

Gies, H.P., Herlihy, E. and Rivers, J. (1992) *Personal Dosimetry of Solar UVB using Polysulphone Film. Proceedings of the IRPA 8 Congress,* Montreal.

Gies, H.P., Roy, C.R., Elliott, G. and Zongli, W. (1994) Ultraviolet radiation protection factors for clothing. *Health Physics*, **67**, 131–9.

Gies, H.P., Roy, C.R., Toomey, S., MacLennan R. and Watson, M. (1995) Solar UVR exposures of three groups of outdoor workers on the Sunshine Coast, Queensland. *Photochemistry and Photobiology*, **62**, 1015–21.

Grob, J.J., Guglielmina, C., Gouvernet, J. *et al.* (1993) Study of sunbathing habits in children and adolescents: application to the prevention of melanoma. *Dermatology*, **186**, 94–8.

Health Council of the Netherlands, Risks of UV Radiation Committee (1994) *UV Radiation from Sunlight,* Health Council of the Netherlands, The Hague.

Herlihy, E., Gies, P.H., Roy, C.R. and Jones, M. (1994) Personal dosimetry of solar UV radiation for different outdoor activities. *Photochemistry and Photobiology*, **60**, 228–94.

Hill, D., White, V., Marks, R. and Borland, R. (1993) Changes in sun-related attitudes and behaviours, and reduced sunburn prevalence in a population at high risk of melanoma. *European Journal of Cancer Prevention*, **2**, 447–56.

Holman, C.D.J., Gibson, I.M., Stephenson, M. and Armstrong, B.K. (1983) Ultraviolet irradiation of human body sites in relation to occupation and outdoor activity: field and studies using personal UVR dosimeters. *Clinical and Experimental Dermatology*, **8**, 269–77.

Hughes, B.R., Altman, D.G. and Newton, J.A. (1993) Melanoma and skin cancer: evaluation of a health programme for secondary school. *British Journal of Dermatology*, **128**, 412–17.

International Radiation Protection Association, International Non-Ionizing Radiation Committee (1991) Health issues of ultraviolet A sunbeds used for cosmetic purposes. *Health Physics*, **61**, 285–8.

Jarrett, P., Sharp, C. and McLelland, J. (1993) Protection of children by their mothers against sunburn. *British Medical Journal*, **306**, 1448..

Knuschke, P. and Barth, J. (1996) Biologically weighted personal UV dosimetry. *Journal of Photochemistry and Photobiology*, **36**, 77–83.

Kricker, A., Armstrong, B.K. and English, D.R. (1994) Sun exposure and non-melanocytic skin cancer. *Cancer Causes and Control*, **5**, 367–92.

Larkö, O. and Diffey, B.L. (1983) Natural UV-B radiation received by people with outdoor, indoor and mixed occupations and UV-B treatment of psoriasis. *Clinical and Experimental Dermatology*, **8**, 279–85.

Larkö, O. and Diffey, B.L. (1986) Occupational exposure to ultraviolet radiation in dermatology departments. *British Journal of Dermatology*, **114**, 468–84.

Leach, J.F., McLeod, V.E., Pingstone, A.R., Davis, A. and Deane, G.H.W. (1978) Measurement of the ultraviolet doses received by office workers. *Clinical and Experimental Dermatology*, **3**, 77–9.

Lillquist, P.P., Baptiste, M.S., Witzikgman, M.A. and Nasca, P.C. (1994) A population-based survey of sun lamp and tanning parlor use in New York State, 1990. *Journal of the American Academy of Dermatology*, **31**, 510–12.

MacKie, R.M. and Rycroft, M.J. (1988) Health and the ozone layer: skin cancers may increase dramatically. *British Medical Journal*, **297**, 369–70.

Madronich, S. (1993) The atmosphere and UV-B radiation at ground level in *Environmental UV Photobiology*, (eds A.R. Young, L.O. Bjorn, J. Moan and W. Multsch), Plenum Press, New York, pp. 1–39.

Martin, P. and Bateson, P. (1993) *Measuring Behaviour: an Introductory Guide*, 2nd edn, Cambridge University Press, Cambridge, pp. 13–14.

McKinlay, A.F. and Whillock, M.J. (1987) Measurement of ultraviolet radiation from fluo-

rescent lamps used for general lighting and other purposes in the UK in *Human Exposure to Ultraviolet Radiation: Risk and Regulations*, (eds W.F. Passchier and B.F.M. Bosnjakovic), Elsevier, Amsterdam, pp. 253–8.

McKinlay, A.F., Whillock, M.J. and Meulemans, C.C.E. (1989) *Ultraviolet Radiation and Blue-light Emissions from Spotlights Incorporating Tungsten Halogen Lamps.* Report NRPB-R228, National Radiological Protection Board, Didcot, UK.

McLaughlan, R. (1989) UK population attitude to tanning. Unpublished market survey.

Melia, J. and Bulman, A. (1995) Sunburn and tanning in a British population. *J Public Health Medicine*, **17**, 223–9.

Melville, S.K., Rosenthal, F.S., Luckmann, R. and Lew, RA. (1991) Quantitative ultraviolet skin exposure in children during selected outdoor activities. *Photodermatology, Photoimmunology and Photomedicine*, **8**, 99–104.

Mermelstein, R.J. and Riesenberg, L.A. (1992) Changing knowledge and attitudes about skin cancer risk factors in adolescents. *Health Psychology*, **11**, 371–6.

Molina, M. and Rowland, F.S. (1974) Stratospheric sink for chlorofluoromethanese-chlorine atom catalyzed destruction of ozone. *Nature*, **249**, 810–12.

Morris, J. and Elwood, M. (1995) *How Effective are Sun Exposure Modification Programmes?* Hugh Adam Cancer Epidemiology Unit, University of Otago, Dunedin, New Zealand.

Mutzhas, M.F. (1986) UVA-emitting light sources in *The Biological Effects of UVA Radiation*, (eds F. Urbach and R.W. Gange), Praeger, New York, pp. 10–23.

Parkin, D.M., Muir, C.S., Whelan, S.L. *et al.* (eds) (1992) *Cancer Incidence in Five Continents, Vol VI*, International Agency for Research on Cancer, Lyon.

Peak, M.J. and Peak, J.G. (1986) Molecular photobiology of UVA. In *The Biological Effects of UVA Radiation*, (eds F. Urbach and R.W. Gange), Praeger, New York, pp. 42–52.

Phillips, R. (1983) *Sources and Applications of Ultraviolet Radiation*, Academic Press, London.

Pratt, K. and Borland, R. (1994) Predictors of sun protection among adolescents at the beach. *Australian Psychologist*, **29**, 135–9.

Rosenthal, F.S., Lew, R.A., Rouleau, L.J. and Thomson, M. (1990) Ultraviolet exposure to children from sunlight: a study using personal dosimetry. *Photodermatology, Photoimmunology and Photomedicine*, **7**, 77–81.

Rosenthal, F.S., West, S.K., Munoz, B. *et al.* (1991) Occular and facial skin exposure to ultraviolet radiation in sunlight: a personal exposure model with application to a worker population. *Health Physics*, **61**, 77–86.

Roy, C.R. and Gies, H.P. (1992) *Results from an Australian Solar UVR Measurement Network and Implications for Radiation Protection Policy.* Proceedings of the 8th International Congress of the International Radiation Protection Association, Montreal. **Vol. 1**, pp. 759–62.

Russell Jones, R. (1987) Ozone depletion and cancer risk. *Lancet*, **ii**, 443–4.

Schothorst, A.A., Slaper, H., Schouten, R. and Suurmond, D. (1985) UVB doses in maintenance psoriasis phototherapy versus solar UVB exposure. *Photodermatology*, **2**, 213–20.

Shehade, S.A., Roberts, P.J., Diffey, B.L. and Foulds, I.S. (1987) Photodermatitis due to spot welding. *British Journal of Dermatology*, **117**, 117–19.

Slaper, H. (1987) Skin cancer and UV exposure: investigations on the estimation of risks. PhD thesis, University of Utrecht, The Netherlands.

Spencer, J.M., and Amonette, R.A. (1995) Indoor tanning: risks, benefits, and future trends. *Journal of the American Academy of Dermatology*, **33**, 188–98.

Tenkate, T.D. and Collins, M.J. (1997) Personal ultraviolet radiation exposure of workers in a welding environment. *American Industrial Hygiene Association Journal*, **58**, 33–8.

United Nations Environment Programme (1991) *Environmental Effects of Ozone Depletion: 1991 Update*, , UNEP,

Vail-Smith, K. and Felts, W.M. (1993) Sunbathing: college students' knowledge, attitudes, and perceptions of risks. *College Health*, **42**,, 21–6.

Van Weelden, H., De Gruijl, F.R., Van Der Putte, S.C.J., Toonstra, J. and Van Der Leun, J.C. (1988) The carcinogenic risks of modern tanning equipment: is UV-A safer than UV-B? *Archives of Dermatology Research*, **280**, 300–7.

Webb, A.R. (1985) Solar ultraviolet radiation and vitamin D synthesis in man. PhD thesis, University of Nottingham, UK.

Wong, J.C.F., Airey, D.K. and Fleming, R.A. (1996) Annual reduction of solar UV exposure ton the facial area of outdoor workers in Southeast Queensland by wearing a hat. *Photodermatology, Photoimmunology and Photomedicine*, **12**, 131–5.

THE MOLECULAR AND GENETIC EFFECTS OF ULTRAVIOLET RADIATION EXPOSURE ON SKIN CELLS

3

Antony R. Young

INTRODUCTION

The ultraviolet (UV) and visible components of solar radiation have a wide range of normal and abnormal effects on human skin, as described elsewhere in this book, although the majority of these are in fact normal. This chapter focuses on some of the molecular events that are thought to initiate or modulate these normal effects, which range from sunburn to skin cancer. However, it is first important to appreciate that the current basis of our understanding of these effects has been derived largely from studies on *in vitro* and animal models and whilst these provide obvious advantages, it is clearly important to confirm such model observations in human tissue, preferably *in vivo*, whenever possible. It is also important the observations be based on work with environmentally relevant wavelengths (i.e. ≥ 295 nm) at doses that have clinical significance (i.e. ≤ 3–4 minimal erythemal doses (MED)).

EPIDERMAL CHROMOPHORES AND ACTION SPECTRA

The clinical features of cutaneous solar exposure, whether acute or chronic, are the consequences of a usually complex series of

photochemical and photobiological events. Of these, the most fundamental is the absorption of solar UV or visible radiation by skin chromophores (see Young (1997) for review), the term chromaphore relates in a strict sense only to the conjugated multiple bonded (unsaturated) atoms of the molecule in question although usually used loosely to describe the whole molecule. A chromophore in solution has a very characteristic UV/visible radiation absorption spectrum, the energy from such absorption potentially enabling it to undergo chemical reactions within itself or with other molecules in the immediate subcellular environment. Such a chromophore may itself be a target biomolecule (e.g. DNA or urocanic acid), its direct structural alteration by UV or visible radiation absorption initiating the biological response. Alternatively, it may be a normal endogenous molecule (e.g. a porphyrin), causing indirect photosensitized damage to adjacent biomolecules (e.g. strand breaks in DNA) by the generation of, for example, reactive oxygen species (ROS) such as singlet oxygen or the superoxide anion (see UVR-induced oxidative stress, below); in fact, the accumulation of abnormally high levels of endogenous chromophores such as porphyrins because of congenital or acquired metabolic disorders may lead to certain photosensitivity disorders such as the porphyrias.

Photodermatology. Edited by J.L.M. Hawk. Published in 1998 by Chapman & Hall, London. ISBN 0 412 72460 X.

It is therefore clear that a detailed understanding of the mechanisms of the effects of UVR on skin is not possible without knowledge of the specific chromophores in question but, perhaps surprisingly, we will lack this knowledge in most cases. Clearly, DNA is one chromophore, UV absorption leading to mutagenic alterations in its structure, but indirect oxidative damage to the molecule may also occur following radiation absorption by other, as yet undefined molecules (see UVR-induced oxidative stress, below). However, since the absorption spectrum of the initiating chromophore determines the wavelength dependence, or **action spectrum**, of a given photobiological endpoint, this action spectrum can be used under ideal conditions to identify the chromophore, in that the two curves should overlap, as shown by a comparison of the spectrum of DNA absorption and that for the formation of thymine dimers *in vitro* in Figure 3.1(b). On the other hand, such conditions almost never occur in human skin and action spectra thus usually require correction, for example with epidermal transmission spectra, before definite mechanistic conclusions can be made.

UROCANIC ACID

Urocanic acid (UCA) is a deamination product of histidine, being formed in the stratum corneum by the enzyme histidine ammonia-lyase (histidase) but not broken down there because of a lack of urocanase at that site. Consequently, UCA is found at uniquely high concentrations in the stratum corneum. These are fairly constant in a range of body sites at about 6–12 nmol/cm^2 but are much higher, as might be expected, in the sole at 62 nmol/cm^2 (Kavanagh *et al.*, 1995). UCA may occur as either a trans- or cis-isomer, the former being the natural form in normal unirradiated skin before UVR exposure results in trans $\rightarrow$ cis photoiseomerization (Fig. 3.2). Both forms show broadly similar UVR absorption profiles, with absorption

peaks at about 268 nm (Fig. 3.2), and it was originally believed that UCA was a natural sunscreen. However, an action spectrum for the inhibition of normal immune function, derived from a mouse contact hypersensitivity (CHS) model, demonstrated a similar peak at 270 nm, thus providing a basis for proposing UCA as a possible chromophore for UVR-induced immunosuppression (De Fabo and Noonan, 1983). Since then, other experiments with a range of methodologies have supported this hypothesis, suggesting that cis-UCA may modulate many UVR-induced immunological responses (see Norval *et al.*, (1995) for recent review), although a recent study failed to confirm it as a mediator for the inhibition of CHS (El-Ghorr and Norval, 1995) while supporting its role in the suppression of a different model of immune function, namely delayed-type hypersensitivity. However, *in vitro* studies of the action spectrum for trans- $\rightarrow$ cis-UCA photoisomerization now show a maximum at about 280 nm, which demonstrates a 12 nm red-shift between absorption and action spectra (Jones *et al.*, 1966), but the authors suggest that this may be due to differences in the quantum yields for isomerization over the waveband range studied. In mouse skin *in vivo*, on the other hand, the action spectrum is shifted yet again, with a peak at 310–315 nm (Gibbs *et al.*, 1993), perhaps because of 270–280 nm screening by stratum corneum protein chromophores.

DNA

DNA, with an absorption maximum in the UVC region at about 260 nm (see Fig. 3.1(a)), also shows significant absorption in the solar UVB region as well as some UVA-absorbing properties (Sutherland and Griffin, 1981). Such absorption results in the formation of characteristic photoproducts, as shown in Figure 3.1(a), the most widely studied of which are cyclobutane pyrimidine dimers (CPD), which may be thymine-thymine

(a)

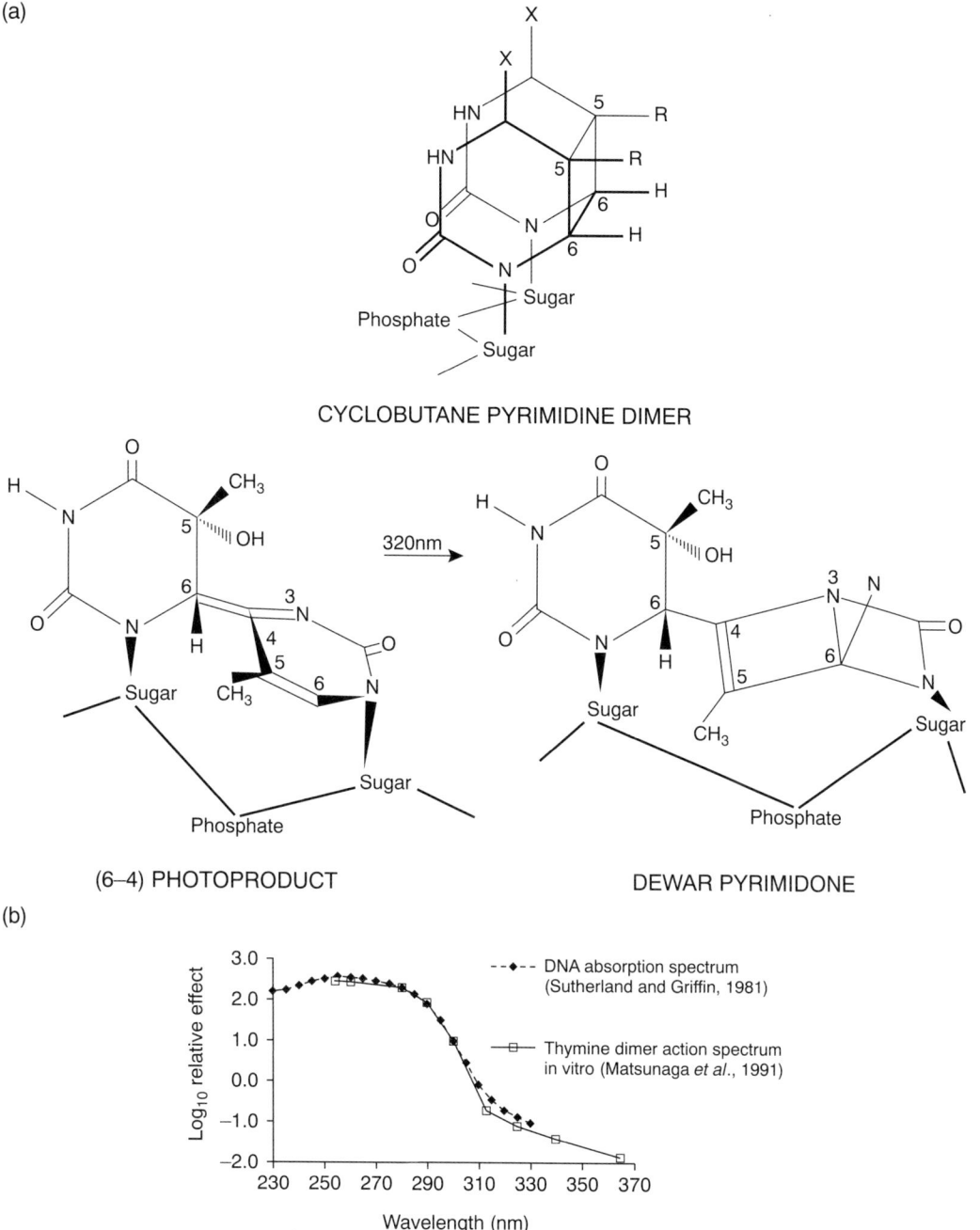

Figure 3.1 (a) Characteristic DNA photolesions resulting from direct absorption of UVR by DNA. (b) Quantum-corrected action spectrum for formation of thymine dimers *in vitro* shows good correlation with absorption spectrum of DNA. Action spectrum for formation of thymine dimers in human skin, especially at wavelengths of less than 300 nm, is different because of absorption by other chromophores, e.g. urocanic acid. (Author thanks Dr John Sutherland and Dr Tsukasa Matsunaga for generously providing raw data.)

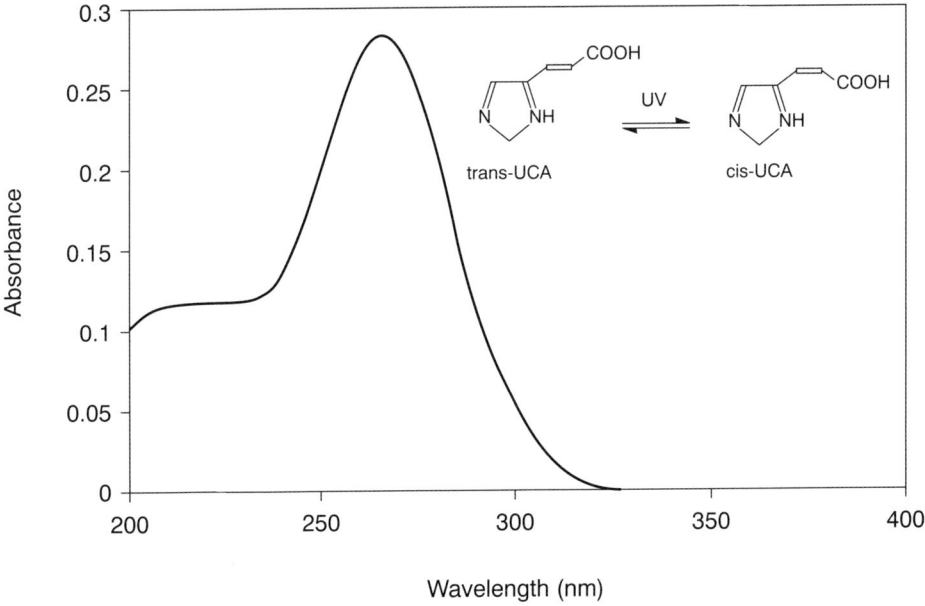

Figure 3.2 Molecular structure and absorption spectrum of urocanic acid. Several studies have implicated trans → cis photoisomerization as an initiating photochemical reaction for some models of UVR-induced immunosuppression. However, other studies have implicated DNA as chromophore. (Data generously provided by Dr N.K. Gibbs.)

(T = T), cytosine-cytosine (C = C), thymine-cytosine (T = C) or cytosine-thymine (C = T); recent studies on human skin explants with sensitive ^{32}P-high pressure liquid chromatography techniques, which recognize trinucleotides, have shown the rank order for formation of these lesions by UVB TT = C > TT = T > ΛT = T (Bykov and Hemminki, 1996). However, at an approximately erythemogenic UVB dose (20 mJ/cm^2), there is only a small difference between the levels of TT = C and TT = T. These authors also found higher levels of UVB- but not UVC-induced CPD in skin as compared to those occurring in naked DNA, suggesting that skin CPD may be induced partly by UVB photosensitizing reactions. Further, Mitchell *et al.* (1992) have reported a UVB-induced ratio in naked DNA for T = T : C = T : T = C : C = C of 52 : 19 : 21 : 7 and for UVC of 68 : 13 : 16 : 3, indicating also that CPD formation is spectrally dependent

overall. In addition, CPD may be induced by UVA irradiation in human skin *in vivo* (Freeman *et al.*, 1987, 1989; Young *et al.*, 1997) and in cells in culture (Matsunaga *et al.*, 1991). Apart from the formation of CPD, adjacent pyrimidines may also form the pyrimidine (6-4) pyrimidine photoproducts, or photoproducts (6-4) (see Fig. 3.1), generally at a lower frequency than CPD (Bykov and Hemminki, 1996; Mitchell and Nairn, 1989); these lesions, which show an absorption maximum at about 320 nm, may then be photoisomerized to the Dewar photoproduct following UVA irradiation (see Fig. 3.1). As expected, the *in vitro* action spectra for the formation of CPD and 6-4 are very similar (Matsunaga *et al.*, 1991), correlating well with the absorption spectrum of DNA (see Fig. 3.1), while the action spectrum for Dewar photoproduct formation from 6-4 correlates well with the absorption spectrum of 6-4

(Matsunaga *et al.*, 1991; Mitchell and Rosenstein, 1987). Although radiation of around 320 nm is the most efficient for 6-4 to Dewar conversion, the Dewar photoproduct *per se* is the more efficiently produced at shorter wavelengths because they are much more effective at inducing the 6-4 precursor (Matsunaga *et al.*, 1993).

DNA may be damaged by UVR-induced oxidative reactions, as well as by direct radiation absorption, although much less is known about the chromophores, photochemistry and photobiology involved in such damage (Cadet *et al.*, 1997). In fact, there is as yet limited direct evidence for such damage, although it may be expected from the production of UVR-induced ROS. DNA lesions likely to be caused by ROS include strand breaks and protein crosslinking (Peak and Peak, 1991), as well as the formation of 8-hydroxy-deoxyguanisine (8-OHdG) (Beehler *et al.*, 1991; Hattori *et al.*, 1997).

DNA PHOTOLESIONS IN THE SKIN *IN VIVO* AND THEIR REPAIR

During the past decade, several studies have reported the presence of CPD in human epidermis after its *in vivo* exposure to UVR. However, for the most part, these have used endonuclease-sensitive site (ESS) techniques which require epidermal disaggregation prior to analysis. Thus, the relatively recent development of monoclonal antibodies highly specific for DNA photolesions, in association with quantitative image analysis techniques, provides another approach for the study of DNA photodamage and its repair. For example, Chadwick *et al.* (1995) and Young *et al.* (1996) have demonstrated the presence of thymine dimers and 6-4 in human epidermis *in situ*, while the Dewar photoisomer was detected with a UVC + UVA irradiation protocol (Chadwick *et al.*, 1995) but not, surprisingly, after exposure to 4 MED of solar simulating radiation (SSR) (Young *et al.*, 1996). However, Clingen *et al.* (1995) did

detect the Dewar product in human mononuclear cells exposed to natural summer UK (50°N) sunlight.

Young *et al.* (1996) have investigated the decay kinetics of thymine dimers and 6-4 in human epidermis of skin types I and II exposed to SSR. Repair of the latter is rapid with the half-life of 2.3 hours, consistent with the results of comparable studies *in vitro* and in animal models (see Young *et al.*, 1996); however, the thymine dimer decay curve showed a half-life of 33.3 hours, suggesting a much slower repair, and much slower than has previously been reported for CPD. However, although thymine dimers represent a major CPD fraction (Bykov and Hemminki, 1996; Mitchell *et al.*, 1992), it is possible that the repair rates for different CPD types are different. On the other hand, some evidence suggests that slow DNA repair may be a factor in the causation of skin cancer. Young adults with basal cell carcinoma and skin type 1 basal cell carcinoma patients show reduced overall DNA photolesion repair capacity in peripheral lymphocytes when compared with age-matched controls, suggesting, as is the case with xeroderma pigmentosum patients (see Chapter 11), that poor DNA repair capacity is a skin cancer risk factor (Wei *et al.*, 1993, 1995). However, a comparison of the repair kinetics of epidermal thymine dimers and 6-4 has shown no differences between the skin cancer-prone types I/II and the more resistant types III/IV (author's unpublished data).

It is apparent from the foregoing that the global measurement of DNA repair gives an incomplete and misleading picture of events at the gene level. Thus, several *in vitro* studies have shown transcription-coupled repair in which the transcribed strand shows faster CPD repair than the non-transcribed strand (for review, see Hanawalt (1996)). For example, *in vitro* studies with human cells have shown preferential repair of the p53 gene in the transcribed strand (Ford *et al.*, 1994), as have studies in mouse skin demonstrating about 80% lesion loss in 24 hours, whereas almost no such repair was seen in non-transcribed strands (Ruven *et al.*, 1994). Further, another mouse study showed that 60% of CPD repair in actively transcribed genes occurred within the first four hours after exposure, with no repair at all in the inactive c-mos proto-oncogene (Ruven *et al.*, 1993). In addition, CPD repair rates may vary within a given gene; for example, more than 50% of CPDs were still present 24 hours after $20 \, \text{mJ/cm}^2$ of UVC in the promoter region of the human c-jun gene, but repair was tenfold faster near the transcription initiation site on both transcribed and non-transcribed strands (Tu *et al.*, 1996). However, a repair gradient was seen on the transcribed strand, with more efficient repair at the 5′ end of the gene. It is not known if this phenomenon is c-jun specific, shared with other UVR-inducible genes or common to all genes. In addition, some *in vitro* studies now suggest that rapid CPD repair is not invariably confined to the transcribed gene and that 6-4 repair lacks strand specificity (Mullenders *et al.*, 1993; Vreeswijk *et al.*, 1994); however, more recent data again appear to show transcription-coupled 6-4 repair (Van Hoffen *et al.*, 1995).

LOCATION OF DNA PHOTOLESIONS WITHIN THE EPIDERMIS

It is reasonable to assume that unrepaired DNA damage is unlikely to have long-term genetic consequences unless it is in the proliferative basal layer of the epidermis. Thus, a specific and important advantage of the use of monoclonal antibody techniques over previous ones is that lesion location within the epidermis, or dermis, can be identified; furthermore, damage to specific cell types such as melanocytes can be shown with double-staining techniques (Potten *et al.*, in press). By these means, Chadwick *et al.* (1995) have shown that non-solar UVC-induced human DNA photodamage is confined

mainly to the suprabasal layers. In addition, perhaps surprisingly, an assessment of thymine dimer levels at various epidermal layers showed a lack of damage gradient with depth for UVB at 300 nm, an observation recently confirmed in a more comprehensive analysis of the action spectra for thymine dimer formation in human skin *in vivo* (Young *et al.*, 1997). These data further suggest that the potential effects of ozone layer depletion on human non-melanoma skin cancer may have been underestimated from UVR transmission measurements on *ex vivo* epidermal samples (De Gruijl and van der Leun, 1994).

The mouse model has been used to study CPD formation in antigen-presenting cells (Vink *et al.*, 1996) and such cells containing CPD have been recovered from draining lymph nodes at least four days after skin irradiation; thus cutaneous DNA damage can be transferred via cell trafficking to other parts of the body.

UVR-INDUCED MUTATIONS IN KERATINOCYTES AND MELANOCYTES AND THEIR CONSEQUENCES

The mutagenic potential of DNA photolesions has long been established in *in vitro* systems, while their significance in animal and human skin has also become apparent over the past few years.

UVR-induced mutations are highly specific to dipyrimidine sites and this characteristic, a direct consequence of photoproduct formation at such sites, provides an important means of identifying genes. The UVR-induced mutation in relevant mutations mainly involved guanine (C) cytosine to adenine (A) thymine transitions, almost invariably from C → T or CC → TT (tandem) base changes. It has recently been suggested that such mutations are mediated via the deamination of cytosine to uracil (Peng and Shaw, 1996). Further, the apparently low mutagenic potential of T = T lesions (Ziegler *et al.*, 1993), and possibly their slow repair in comparison to overall CPD, may be due to the so-called A rule, which states that only adenine is incorporated opposite any unrecognized lesions. It is now widely accepted that one of the most important mutations in human cancer is that of the p53 gene and several recent studies have provided compelling evidence that a characteristic UVR-induced mutation of this type plays a major role in the initiation of non-melanoma skin cancer and actinic keratoses (Daya-Grosjean *et al.*, 1995; Ziegler *et al.*, 1993). Thus, tandem dipyrimidine p53 mutations are very rare (less than 1%) in internal tumours but occur in 14% and 53% of non-melanoma skin tumours from normal and xeroderma pigmentosum patients respectively, while only 61% of p53 base substitutions in internal tumours are opposite dipyrimidine sequences compared with more than 90% in non-melanoma skin cancers (Daya-Grosjean *et al.*, 1995). In addition, p53 mutation hotspots in skin cancers are different from those of internal tumours (Ziegler *et al.*, 1993).

Other recent evidence now indicates that intermittent or chronic solar exposure favours clonal expansion of p53 mutated human keratinocytes *in situ* in normal skin (Jonason *et al.*, 1996). Thus, three-dimensional morphological analysis has shown conically shaped clones originating from the dermoepidermal junction, apparently indicative of stem cell origins. The frequencies and sizes of such clones were much greater in chronically sun-exposed skin but the average clone size was age independent. These observations therefore suggest that, in addition to inducing p53 mutations, solar exposure may continue to act as a so-called tumour promoter.

There are different types of UVR-induced mutation with varying prevalences and these have been assessed at the APRT locus in CHO cells (Drobetsky *et al.*, 1995), $C \rightarrow T$ base changes accounting for 57%, 67% and 22% of UVC-, UVB- and UVA-induced mutations respectively; on the other hand, $CC \rightarrow TT$ changes were fewer but of equal prevalence (5%) for all three spectral regions. Further,

37% of UVA-induced lesions were $T \rightarrow G$ transversions compared with 9% for UVB, suggesting this may be useful in identifying UVA-induced genetic damage. However, this observation was not confirmed in a human cell line by Robert *et al.* (1996), who instead found some $A \rightarrow T$ transversions. Nevertheless, these data do indicate that UVA, which accounts for more than 95% of solar UVR, may also play an important role in human skin cancer. As far as malignant melanoma is concerned, p53 mutation does not seem to play a major inducing role, although UVR-specific mutations of this type have been reported in metastatic melanoma (Hartmann *et al.*, 1996). However, charac-teristic UVR-induced mutations of the CDKN2 gene, which codes for the cyclin-dependent kinase inhibitor p16, have instead been implicated in this condition (Pollack *et al.*, 1995).

NON-GENETIC CONSEQUENCES OF DNA PHOTODAMAGE IN RELATION TO SKIN CANCER

There is considerable evidence that UVR-induced mutation is important in skin cancer. However, DNA photodamage may also lead to other consequences with important roles in skin cancer, as shown in Figure 3.3, but whereas mutations leave characteristic signatures, it is often difficult to establish a link between photolesions and non-genetic biological outcomes. Nevertheless, a general approach to this problem has been to enhance CPD repair, either by the photoactivation of photolyase, which monomerizes CPD, or by the addition of endonucleases, which recognize CPD. Thus, animal studies in which DNA repair has been so enhanced have shown an important role for CPD in the induction of both non-melanoma (Yarosh *et al.*, 1992) and melanoma (Ley *et al.*, 1989) skin cancer, but it must also be borne in mind that the excision repair process, as well as the lesion *per se*, may conceivably initiate contributory biological responses.

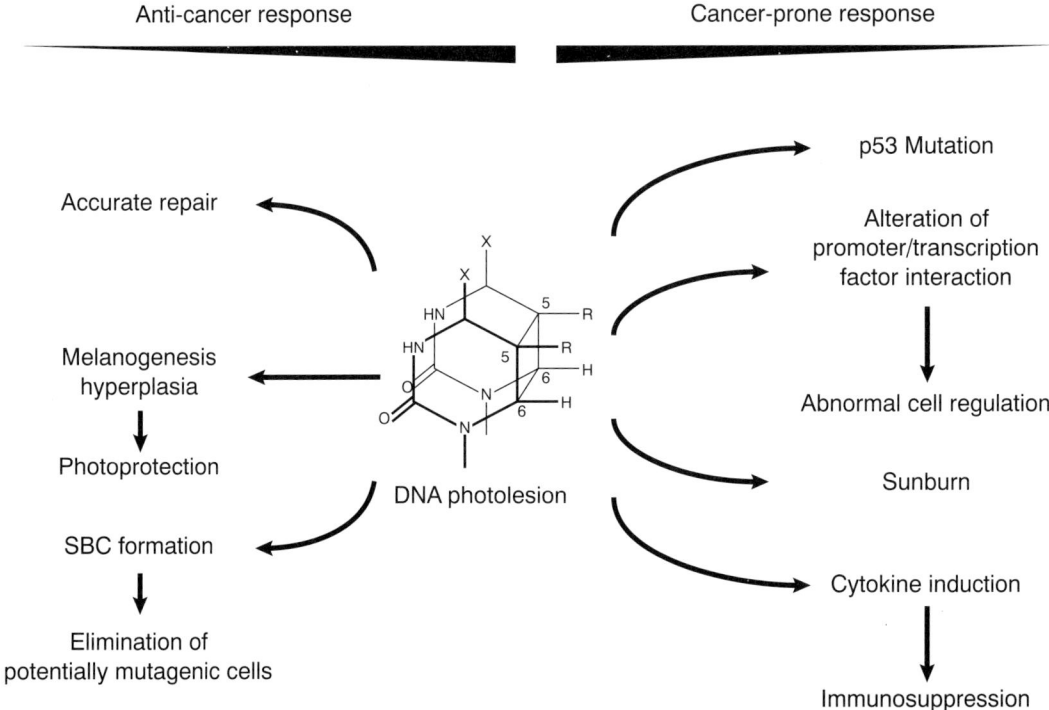

Anti-cancer response   Cancer-prone response

Accurate repair

Melanogenesis
hyperplasia

Photoprotection

SBC formation

Elimination of
potentially mutagenic cells

DNA photolesion

p53 Mutation

Alteration of
promoter/transcription
factor interaction

Abnormal cell regulation

Sunburn

Cytokine induction

Immunosuppression

Figure 3.3 Possible relationships between DNA photoproducts (e.g. CPD) and skin cancer. Scheme shows that single type of photolesion may induce multiple biological responses which contribute to skin cancer.

INFLAMMATION (SUNBURN, ERYTHEMA)

UVR-induced inflammation (sunburn, erythema) is the most widely used clinical endpoint for clinical and experimental photobiological investigations in general and, in particular, is the standard endpoint for sunscreen sun protection factor (SPF) determinations. In addition, epidemiological evidence suggests a link between malignant melanoma and basal cell carcinoma and sunburning episodes (Elwood, 1996; Kricker et al., 1995; Whiteman and Green, 1994). As yet, the chromophore for UVR inflammation has not been unequivocally established, but UVA-induced activation of endogenous CPD repair enzyme, photolyase, in the marsupial *Monodelphis domestica* has been shown to inhibit UVB-induced inflammation (Ley,

1985), thus providing strong evidence that CPD formation is directly associated with initiating the response. More recently, comparisons of the action spectra for thymine dimer formation in human skin *in vivo* and in inflammatory erythema, in the same volunteers, have also provided evidence, this time indirect, to support a role for DNA photodamage, but not necessarily the CPD, in the erythema induction (Young *et al.*, 1997). Beyond this, there is further evidence that topical application of liposome-encapsulated endonuclease DNA repair enzyme increases the 48-hour MED in Japanese xeroderma pigmentosum patients (Yarosh *et al.*, 1996), while Young *et al.* (1996) have observed that the loss of 6-4 correlated with the simultaneous onset of SSR-induced erythema in human skin, thus suggesting that the 6-4 repair itself may initiate the erythema response. Overall, these data therefore strongly suggest that erythema may be regarded as a clinical surrogate for DNA photodamage, but it must also be clearly remembered that thymine dimers and 6-4 are also induced in human epidermis, albeit in proportionally smaller amounts by sub-erythemal SSR exposures (Young *et al.*, 1996).

MELANOGENESIS

The addition of the DNA repair enzyme, endonuclease, to UV-irradiated cultured melanocytes enhances melanogenesis, suggesting that DNA excision repair may initiate this process (Gilchrest *et al.*, 1993), a hypothesis which has now been further evaluated by the addition of synthetic thymidine dinucleotides, which mimic dimer excision fragments, to cultured mouse melanoma cells and human melanocytes in the absence of UVR exposure (Eller *et al.*, 1994). Such cells showed an increase in melanin content and tyrosinase mRNA concentrations as a result, while the topical application of thymidine dinucleotide to guinea pig skin also induced melanogenesis with a time course similar to that observed after UVR.

Little is known about the photoprotective properties of human pigmentation although epidemiological data indicate that constitutive pigmentation protects against skin cancer. Furthermore, 'white' skin types III/IV who tan well are at less risk than skin types I/II who tan poorly if at all. One study showed that SSR-induced tanning in skin types III/IV resulted in a protection factor of about 2 against DNA photodamage but no photoprotection was seen in skin types I/II despite SSR-induced pigmentation which was seen at the histological level only in skin type I. (Young *et al.*, 1991; Potten *et al.*, 1993). Although modest, a persistent protection factor of 2 could result in a 50% reduction of cumulative UVR dose and significantly delay the onset of skin cancer.

HYPERPLASIA

Cutaneous hyperplasia lasting for some weeks follows most UVR, although generally not UVA, exposure, as a result of markedly increased cellular DNA, RNA and protein synthesis and mitosis, after some hours of cessation of such activity (Hawk and Parrish, 1982). At least in animals, this follows the induction of DNA damage and may be related to it, as for melanogenesis and perhaps inflammation, although its degree correlates better with the tendency to later carcinogenesis (Berton *et al.*, 1997). This several-fold, particularly stratum corneum, cutaneous thickening may then perhaps give some protection against later photodamage, in association with that provided by melanogenesis.

CYTOKINE AND ADHESION MOLECULE INDUCTION AND IMMUNOSUPPRESSION

The exposure of keratinocytes to UVR modulates the synthesis and release of a wide range of cytokines, for example tumour necrosis factor alpha (TNF-α) and interleukin (IL)-10 (Ullrich, 1995), and of adhesion molecules (Krutmann *et al.*, 1994), some of which are thought to play a major role in UVR-induced inflammation and immunosuppression (see Chapter 5). Yarosh (1992) and Yarosh and Kripke (1996) have speculated that such cytokine induction is mediated through DNA photodamage, but the precise chromophore initiating the actual immunosuppression itself remains controversial, both DNA and urocanic acid being considered as candidate molecules (see Urocanic acid and DNA, above). Thus, mouse studies have suggested that post-UVR topical application of the liposome-encapsulated CPD repair enzyme, completely or partially abrogates normal UVR-induced inhibition of contact hypersensitivity (CHS) and delayed-type hypersensitivity (DTH) (Kripke *et al.*, 1992; Wolf *et al.*, 1993), restores the antigen-presenting function of Ia+ cutaneous dendritic cells recovered from draining lymph nodes (Vink *et al.*, 1996). More recent studies again, once more in association with enhanced CPD repair, have provided evidence that DNA is also the chromophore for IL-10 production *in vitro* and in mouse skin *in vivo* (Nichigori *et al.*, 1996), while others *in vitro* suggest the same for TNF-α, the enhanced repair of CPD inhibiting transcription of the TNF-α promoter (Heymadi *et al.*, 1996). However, this is not in accord with our own recent *in vivo* data (unpublished), in which CPD repair was independent of skin type but more TNF-α release per MED was observed in sun-sensitive people. Nevertheless, the UVR-induced inhibition of intercellular adhesion molecule-1 (ICAM-1) gene expression in fibroblasts again appears to be mediated through DNA photodamage (Krutmann *et al.*, 1994, 1996; Krutmann and Grewe, 1995).

SUNBURN CELL FORMATION

Characteristic eosinophilic cells with shrunken cytoplasm and pyknotic nuclei are observed in the epidermis after UVR exposure (Young, 1987); these are known as sunburn cells (SBC) and now widely recognized as apoptotic epidermal cells. Animal studies in which CPD repair has been enhanced have provided evidence that DNA is a major chromophore for their formation (Applegate *et al.*, 1985; Wolf *et al.*, 1995) although oxidative damage has also been implicated (Hanada *et al.*, 1997). Young (1987) speculated that the formation of such cells was an active process directed at preventing later carcinogenesis, a concept now supported by studies showing their decreased formation in p53-deficient mice (Ziegler *et al.*, 1994), thus suggesting that p53 induction initiates SBC formation. Further, the localisation of p53 protein and frequency of apoptosis have been shown to correlate directly with UVB irradiation dose in human keratinocytes *in vitro* (Cotton and Spandau, 1997), observations consistent with the role of p53 as genomic guardian and the hypothesis that p53 mutation spares DNA-damaged keratinocytes and permits their progression by clonal expansion to malignancy (see UVR-induced mutations, above).

EFFECTS OF UVR EXPOSURE ON INTRACELLULAR SIGNAL TRANSDUCTION

Exposure to adverse external stimuli, including UVR, is known to modify gene transcription and many of the clinical effects of cutaneous solar exposure are almost certainly the consequence of such UVR-induced changes which have been documented for at least 100 mammalian genes both *in vitro* and *in vivo* (Keyse, 1993; Tyrrell, 1996). Such genes with particular relevance to skin are, for example, those associated with collagenase and other matrix metalloproteinases (MMPs) (Fisher *et al.*, 1996; Brenneisen *et al.*, 1996; Wlaschek *et al.*, 1995), elastin and fibrillin (Bernstein *et al.*, 1994), collagen types I and III (Neocleous *et al.*, 1997) and haem oxygenase 1 (Tyrrell, 1996).

MECHANISMS OF UVR-INDUCED ALTERATIONS IN GENE TRANSCRIPTION

The mechanisms by which incident UVR interacts with gene expression are very complex but are gradually becoming understood. Thus, there are cascades of molecular events initiated by signals resulting from the absorption of UVR by cellular chromophores; multiple transduction of these signals then ultimately often rapidly interferes with transcription factors, pre-existing proteins which after undergoing post-translational modification, can in turn enhance gene expression. A more detailed account of the current understanding of these mechanisms is outside the scope of this chapter, however, and interested readers are therefore referred to the excellent recent reviews by Bender *et al.* (1997) and

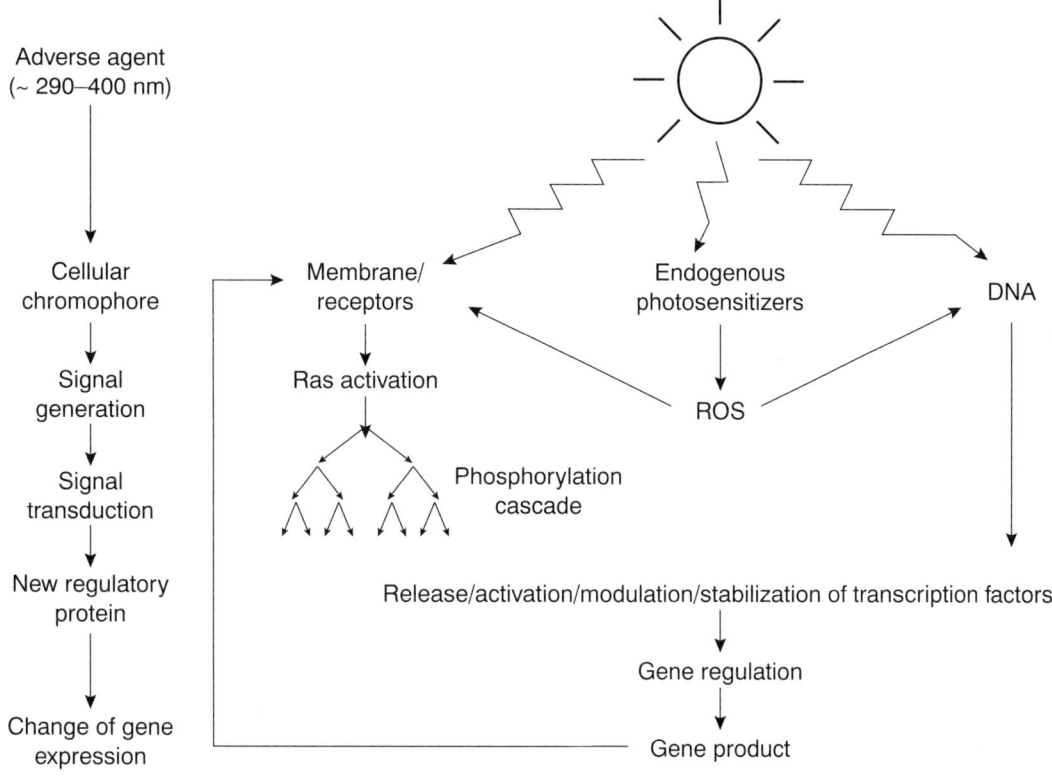

Figure 3.4 Simplified account of possible mechanisms of UVR-induced gene expression determined in *in vitro* systems, often after genetic manipulation. (See Bender *et al.* (1997) for recent comprehensive review.) ROS, reactive oxygen species.

Pentland (1996), the latter in summary form. Nevertheless, a simplistic account of some of the mechanistic events involved is given in Figure 3.4. Further, UVC irradiation has been shown to activate tyrosine kinase activity in the epidermal growth factor and insulin receptors of cultured cells with a functional kinase domain (Coffer *et al.*, 1995) while neither the kinase activity nor a panel of downstream events, for example leukotriene synthesis and transcriptional induction, was observed in mutant cells with a 'Rinasededd' receptor. These studies thus suggest a major role for receptor-mediated events in the cellular response to UVR exposure, as well as providing indirect evidence that this response also shares many of the pathways of growth factor-induced signal transduction.

To date, UVR-related research has focused on three transcription factors, namely activator protein (AP)-1 complexes, tumour suppressor gene p53 and nuclear factor kappa B (NFκB).

AP-1

A complex of c-jun and c-fos oncogene products form one of the AP-1 transcription factors. The c-jun gene is itself autoregulated by its own product within a heterdimeric complex with ATF-2. Relatively small doses of UVC (30 mJ/cm^2) rapidly induce transcription of the c-jun and c-fos genes with maximal levels about 30 minutes after exposure

(Herrlich *et al.*, 1994). However, inhibition of protein synthesis by the addition of cycolheximide does not inhibit UV-induced transcription of genes that depend on c-jun/c-fos products, demonstrating the importance of post-translational modification of pre-existing AP-1.

p53

The consequences of p53 mutation have been described above, but otherwise UVR exposure results in enhanced normal p53 expression after the stabilization of a previously unstable protein, rather than after increased p53 transcription. Further immunocytochemical staining has shown increased p53 levels in human skin *in vivo* after solar simulating (Hall *et al.*, 1993) and UVA, UVB and UVC (Campbell *et al.*, 1993) irradiation. The UVC staining was confined to the upper epidermis, consistent with the location of DNA photolesions such as CPD (Chadwick *et al.*, 1995), while the UVB (300 nm) changes occurred evenly throughout the epidermis, again consistent with their being at CPD locations (Chadwick *et al.*, 1995; Young *et al.*, 1997). However, the UVA-induced accumulation of p53 were in the basal layer only, in contrast with the presence of CPD in all epidermal layers (Young *et al.*, 1997), thus perhaps suggesting the possibility of p53 induction also by methods other than those associated with CPD formation, for example, by an endogenous photosensitizer in the basal layer.

NFκB

NFκB is a cytoplasmic factor normally kept inactive by its complexation with the protein IκB. Dissociation of this complex is then a prerequisite for migration of the factor to the nucleus and its consequent transcriptional activity. UVB and UVC irradiation have been shown to induce this activity independently of nuclear DNA photodamage (Devary *et al.*, 1993; Simon *et al.*, 1994), thus suggesting that membrane-related chromophores may initiate the transduction cascade, but a recent study now suggests that NFκB may be activated by photo-oxidative damage to DNA (Legrand-Poels *et al.*, 1995).

Recent *in vivo* skin data have shown that 2 MED of UVB irradiation may upregulate AP-1 and NFκB DNA binding within 15 minutes of exposure (Fisher *et al.*, 1996), while substantial increases in binding of up to half the maximum observed with 2 MED were also seen within 30 minutes with doses as low as 0.1 MED. Dose–response and time course studies for the production of some metalloproteinase proteins and their corresponding mRNAs also correlated well with this upregulation, thus suggesting a causal relationship, although *in vitro* wavelength dependence studies suggested that DNA was not the chromophore (Brenneisen *et al.*, 1996). Overall, however, the studies above of Fisher *et al.* (1996) suggest that a few minutes' sun exposure may have profound molecular and possibly clinical consequences, metalloproteinases perhaps playing a major role in skin photoageing (Fisher *et al.*, 1996). In addition, these enzymes may also have a crucial role in skin carcinogenesis, a recent study having shown no UVB-induced tumours in elastase-deficient mice but a 100% prevalence in genetically related normal animals (Starcher *et al.*, 1996); however, the precise explanation for this observation remains uncertain.

UVR-induced CPD and 6-4 have been demonstrated at specific transcription factor binding sites in the promoter region of human genes such as c-jun, c-fos and proliferating cell nuclear antigen (PCNA) (Tornaletti and Pfeifer, 1995), the level of such photodamage is dependent on the presence or absence of transcription factor complexation.

Thus, the presence of CPD in DNA oligonucleotide sequences specifically recognized by transcription factors such as AP-1, p53 and NFκB, all synthetic promoters, has major inhibitory effects on their binding (Tommasi *et al.*, 1996). This observation, therefore, coupled with the known occurrence of slow DNA repair in the promoter regions of genes (Gao *et al.*, 1994; Tu *et al.*, 1996), gives rise to the possibility that photodamage at such sites, sustained with or without transcription factor complexation, may interfere with normal cell regulation.

UVR-INDUCED OXIDATIVE STRESS

There is considerable evidence that the cutaneous effects of UVC and UVB irradiation are mediated by different molecular mechanisms from those of UVA. Thus, *in vitro* studies have shown that the former are largely initiated by direct DNA chromophore damage as a result of UVR absorption; in contrast, however, the UVA effects are mainly from indirect damage by reactive oxygen species (ROS), generated following radiation absorption by other, as yet poorly defined chromophores. In view of these differences, there is an increasing trend to subdivide the UVA spectrum into UVAI (340–400 nm) and UVAII (320–340 nm), to take into account the fact that UVAII-induced damage is generally similar to that caused by UVB; however, it must also be stressed that there is no absolute cut-off wavelength between the two mechanisms as the absorption spectra for different chromophores appear to overlap. Thus, UVB irradiation may also induce the oxidative damage normally associated with UVA, the characteristic lesion 8-hydroxydeoxyguanisine (8-OHdG) having been demonstrated in UVB-irradiated mouse keratinocytes both *in vitro* (Beehler *et al.*, 1992) and *in vivo* (Hattori *et al.*, 1997), while there is also good *in vitro* evidence that much UVB-induced cytotoxic damage may be of a similar nature (Beehler *et al.*, 1992; Punnonen *et al.*, 1991; Tyrrell and Pidoux, 1988; Vile *et al.*, 1995).

The contribution of ROS-associated effects of mammalian skin responses *in vivo*, including in particular to solar UVR-induced inflammation, is poorly understood. However, action spectrum studies for the induc-tion of squamous cell carcinoma in the mouse suggest the presence of a related UVA-absorbing chromophore (De Gruijl and van der Leun, 1994), supporting a possible role for ROS. In addition, studies in human skin *in vivo* have shown that hypoxia suppresses UVA- but not UVB-induced inflammation (Auletta *et al.*, 1986), while recent inflammation action spectrum studies also suggest the involvement of a UVA-absorbing chromophore in the reaction (Anders *et al.*, 1995). Further, antioxidants have been shown to inhibit the human sunburn response (Montenegro *et al.*, 1995) and the development of skin cancer in mice (Black, 1993) and perhaps man (Haegerty, 1994). Recent work also demonstrates that the production of ROS is a common step in the induction of cytoplasmic transcription factors, such as, for example, NFκB which plays a key role in controlling inflammation in endothelial cells (Manning and Anderson, 1994), and in cultured human fibroblasts (Vile *et al.*, 1995), this latter was an important study in that it showed UVB ROS induction required very cytotoxic doses. Such activation of NFκB may then lead to many important cellular and tissue events, including induction of inflammatory mediators such as cytokines (for example, TNF-α, IL-1, IL-6, IL-8), haemopoietic growth factors, activated cell adhesion molecules, inflammatory enzymes (for example, nitric oxide synthetase and cyclo-oxygenase), and degenerative enzymes such as metalloproteinases.

Action spectra for a given outcome may be used as biological weighting functions to determine the relative effects on that outcome of the different UVR wavelengths. With such an approach, almost all calculations have implicated UVB as the major cause of both acute and long-term solar UVR effects, despite the fact that more than 95% of such UVR is in the UVA region. Nevertheless, the determination of an action spectrum for malignant melanoma induction in a fish model has recently suggested that UVA may be of possible major importance in the causation of this tumour (Setlow *et al.*, 1993), and this controversial analysis, although based on a fish but nevertheless supported by some human epidemiological data (Young, 1996), thus suggests a greater role for UVR-induced oxidative damage, at least in producing this outcome, than hitherto suspected. In addition, an ongoing study on melanoma causation in the opossum *Monodelphis domestica* also suggests that UVA may have a greater role in inducing melanoma or its precursors than non-melanoma skin cancer (Ley, 1997).

CONCLUSION

UVR exposure leads to a wide range of acute and long-term normal effects on human skin and research during the past decade has seen considerable progress in our understanding of the molecular basis of these effects. However, these studies have also demonstrated an extreme and perhaps unexpected complexity to these mechanisms. Further, much of the work undertaken has been *in vitro* and thus now requires *in vivo* confirmation in human skin. However, the available evidence increasingly suggests that all cutaneous UVR effects are mediated through a variety of chromophores and in a variety of cellular targets. Furthermore, it is also now clear that damage to one of these chromophores, namely nuclear DNA, can result in several quite different types of adverse acute biological event which, when combined and frequently repeated over many years, may eventually give rise to the outcomes of skin ageing and cancer.

ACKNOWLEDGEMENT

I thank John Sheehan for his help in preparing the figures and references.

REFERENCES

Anders, A., Altheide, H.J., Knalmann, M. *et al.* (1995) Action spectrum for erythema in humans investigated with dye lasers. *Photochemistry and Photobiology*, **61** (2), 200–5.

Applegate, L.A., Stuart, T.D. and Ley, R.D. (1985) Ultraviolet radiation-induced histopathological changes in the skin of the marsupial Monodelphis domestica. I. The effects of acute and chronic exposures and of photoreactivation treatment. *British Journal of Dermatology*, **113** (2), 219–27.

Auletta, M., Gange, R.W., Tan, O.T. *et al.* (1986) Effect of cutaneous hypoxia upon erythema and pigment responses to UVA, UVB, and PUVA (8-MOP + UVA) in human skin. *Journal of Investigative Dermatology*, **86** (6), 649–52.

Beehler, B.C., Przybyszewski, J., Box, H.B. *et al.* (1992) Formation of 8-hydroxydeoxyguanosine within DNA of mouse keratinocytes exposed in culture to UVB and H_2O_2. *Carcinogenesis*, **13** (11), 2003–7.

Bender, K., Blattner, C., Knebel, A. *et al.* (1997) UV-induced signal transduction. *Journal of Photochemistry and Photobiology* (B-Biology), **37** (1-2), 1–17.

Bernstein E.F., Chen, Y.Q., Tamai, K. *et al.* (1994) Enhanced elastin and fibrillin gene expression in chronically photodamaged skin. *Journal of Investigative Dermatology*, **103** (2), 182–6.

Berton, T.R., Mitchell, D.L., Fischer, S.M. and Locniskar, M.F. (1997) Epidermal proliferation but not quantity of DNA photodamage is correlated with UV-induced mouse skin carcinogenesis. *Journal of Investigative Dermatology*, **109** (3), 340–7.

Black, H.S. (1993) The defensive role of antioxidants in skin carcinogenesis, in *Oxidative Stress Dermatology*, (eds J. Fuchs and L. Packer), Marcel Dekker, New York, pp. 243–69.

Brenneisen, P., Oh, J., Wlaschek, M. *et al.* (1996) Ultraviolet B wavelength dependence for the regulation of two major matrix-metalloproteinases and their inhibitor TIMP-1 in human dermal fibroblasts [corrected and republished article originally printed in 1996, 64 (4): 649–57]. *Photochemistry and Photobiology*, **64**, 877–85.

Bykov, V.J. and Hemminki, K. (1996) Assay of different photoproducts after UVA, B and C irradiation of DNA and human skin explants. *Carcinogenesis*, **17** (9), 1949–55.

Cadet, J., Berker, M., Douki, T. *et al.* (1997) Effects of UV and visible radiations on DNA- final base damage (Review). *Biological Chemistry*, **378** (11), 1275–86.

Campbell, C., Quinn, A.G., Angus, B. *et al.* (1993) Wavelength specific patterns of p53 induction in human skin following exposure to UV radiation. *Cancer Research*, **53**, 2697–9.

Chadwick, C.A., Potten, C.S., Nikaido, O. *et al.* (1995) The detection of cyclobutane thymine dimers (6-4) photolesions and the Dewar photisomers in sections of UV-irradiated human skin using specific antibodies, and the demonstration of depth penetration effects. *Journal of Photochemistry and Photobiology* (B-Biology), **28** (2), 163–70.

Clingen, P.H., Arlett, C.F., Roza, L. *et al.* (1995) Induction of cyclobutane pyrimidine dimers, pyrimidine (6-4) pyrimidone photoproducts, and Dewar valence isomers by natural sunlight in normal human mononuclear cells. *Cancer Research*, **55** (11), 2245–8.

Coffer, P.J., Burgering, B.M., Peppelenbosch, M.P. *et al.* (1995) UV activation of receptor tyrosine kinase activity. *Oncogene*, **11** (3), 561–9.

Cotton, J. and Spandau, D.F. (1997) Ultraviolet B-radiation dose influences the induction of apoptosis and p53 in human keratinocytes. *Radiation Research*, **147** (2), 148–55.

Daya-Grosjean, L., Dumaz, N. and Sarasin, A. (1995) The specificity of p53 mutation spectra in sunlight induced human cancers. *Journal of Photochemistry and Photobiology*, (B-Biology), **28** (2), 115–24.

De Fabo, E.C. and Noonan, F.P. (1983) Mechanism of immune suppression by ultraviolet irradiation in vivo. I. Evidence for the existence of a unique photoreceptor in skin and its role of photoimmunology. *Journal of Experimental Medicine*, **158** (1), 84–98.

De Gruijl, F.R., and van der Leun, J.C. (1994) Estimate of the wavelength dependency of ultraviolet carcinogenesis in humans and its relevance to the risk assessment of a stratospheric ozone depletion. *Health Physics*, **67** (3), 1–8.

Devary, Y., Rosette, C., DiDonato, J.A. and Karin, M. (1993) NF-κB Activation by ultraviolet light not dependent on a nuclear signal. *Science* **261**, 1442–5.

Drobetsky, E.A., Turcotte, J. and Chateauneuf, A. (1995) A role for ultraviolet A in solar mutagenesis. *Proceedings of the National Academy of Sciences of the USA*, **92** (6), 2350–4.

El-Ghorr, A.A. and Norval, M. (1995) A monoclonal antibody to cis-urocanic acid prevents the ultraviolet-induced changes in Langerhans cells and delayed hypersensitivity responses in mice, although not preventing dendritic cell accumulation in lymph nodes draining the site of irradiation and contact hypersensitivity responses. *Journal of Investigative Dermatology*, **105** (2), 264–8.

Eller, M.S., Yaar, M. and Gilchrest, B.A. (1994) DNA damage and melanogenesis. *Nature*, **372** (6506), 413–14.

Elwood, J.M. (1996) Melanoma and sun exposure. *Seminars in Oncology*, **23** (6), 650–66.

Fisher, G.J., Datta, S.C., Talwar, H.S. *et al.* (1996) Molecular basis of sun-induced premature skin ageing and retinoid antagonism. *Nature*, **379** (6563), 335–9.

Freeman, S.E., Gange, R.W., Sutherland, J.C. *et al.* (1987) Production of pyrimidine dimers in DNA of human skin exposed in situ to UVA radiation. *Journal of Investigative Dermatology*, **88** (4), 430–3.

Freeman, S.E., Hacham, H., Gange, R.W. *et al.* (1989) Wavelength dependence of pyrimidine dimer formation in DNA of human skin irradiated in situ with ultraviolet light. *Proceedings of the National Academy of Sciences of the USA*, **86** (14), 5605–9. xxxxx ???

Gao, S., Drouin, R. and Holmquist, G.P. (1994) DNA repair rates mapped along the human PGK-1 gene at nucleotide resolution. *Science*, **263**, 1438–40.

Gibbs, N.K., Norval, M., Traynor, N.J. *et al.* (1993) Action spectra for trans to cis photoisomerisation of urocanic acid in vitro and in mouse skin [published erratum appears in *Photochem Photobiol* (1993) **58** (5), 769]. *Photochemistry and Photobiology*, **57** (3), 584–90.

Gilchrest, B.A., Zhai, S., Eller, M.S. *et al.* (1993). Treatment of human melanocytes and S91 melanoma cells with the DNA repair enzyme T4 endonuclease V enhances melanogenesis after ultraviolet irradiation. *Journal of Investigative Dermatology*, **101**, 666–72.

Hall, P.A., McKee, P.H., Menage, H.D. *et al.* (1993) High levels of p53 protein in UV-irradiated normal human skin. *Oncogene*, **8** (1), 203–7.

Hanada, K., Sawamura, D., Tamai, K. *et al.* (1997) Photoprotective effect of esterified glutathione against ultraviolet B-induced sunburn cell formation in the hairless mice. *Journal of Investigative Dermatology*, **108** (5), 727–30.

Hanawalt, P.C. (1996) Role of transcription-coupled DNA repair in susceptibility to environmental carcinogenesis [review]. *Environmental Health Perspectives*, **104** (Suppl 3), 547–51.

Hartmann, A., Blaszyk, H., Cunningham, J.S. *et al.* (1996) Overexpression and mutations of p53 in metastatic malignant melanomas. *International Journal of Cancer*, **67** (3), 313–17.

Hattori, Y., Nishigori, C., Tanaka, T. *et al.* (1997) 8-hydroxy-2'-deoxyguanosine is increased in epidermal cells of hairless mice after chronic ultraviolet B exposure. *Journal of Investigative Dermatology*, **107**, 733–7.

Hawk, J.L.M. and Parrish, J.A. (1982) Responses of normal skin to ultraviolet radiation, in *The Science of Photomedicine*, (eds J.D. Regan and J.A. Parrish), Plenum Press, New York, pp. 219–60.

Haegerty, A.H.M. (1994) Glutathione S-transferase GSTM1 phenotypes and protection against cutaneous tumours. *Lancet*, **343**, 266–7.

Hejmadi, V., Kibitel, J. O'Connor, A. *et al.* (1996) DNA damage induced by UV is a signal for increased TNFα expression in human cells [abstract]. *Photochemistry and Photobiology*, , **63S**, 110S.

Herrlich, P., Sachsenmaier, C., Radler-Pohl, A. *et al.* (1994) The mammalian UV response: mechanism of DNA damage induced gene expression. *Advances in Enzyme Regulation*, **34**, 381–95.

Jonason, A.S., Kunala, S., Price, G.J. *et al.* (1996) Frequent clones of p53-mutated keratinocytes in normal human skin. *Proceedings of the National Academy of Sciences of the USA*, **93** (24), 14025–9.

Jones, C.D., Barton, A.K., Crosby, J. *et al.* (1996) Investigating the red shift between in vitro and in vivo urocanic acid photoisomerization action spectra. *Photochemistry and Photobiology*, **63** (3), 302–5.

Kavanagh, G., Crosby, J. and Norval, M. (1995) Urocanic acid isomers in human skin: analysis of site variation. *British Journal of Dermatology*, **133** (5), 728–31.

Keyse, S.M. (1993) The induction of gene expression in mammalian cells by radiation [review]. *Seminars in Cancer Biology*, **4** (2), 119–28.

Kricker, A., Armstrong, B.K., English, D.R. *et al.* (1995) Does intermittent sun exposure cause basal cell carcinoma? A case-control study in Western Australia. *International Journal of Cancer*, **60** (4), 489–94.

Kripke, M.L., Cox, P.A., Alas, L.G. *et al.* (1992) Pyrimidine dimers in DNA initiate systemic immunosuppression in UV-irradiated mice. *Proceedings of the National Academy of Sciences of the USA*, **89** (16), 7516–20.

Krutmann, J. and Grewe, M. (1995) Involvement of cytokines, DNA damage, and reactive oxygen intermediates in ultraviolet radiation-induced modulation of intercellular adhesion molecule-1 expression. *Journal of Investigative Dermatology*, **105** (Suppl 1), 67S–670S.

Krutmann, J., Bohnert, E. and Jung, E.G. (1994) Evidence that DNA damage is a mediate in ultra-violet B radiation-induced inhibition of human gene expression: ultraviolet B radiation effects on intercellular adhesion molecule-1(ICAM-1) expression. *Journal of Investigative Dermatology*, **102** (4), 428–32.

Krutmann, J., Ahrens, C., Roza, L. *et al.* (1996) The role of DNA damage and repair in ultra-violet B radiation-induced immunomodulation: relevance for human photocarcinogenesis. *Photochemistry and Photobiology*, **63** (4), 394–6.

Legrand-Poels, S., Bours, V., Piret, B. *et al.* (1995) Transcription factor NF-kappa B is activated by photosensitization generating oxidative DNA damages. *Journal of Biological Chemistry*, **270** (12), 6925–34.

Ley, R.D. (1985) Photoreactivation of UV-induced pyrimidine dimers and erythema in the marsupial Monodelphis domestica *Proceedings of the National Academy of Sciences of the USA*, **82** (8), 2409–11.

Ley, R.D. (1997) (UV-A)-induced precursors of melanoma in Monodelphis domestica [abstract]. *Photochemistry and Photobiology*, **65S**, 74S.

Ley, R.D., Appelgate, L.A., Padilla, R.S. *et al.* (1989) Ultraviolet radiation-induced malignant melanoma in Monodelphis domestica. *Photochemistry and Photobiology*, **50** (1), 1–5.

Manning, A.M., Beth, F.P., Rosenbloom, C.L. *et al.* (1995) NF-kB is activated during acute inflammation *in vivo* in association with elevated endothelial cell adhesion moleallegene expression and leukocyte recruitment. *Journal Inflammation*, C (45), 243–296.

Matsunaga, T., Hatakeyama, Y., Ohta, M. *et al.* (1993) Establishment and characterization of a monoclonal antibody recognizing the Dewar isomers of (6-4) photoproducts. *Photochemistry and Photobiology*, **57** (6), 934–40.

Matsunaga, T., Hieda, K. and Nikaido, O. (1991) Wavelength dependent formation of thymine dimers and (6-4) photoproducts in DNA by monochromatic ultraviolet light ranging from 150 to 365 nm. *Photochemistry and Photobiology*, **54** (3), 403–10.

Mitchell, D.L. and Nairn, R.S. (1989) The biology of the (6-4) photoproduct. *Photochemistry and Photobiology*, **49** (6), 805–19.

Mitchell, D.L. and Rosenstein, B.S. (1987) The use of specific radioimmunoassays to determine action spectra for the photolysis of (6-4) photoproducts. *Photochemistry and Photobiology*, **45** (6), 781–6.

Mitchell, D.L., Jen, J. and Cleaver, J.E. (1992) Sequence specificity of cyclobutane pyrimidine dimers in DNA treated with solar (ultraviolet B) radiation. *Nucleic Acids Research*, **20** (2), 225–9.

Montenegro, L., Bonina, F., Rigano, L. *et al.* (1995) Protective effect evaluation of free radical scavengers on UVB induced human cutaneous erythema by skin reflectance spectrophotometry. *International Journal of Cosmetic Science*, **17**, 91–103.

Neocleous, V., Young, A.R. and Brownson, C. (1997) UVR modulates the steady state levels of skin collagen transcripts in hairless mice. *Photochemistry and Photobiology*, **66**, 676–682.

Nishigori, C., Yarosh, D.B., Ullrich, S.E. *et al.* (1996) Evidence that DNA damage triggers interleukin 10 cytokine production in UV-irradiated murine keratinocytes. *Proceedings of the National Academy of Sciences of the USA*, **93** (19), 10354–9.

Norval, M., Gibbs, N.K. and Gilmour, J. (1995) The role of urocanic acid in UV-induced immunosuppression: recent advances (1992–1994). *Photochemistry and Photobiology*, **62** (2), 209–17.

Peak, J.G. and Peak, M.J. (1991) Comparison of initial yields of DNA-to-protein crosslinks induced in human cells in culture by X-rays, gamma rays, 0.05 McV neutrons, light photons in the UVC, UVB, UVA regions, and blue light. *Mutation Research*, **246** (1), 187–91.

Peng, W. and Shaw, B.R. (1996) Accelerated deamination of cytosine residues in UV-induced cyclobutane pyrimidine dimers leads to CC → TT transitions. *Biochemistry*, **35** (31), 10172–81.

Pentland, A.P. (1996) Signal transduction mechanisms in photocarcinogenesis. *Photochemistry and Photobiology*, **63** (4), 379–80.

Pollock, P.M., Yu, F., Qiu, L. *et al.* (1995) Evidence for UV induction of CDKN2 mutations in melanoma cell lines. *Oncogene*, **11** (4), 663–8.

Potten, C.S., Chadwick, C.A., Cohen, A.J. *et al.* (1993) DNA damage in UV-irradiated skin in vivo: automated direct measurement by image analysis (thymine dimers) compared with indirect measurement (unscheduled DNA synthesis) and protection by 5-methoxypsoralen. *International Journal of Radiation Biology*, **63** (3), 313–24.

Potten, C.S., Young, A.R., Nikaido, O. *et al.* (1998) Human melanocytes and keratinocytes exposed to UVB or UVA *in vivo* show comparable levels of thymine dimers. *Sound of Investigative Dermatology* (in press).

Punnonen, K., Puntala, A., Jansen, C.T. *et al.* (1991) UVB irradiation induces lipid peroxidation and reduces antioxidant enzyme activities in human keratinocytes in vitro. *Acta Dermatolo-Venereologica*, **71** (3), 239–42.

Robert, C., Muel, B., Benoit, A. *et al.* (1996) Cell survival and shuttle vector mutagenesis induced by ultraviolet A and ultraviolet B radiation in a human cell line. *Journal of Investigative Dermatology*, **106** (4), 721–8.

Ruven, H.J., Berg, R.J., Seelen, C.M. *et al.* (1993) Ultraviolet-induced cyclobutane pyrimidine dimers are selectively removed from transcriptionally active genes in the epidermis of the hairless mouse. *Cancer Research*, **53** (7), 1642–5.

Ruven, H.J., Sellen, C.M., Lohman, P.H. *et al.* (1994) Strand-specific removal of cyclobutane pyrimidine dimers from the p53 gene in the epidermis of UVB-irradiated hairless mice. *Oncogene*, **9** (12), 3427–32.

Setlow, R.B., Grist, E., Thompson, K. *et al.* (1993) Wavelengths effective in induction of malignant melanoma. *Proceedings of the National Academy of Sciences of the USA,*, **90** (14), 6666–70.

Simon, M.M., Aragane, Y., Schwarz, A. *et al.* (1994) UVB light induces nuclear factor kB (NFkB) activity independently from chromosomal DNA damage in cell-free extracts. *Journal of Investigative Dermatology*, **102**, 422–7.

Starcher, B., O'Neal, P., Granstein, R.D. *et al.* (1966) Inhibition of neutrophil elastase suppresses the development of skin tumours in hairless mice. *Journal of Investigative Dermatology*, **107** (2), 159–63.

Sutherland, J.C. and Griffin, K.P. (1981) Absorption spectrum of DNA for wavelengths greater than 300 nm. *Radiation Research*, **86** (3), 399–409.

Tommasi, S., Swiderski, P.M., Tu, Y. *et al.* (1996) Inhibition of transcription factor binding by ultraviolet-induced pyrimidine dimers. *Biochemistry*, **35** (49), 15693–703.

Tornaletti, S. and Pfeifer, G.P. (1995) UV light as a footprinting agent: modulation of UV-induced DNA damage by transcription factors bound at the promoters of three human genes. *Journal of Molecular Biology*, **249** (4), 714–28.

Tu, Y., Tornaletti, S. and Pfeifer, G.P. (1996) DNA repair domains within a human gene: selective repair of sequences near the transcription initiation site. *EMBO Journal*, **15** (3), 675–83.

Tyrrell, R.M. (1996) Activation of mammalian gene expression by the UV component of sunlight – from models to reality. *BioEssays*, **18** (2), 139–48.

Tyrrell, R.M. and Pidoux, M. (1988) Correlation between endogenous glutathione content and sensitivity of cultured human skin cells to radiation at different wavelengths in the solar ultraviolet range. *Photochemistry and Photobiology*, **47** (3), 405–12.

Ullrich, S.E. (1995) The role of epidermal cytokines in the generation of cutaneous immune reactions and ultraviolet radiation-induced immune suppression. *Photochemistry and Photobiology*, **62** (3), 389–401.

van Hoffen, A., Venema, J., Meschini, R. *et al.* (1995) Transcription-coupled repair removes both cyclobutane pyrimidine dimers and 6-4 photoproducts with equal efficiency and in a sequential way from transcribed DNA in xeroderma pigmentosum group C fibroblasts. *EMBO Journal*, **14** (2), 360–7.

Vile, G.F., Tanew-Ilitschew, A. and Tyrell, R.M. (1995) Activation of NF-kappa B in human skin fibroblasts by the oxidative stress generated by UVA radiation. *Photochemistry and Photobiology*, **62** (3), 463–8.

Vink, A.A., Strickland, F.M., Bucana, C. *et al.* (1996) Localization of DNA damage and its role in altered antigen-presenting cell function in ultraviolet-irradiated mice *Journal of Experimental Medicine*, **183** (4), 1491–500.

Vreeswijk, M.P., van Hoffen, A., Westland, B.E. *et al.* (1994) Analysis of repair of cyclobutane pyrimidine dimers and pyrimidine 6-4 pyrimidone photoproducts in transcriptionally active and inactive genes in Chinese hamster cells. *Journal of Biological Chemistry*, **269** (50), 31858–63.

Wei, Q., Matanoski, G.M., Farmer, E.R. *et al.* (1993) DNA repair and aging in basal cell carcinoma: a molecular epidemiological study. [published erratum appears in *Proc Natl Acad Sci USA* (1993) **90** (11):5378]. *Proceedings of the National Academy of Sciences of the USA*, **90** (4), 1614–18.

Wei, Q., Matonski, G.B., Farmer, E.R. *et al.* (1995) DNA repair capacity for ultraviolet light-induced damage is reduced in peripheral lymphocytes from patients with basal cell carcinoma. *Journal of Investigative Dermatology*, **104** (6), 933–6.

Whiteman, D. and Green, A. (1994) Melanoma and sunburn. *Cancer Causes and Control*, **5** (6), 564–72.

Wlaschek, M., Briviba, K., Stricklin, G.P. *et al.* (1995) Singlet oxygen may mediate the ultraviolet A-induced synthesis of interstitial collagenase. *Journal of Investigative Dermatology*, **104** (2), 194–8.

Wolf, P., Yarosh, D.B. and Kripke, M.L. (1993) Effects of sunscreens and a DNA excision repair enzyme on ultraviolet radiation-induced inflammation, immune suppression, and cyclobutane pyrimidine dimer formation in mice. *Journal of Investigative Dermatology*, **101** (4), 523–7.

Wolf, P., Cox, P., Yarosh, D.B. *et al.* (1995) Sunscreens and T4N5 liposomes differ in their ability to protect against ultraviolet-induced sunburn cell formation, alterations of dendritic epidermal cells, and local suppression of contact hypersensitivity. *Journal of Investigative Dermatology*, **104** (2), 287–92.

Yarosh, D.B. (1992) The role of DNA damage and UV-induced cytokines in skin cancer [review]. *Journal of Photochemistry and Photobiology* (B-Biology), **16** (1), 91–4.

Yarosh, D.B. and Kripke, M.L. (1996) DNA repair and cytokines in antimutagenesis and anticarcinogenesis [review]. *Mutation Research*, **350** (1), 255–60.

Yarosh, D.B., Alas, L.G., Yee, V. *et al.* (1992) Pyrimidine dimer removal enhanced by DNA repair liposomes reduces the incidence of UV skin cancer in mice. *Cancer Research*, **52** (15), 4227–31.

Yarosh, D.B., Klein, J., Kibitel, J. *et al.* (1996) Enzyme therapy of xeroderma pigmentosum: safety and efficacy testing of T4N5 liposome lotion containing a prokaryotic DNA repair enzyme. *Photodermatology, Photoimmunology and Photomedicine*, **12** (3), 122–30.

Young, A.R. (1987) The sunburn cell. *Photodermatology*, **4** (3), 127–34.

Young, A.R. (1996) Does UVA exposure cause human malignant melanoma? *European Journal of Dermatology*, **6** (3), 225–6.

Young, A.R. (1997) Chromophores in human skin. *Physics in Medicine and Biology*, **42**, 789–802.

Young, A.R., Potten, C.S., Chadwick, C.A. *et al.* (1991) Photoprotection and 5-MOP photochemoprotection from UVR-induced DNA damage in humans: the role of skin type. *Journal of Investigative Dermatology*, **97** (5), 942–8.

Young, A.R., Chadwick, C.A., Harrison, G.I. *et al.* (1996) The in situ repair kinetics of epidermal thymine dimers and 6-4 photoproducts in human skin types I and II. *Journal of Investigative Dermatology*, **106** (6), 1307–13.

Ziegler, A., Leffell, D.J., Kunala, S. *et al.* (1993) Mutation hotspots due to sunlight in the p53 gene of nonmelanoma skin cancers. *Proceedings of the National Academy of Sciences of the USA*, **90** (9), 4216–20.

Ziegler, A., Jonason, A.S., Leffell, D.J. *et al.* (1994) Sunburn and p53 in the onset of skin cancer. *Nature*, **372** (6508), 773–6.

4

THE ACUTE EFFECTS OF ULTRAVIOLET RADIATION ON THE SKIN

Gillian M. Murphy

The predominant early responses of human skin to ultraviolet (UV) irradiation are inflammation, tanning and thickening of the epidermis, although the important effects of vitamin D synthesis and immunological change also occur. The mechanisms underlying these processes and their clinical relevance are summarized in this chapter.

ACUTE EFFECTS OF UVB ON THE SKIN

UVB irradiation leads to acute inflammation, tanning and thickening of the skin together with vitamin D synthesis and immunosuppression, the action spectra for such inflammation and tanning incriminating UVB as most efficient at producing these effects (Parrish *et al.*, 1982).

Clinically evident inflammation caused by UVB is a delayed event, the first measurable change being vasodilatation identifiable within 1–5 hours by a reflectance device. Depending on the UV dose and skin type, erythema then gradually becomes visible, reaching maximal intensity by 24 hours and fading within three days. This inflammation persists longer in older individuals and those with defective DNA repair mechanisms. Pigmentation of the skin, or tanning, is also a delayed effect, mediated by melanocyte melanin synthesis. Melanocyte stimulating

hormone (MSH) receptors on melanocytes are upregulated during this process and a human skin equivalent model demonstrates the paracrine function of keratinocytes (Archambault *et al.*, 1982) which release several factors including MSH to stimulate the melanogenesis. Melanin absorbs and scatters UV radiation and also acts as a free radical scavenger. Melanosomes containing newly synthesized melanin are thus distributed throughout the epidermis, but particularly over the nuclei of the basal keratinocytes through the dendritic processes of the melanocytes, so as to minimize further UV damage to the epidermis and especially its stem cells. Evidence now implicates DNA damage and the excision of pyrimidine dimers as the initiating stimulus to the process (Eller *et al.*, 1996). Thus, tanning apparently occurs as a response to DNA damage and, although primarily a reaction to such cellular injury, leads as a result to a photoprotective outcome.

Epidermal proliferation, leading to epidermal thickening, also begins within hours and is histologically evident within days, while clinically evident desquamation of skin, a further delayed effect of acute UVB injury, is evident 2–3 weeks later, proportional to the degree of UV injury. UVB exposure also induces protein degrading enzymes (proteinases) at low doses, collagenase, stromelysin and gelatinase mRNA and protein being induced by UVB irradiation

Photodermatology. Edited by J.L.M. Hawk. Published in 1998 by Chapman & Hall, London. ISBN 0 412 72460 X.

corresponding to 2–3 minutes of sun exposure (Fisher *et al.*, 1996). This acute response perhaps contributes to the long-term effects of UV irradiation on dermal collagen and elastin, an outcome observed clinically as photo-ageing (Brash and Gilchrest, 1996).

UVB-INDUCED CYTOKINES

The proinflammatory effects of UVB have been well studied by means of *in vivo* tech-niques, including in particular suction blisters and skin chambers affixed to abraded irradi-ated skin. With appropriate controls, the mediators of UV-induced inflammation have been defined in this way. Histamine release is an early event, suggesting that mast cells are involved in the initial phase of the inflam-matory response, while important proinflam-matory prostaglandins are PGD_2 and PGI_2 peaking at six hours and PGE_2 and $PGF_{2\alpha}$ peaking at 24 hours (Black *et al.*, 1978). 12-Hydroxyeicosatetraenoic acid (12-HETE) is also a powerful proinflammatory compound and appears to have a similar time course for release as PGE_2 (Black *et al.*, 1980), but leukotrienes do not appear to be involved. In addition to these, the interleukin cytokine family is a powerful group of compounds with many overlapping effects. For example, interleukin-1 like activity has been detected *in vivo* in human skin (Murphy *et al.*, 1989) within 30 minutes of UVB irradiation, with a biphasic time course suggesting the release of preformed IL-like activity as well as subse-quent IL-1 synthesis. IL-1 then leads to release of IL-6, both IL-1 and IL-6 being found in serum, with IL-1 detectable 1–4 hours after irradiation but returning to baseline levels within eight hours (Granstein and Sauder, 1987). IL-6 reaches peak values by 12 hours and persists for more than 72 hours, appearing to be a main mediator of the human sunburn reaction, with fever peaking at the time of its maximum serum concen-tration (Urbanski *et al.*, 1990). Thus, these compounds seem likely to be important in the continuation of the inflammatory cascade as compared with histamine and the prostaglandins, which may assist in initiating it. This contention is supported by the fact that antihistamines and drugs with anti prostaglandin activity lead to partial blocking of the early phase of the erythemal response but fail to prevent it after 24 hours. Further work has shown that UVB exposure of cultured keratinocytes leads to IL-1α and IL-1β mRNA detectable at six hours, the simul-taneously expressed IL-1 inhibitor IL-1RA having a similar time course for release as that of IL-1α (Kupper *et al.*, 1987), while IL-10, granulocyte macrophage colony-stimulating factor (GM-CSF) and tumour necrosis factor (TNF)-α and -β are also increased. The func-tional relevance of these various cytokines is slowly being disentangled, blocking anti-bodies to IL-10 indicating that this substance plays an important role in the development of immunosuppression, while recent experi-ments further suggest that it may inhibit Langerhans cell antigen presentation (Enk *et al.*, 1993). IL-12, on the other hand, is a recently reported compound likely to be crit-ical in overcoming such immune suppression, its injection into mice after UV irradiation abrogating the immunosuppressive effect of UVB on cutaneous sensitization with a universal sensitizer, an effect prevented by the use of IL-12 blocking antibodies (Riemann *et al.*, 1996). A final possible mediator, recently incriminated as perhaps involved in the whole erythemal response, is nitric oxide, maybe by directly affecting the irradiated vasculature (Deliconstantinos *et al.*, 1995).

Adhesion molecule expression is another modality altered by UVB irradiation, intercel-lular adhesion molecule-1 (ICAM-1) being expressed on epidermal cells for 16 hours thereafter (Krutmann *et al.*, 1990; Norris *et al.*, 1990). E-selectin, formerly known as endothe-lial cell adhesion molecule (ELAM-1), is also upregulated by six hours, peaking by 24 and then diminishing. By contrast, in another study, ICAM-1, as well as vascular cell adhesion molecule-1 (VCAM-1), was unaffected (Norris *et al.*, 1991) and UVB exposure may apparently inhibit interferon (IFN-γ)-induced ICAM-1 expression. In addition, evidence now indicates that cytokines modulate ICAM-1 expression on melanocytes also (Kirbauer *et al.*, 1992). UVB irradiation also inhibits IFN-γ-induced release of IL-7, which promotes T cell growth, an effect reversed by exogenous IL-7. There are a number of possible mechanisms whereby UVB may induce these effects on IFN-γ, not apparently at the receptor level, however, but by IRF-1 expression inhibition, a transcriptional effect. This complex series of cell signalling effects following UVB exposure then determines the clinical, histological and immunological outcomes.

HISTOLOGICAL EFFECTS OF UVB

The histological effects of UVR exposure in part reflect the depth of penetration of the various wavelengths, UVC being mainly absorbed by the stratum corneum although sufficient penetrates to the viable epidermis and possibly the upper dermal papillary vessels to elicit erythema. UVB, on the other hand, exerts its effects predominantly on the epidermis (Gilchrest *et al.*, 1981; Rosario *et al.*, 1979), while UVA penetrates to the dermis with little histological evidence of epidermal effects. UVB-mediated damage to keratinocytes may be observed as early as 30 minutes after irradiation, as the so-called sunburn cells, with a striking appearance comprising shrunken chromatin and eosinophilic cytoplasm, begin to appear. Such cells have sustained significant DNA damage and been eliminated by an active gene-regulated process termed **apoptosis**, a protective mechanism preventing DNA with excessive UV-induced errors from replicating and an efficient method of error-free repair after UV injury. The tumour suppressor gene, p53 and a number of downstream genes such as WAF1 and Bcl2/Bax appear to be important in apoptosis control, as does TNF-α (Schwartz *et al.*, 1995), although blocking antibodies to TNF-α only partially inhibit apoptosis (Schwartz *et al.*, 1995). Sunburn cell numbers peak by 24 hours and by three days postirradiation are found within the stratum corneum. The commonest location for such cells is the lower portion of the epidermis just above the basal layer and it therefore seems that moderately differentiated cells are most susceptible to the apoptotic process.

Endothelial cell swelling occurs within 30 minutes of irradiation, reaching a maximum by 24 hours and persisting for 3 days postirradiation (Gilchrest *et al.*, 1981). Mast cell degranulation occurs within 3–5 hours with depletion of mast cell numbers. Perivascular dermal neutrophils appear immediately postirradiation, reach peak numbers by 14 hours, decline by 48 hours and are replaced by a mononuclear infiltrate which reaches a plateau by 14–21 hours and gradually decreases by two days (Hawk *et al.*, 1988). UVB causes spongiosis of the epidermis, evident 24 hours after irradiation, while antigen-specific T lymphocytes are found there within 24–72 hours and epidermal macrophages with the phototype CDIa-DR + by 72 hours (Cooper *et al.*, 1992). Langerhans cell (LC) numbers, however, decrease rapidly, even doses less than one minimal erythema dose (MED) being sufficient to have a significant effect, whether the dose is given over a prolonged period with low irradiance or is fractionated (Murphy *et al.*, 1993); the decrease begins within an hour, with complete LC disappearance by 24 hours, persistence at low levels for 72 hours and return to baseline by 2–3 weeks (Parles *et al.*, 1989). Many of the histological effects of UVB may be related to the effects of the concomitant cytokine expression.

ACUTE EFFECTS OF UVB ON CELLULAR IMMUNE RESPONSIVENESS

The immunological consequences of acute UVB irradiation are in part due to the accompanying DNA damage but nevertheless are also cytokine mediated. For example, prevention of UV-mediated immune suppression was achieved by the induction of DNA damage repair by photoreactivation in the animal model, *Monodelphis domestica* (Applegate *et al.*, 1989), while secondly, the use of the thymine dimer-specific repair enzyme, T4 endonuclease, decreased the number of cyclobutane pyrimidine dimers in irradiated epidermis. Further, acute UVB irradiation in 40–45% of the population leads to a failure of the immune system to recognize a universal allergen regardless of skin colour (Vermeer *et al.*, 1991), this phenomenon occurring in 100% of those with skin cancer. Initial studies suggested that this reaction was absolute and that those who were susceptible could not subsequently be sensitized to the same allergen applied to non-irradiated skin, though a different allergen might induce a reaction, thus implying that UVB-induced hapten-specific tolerance might occur in some individuals in the population and in most patients with non-melanoma skin cancer. Subsequent dose–response studies, however, suggest that this effect may be overcome by increasing the concentration of allergen and thus that UV resistance or susceptibility appears to be a relative phenomenon (McKenna *et al.*, 1996), studies with erythemogenic UVB administered to immunization sites prior to exposure to the universal allergen dinitrochlorobenzene (DNCB) showing a dose-related reduction in the degree of sensitization and one third of those immunized initially through skin and receiving erythemogenic UV becoming tolerant to DNCB (Cooper *et al.*, 1992). Examination of the antigen-presenting cells in the skin showed a reduction in Langerhans cell numbers and induction of CD1a-DR+ macrophages.

Urocanic acid (UCA) is a chromophore found in the stratum corneum in its trans isomer form. The first clue that this might be relevant is the immunosuppression induced by UV irradiation came from evidence that the absorption spectrum for trans-UCA was identical to that for UV-induced suppression of contact sensitization (De Fabo and Noonan, 1983) and the cis-UCA photoisomer of trans-UCA is highly effective in producing immunosuppression *in vivo*, independent of Langerhans cells. The UV effects on epidermal Langerhans cells and the UV-induced suppression of contact hypersensitivity also have different wavelength dependencies, further indicating that the UCA effect may be independently mediated (Noonan *et al.*, 1984). UCA has also been shown not to bind to DNA and it has been postulated that cis-UCA may act by inducing intraepidermal accumulation of TNF-α, which then prevents epidermal Langerhans cells from carrying hapten to draining lymph nodes where activation of naive hapten-specific T cells must occur (Kurimoto and Streilein, 1993). Polymorphic alleles at the TNF-α and lipopolysaccharide (LPS) genetic loci apparently dictate whether mice are UV susceptible or resistant, that is, whether they develop contact sensitization or not when hapten is painted on to UVB-exposed skin (Streilein, 1993). UCA is, however, proinflammatory when injected intradermally and appears to mediate its effects by a direct effect on PGE_2 (Hart, 1996). However, the exact role of UCA in immunosuppression remains unresolved.

ACUTE EFFECTS OF UVA ON HUMAN SKIN

The importance of understanding UVA radiation effects on skin independently of those induced by UVB stems from the widespread use of UVA sources to induce tanning, the use of UVA, and in particular UVAI, therapeutically and the fact that prolonged sun exposure when using sunscreens with UVB predominating over UVA protection leads to the risk of environmental exposure to large doses of UVA without the warning signs of sunburn. High-output UVA sources now enable precise study of UVA effects.

The action spectra for UVB-induced tanning and erythema are almost identical, but in the UVA range the curves dissociate, the dose of UVA required to induce tanning being less than that which induces erythema. This dissociation has lead to the widespread use of UVA lamps for tanning purposes, thus largely enabling the avoidance of UV-induced inflammation. The time courses for UVA-induced erythema and tanning are both biphasic. Erythema is often evident immediately after UVA irradiation, decreasing by four hours and recrudescing between six and 24 hours. Immediate pigment darkening also occurs after UVA and visible light exposure, apparently the result of photo-oxidation of existing melanin and the redistribution of melanosomes into melanocytic dendritic processes. This phenomenon is most evident in those with constitutive or intrinsically dark skin, but there is little protective effect against erythema induced by UVB irradiation. Genetically susceptible sites in basal layer DNA may, however, be differentially protected by localized nuclear melanin caps. Delayed tanning also occurs with formation of new melanin, peak tanning being evident 72 hours after irradiation, and its main function being protection against further UV damage, although a UVA-induced tan confers a sun protection factor of only 2–11 compared with the overall protection of around 30–40 achieved by repeated UVB irradiation, a difference perhaps due to less stratum corneum thickening with UVA irradiation. As might be expected, however, there is some reduction in epidermal cell damage following further UVB exposure in UVA-tanned skin (Margolis *et al.*, 1989).

EFFECTS OF UVA ON PROINFLAMMATORY MEDIATORS

Though in general the effects of UVAI and UVAII differ, detailed comparisons have not been performed, most studies having used UVA sources encompassing both these wavelengths; some sources emit relatively pure broad-spectrum UVA, for example, UVASUN®, and filtered solar simulators. Therefore, it is important to relate the effects detected to the pureness of the UVA source, as even very small amounts of stray UVB may cause large biological effects (Rivers *et al.*, 1989)

UVA-INDUCED CYTOKINES

Histamine release is later with UVA than after UVB exposure, with concentrations in suction blister fluid rising at 9–15 hours (Hawk *et al.*, 1983), while arachidonic acid and its downstream metabolites PGD_2, PGE_2 and $6\text{-oxo=}F_{1\alpha}$ increase at 5–9 hours after UVA irradiation and return to baseline by 24 hours. Exposure of cultured human keratinocytes to UVA also leads to increased production of $6\text{-keto=}PGF_{1\alpha}$ and PGE_2 1–6 hours after irradiation (Hanson and DeLeo, 1990), but leukotriene B4 and IL-6 appear unaffected.

Adhesion molecule expression is also altered by UVA, *in vivo* work having demonstrated the expression of ICAM-1 and E-selectin on dermal blood vessels. The time course for this expressions has also been studied in cultured human dermal endothelial cells, E-selectin peaking at six hours and ICAM-1 at 24 hours. Chronic exposure of these cells to UVA over six days, however, showed failure of ICAM-1 expression even after additional exposure to the cytokines IL-lα, IL-1β and TNF-α (Heckmann and Pirthauer, 1994). The integrins α1, α3, α5 and β1 are also modulated in expression by single or multiple exposure to UVA (Hogan *et al.*, 1992). Exposure of cultured keratinocytes to UVB and UVA resulted in a biphasic expression of ICAM-1, dose-dependent suppression occurring first at 24 hours and then dose-dependent upregulation from 48–96 hours. IFN-γ normally upregulates ICAM-1 expression, but UVB and UVA irradiation inhibited this upregulation at 24 hours and a dose-dependent effect was then evident from

48–96 hours. These data were interpreted by the authors as possibly explaining the therapeutic effects of UV associated with the suppression of ICAM-1 induction occurring in some photodermatoses, Norris and colleagues (1991) having found that the adhesion molecule expression induced by UVB in normal skin differed from that associated with the delayed hypersensitivity response to injected purified protein derivative. Finally, comparison of the effects of UVB and UVA irradiation on the release of transforming growth factor (TGF)-α showed no change after UVA, though a significant elevation did occur after equally erythemogenic UVB (James *et al.*, 1991; Murphy *et al.*, 1991).

More recent experiments have now differentiated the effects of UVA-I from UVA in general, exposure of cultured keratinocytes to UVAI showing induction of ICAM-1 mRNA expression on normal cells but no or minimal expression on a KB cell line derived from a human epidermoid carcinoma which expresses glutathione fourfold more than normal. Pretreatment of the cells with vitamin E or their irradiation in the presence of a singlet oxygen quencher abrogated the effect, while exposure in the presence of deuterium oxide (which prolongs singlet oxygen half-life) enhanced the ICAM-1 expression. These studies implicate an oxidative mechanism for the induction of ICAM-1 expression by UVAI, probably involving the generation of singlet oxygen (Krutmann and Grewe, 1995; Olaizola-Horn *et al.*, 1993). UVAI irradiation led to the inhibition of IFN-γ-induced ICAM-1 expression for up to 48 hours, when upregulation was observed instead (Christoph *et al.*, 1993; Olaizola-Horn *et al.*, 1994). UVAI-irradiated cultured keratinocytes also release IL-10 in association with enhancement of IL-10 mRNA. TNF-α, IL-1α, IL-6 and IL-8 mRNA and protein expression are also increased by UVAI irradiation of cultured human carcinoma KB calls (Morita *et al.*, 1996), the increased IL-1α and IL-6 expression being observed only in cells where the endogenous

glutathione levels are reduced prior to UVAI irradiation while the TNF-α and IL-8 increases occurred regardless of glutathione level, implying a thiol-dependent IL-1α and IL-6 mechanism. Genetic studies have also demonstrated that the AP-2 binding site of the ICAM-1 gene serves as a UVAI and singlet oxygen-responsive site, suggesting a cause and effect relationship (Krutmann, 1996).

HISTOLOGICAL EFFECTS OF UVA

The histological consequences of exposure of human skin to UVA have been well described (Gilchrest *et al.*, 1983), the changes observed after 2.5 MED of UVA showing a more striking dermal infiltrate than that observed after UVB inflammation. Neutrophils are prominent, intravascular at three hours, extravascular thereafter (Margolis *et al.*, 1989), and present at all time points over 48 hours; however, a far more prominent lymphocytic infiltrate is present in both papillary and reticular dermis throughout. Endothelial cell enlargement occurs immediately after irradiation, becoming more pronounced from 24–48 hours and affecting all dermal venules, while mast cell degranulation and perivenular oedema are also present throughout. Exposure to UVA leads instead to endothelial cell necrosis with an associated prominent neutrophilic upper dermal and mid-dermal infiltrate (Diffey *et al.*, 1987). However, in contrast to UVB injury, UVA induces far less epidermal change (Rosario *et al.*, 1979), sunburn cells not being seen, although keratinocytes appeared variable in size with swollen cells, perinuclear vacuolar change and intercellular oedema evident by three hours. Occasional lymphocytes were also seen in the lower epidermis while Langerhans cells were significantly reduced in number by 15 hours. Stratum corneum thickening did not occur (Rosario *et al.*, 1979). Repeated exposure of human skin to UVA twice weekly for six weeks also resulted in epidermal Langerhans cell depletion, but the lamp source emitted small quantities of UVB sufficient to induce the change and any responses ascribed to UVA should always be considered in the context of the possibility that small amounts of UVB may also be present with biologically relevant activity. Thus, exposure of the buttocks to 1 MED of UVA twice weekly for six months in one study resulted in epidermal thickening, melanization, elastosis and reduced elastin content, changes persisting for three months thereafter (Lowe *et al.*, 1994), while in another, repeated exposure of the skin to 0.5 MED of UVA weekly for six weeks led to epidermal hyperplasia, thickening of the stratum corneum, a dermal inflammatory infiltrate, lysozyme deposition on elastic fibres and Langerhans cell depletion (Lavker *et al.*, 1995). The exact severity of the epidermal changes after UVA exposure may not be unequivocally elucidated until studies with UVAI sources become available.

EFFECTS OF UVA ON
IMMUNOSUPPRESSION

An *in vivo* action spectrum for the induction of photoimmunosuppression has not yet been published, but one for the UV-induced suppression of contact hypersensitivity has, being very similar to the absorption spectrum of UCA and at wavelengths shorter than 290 nm to the DNA absorption spectrum. UVA may also photoisomerize trans- to cis-UCA *in vitro* and *in vivo*, but although UVA irradiation induced cis-UCA, it failed to suppress contact hypersensitivity (Gibbs *et al.*, 1993), and the role of UCA remains uncertain.

Most of the immunosuppressive effects of UV exposure have been ascribed to UVB, but only a few studies have looked at UVA. However, exposure of cultured keratinocytes to UVAI (340–400 nm Sellas lamp) lead to the production of propiomelanocortin-related peptides in one study (Schauer *et al.*, 1994), while endorphin may also be released into the circulation by UVA, perhaps contributing to

the supposed feeling of well-being attributed to UV exposure (Wintzen and Gilchrest, 1996; Wintzen *et al.*, 1996). Finally, slight inhibition of the immune response as measured by the mixed lymphocyte and mixed epidermal cell lymphocyte reactions mediated by cis-UCA may occur *in vivo*.

CONCLUSION

Both UVB and UVA irradiation have profound effects on human skin. These changes, although mainly detrimental to normal skin, may also be used in appropriate circumstances to regulate disease states by the modulation of cellular differentiation and immunological activity. Further exploration of the consequences of such irradiation will now steadily lead to an increasing knowledge of how best to minimize the damaging effects of cutaneous environmental UV exposure, as well as to better therapeutic strategies for cutaneous disease.

REFERENCES

Applegate, L.A., Ley, R.A., Alcalay, K. and Kripke, M.L. (1989) Identification of the molecular target for the suppression of contact hypersensitivity by ultraviolet radiation. *Journal of Experimental Medicine*, **170**, 1117.

Archambault, M., Yaar, M. and Gilchrest, B.A. (1995) Keratinocytes and fibroblasts in a human skin equivalent model enhance melanocyte survival and melanin synthesis after ultraviolet irradiation. *Journal of Investigative Dermatology*, **104**, 859–67.

Black, A.K., Fincham, N., Greaves, M.W. *et al.* (1980) Time course changes in levels of arachidonic acid and prostaglandins D2 E2 F2α in human skin following ultraviolet B irradiation. *British Journal of Clinical Pharmacology*, **10**, 453–7.

Black, A.K., Greaves, M.W., Hensby, C.N. and Plummer, N.A. (1978) Increased prostaglandins E2 and F2α in human skin at 6 and 24 h after ultraviolet B irradiation. *British Journal of Clinical Pharmacology*, **5**, 431–6.

Brash, D.E. and Gilchrest, B.A. (1996) Wrinkles waiting for GODoT. *Nature*, **379**, 301–2.

Christoph, H., Budnik, A., Parlow, F. *et al.* (1993) Ultraviolet (UV) A1 and UVB-radiation affect human keratinocyte (KC) expression of intercellular adhesion molecule-1 (ICAM-I) by different mechanisms. *Journal of Investigative Dermatology*, **100**, 443.

Cooper, K.D., Oberhelman, L., Hamilton, T.A. *et al.* (1992) UV exposure reduces immunization rates and promotes tolerance to epicutaneous antigens in humans: relationship to dose CD1a-DR4 + epidermal macrophage induction, and Langerhans cell depletion. *Proceedings of the National Academy of Science of the USA*, **89**, 8497.

DeFabo, E.C., and Noonan, F.P. (1983) Mechanism of immune suppression by ultraviolet irradiation *in vivo*. 1. Evidence for the existence of a unique photoreceptor in skin and its role in photoimmunology. *Journal of Experimental Medicine*, **158**, 84–9.

Deliconstantinos, G., Villiotou, V. and Stravrides, J.C. (1995) Release by ultraviolet B (UVB) radiation of nitric oxide (NO) from human keratinocytes: a potential role for nitric oxide in erythema production. *Br J. Pharmacol* **114**, 1257–65.

Diffey, B.L., Farr, P.M., Oakly, A.M. (1987) Quantitative studies on UVA-induced erythema in human skin. *British Journal of Dermatology*, **117**, 57–66.

Eller, M.S., Ostrom, K. and Gilchrest, B.A. (1996) DNA damage enhances melanogenesis. *Proceedings of the National Academy of Science of the USA*, **93**, 1087–92.

Enk, A.H., Angeloni, V.L., Udey, M.C., Katz, S.I. (1993) Inhibition of Langerhans cell antigen-presenting function by IL-10. *Journal of Immunology*, **151**, 2390.

Fisher, G.J., Datta, S.C., Talwar, H.S. *et al.* (1996) Molecular basis of sun-induced premature skin ageing and retinoid antagonism. *Nature*, **379**, 335–9.

Gibbs, N.K., Norval, M., Traynor, N.J. *et al.* (1993) Action spectra for the trans to cis photoisomerisation of urocanic acid *in vitro* and in mouse skin. *Photochemistry and Photobiology*, **57**, 584–90.

Gilchrest, B.A., Soter, N.A., Hawk, J.L.M. *et al.* (1983) Histological changes associated with ultraviolet A-induced erythema in normal human skin. *Journal of the American Academy of Dermatology*, **9**, 213–19.

Gilchrest, B.A., Soter, N.A., Stoff, J.S. and Mihm, M.C. Jr. (1981) The human sunburn reaction: histologic and biochemical studies. *Journal of the American Academy of Dermatology*, **5**, 411–22.

Granstein, R.D. and Sauder, D.N. (1987) Whole body exposure to ultraviolet radiation results in increased serum interleukin-1 activity in humans. *Lymphokine Research*, **6**, 193–7.

Hansen and DeLeo, V. (1990) Long-wave ultraviolet light induces phospholipase activation in cultured human epidermal keratinocytes. *Journal of Investigative Dermatology*, **95**, 158–63.

Hart, P. (1996) *Urocanic Acid*. Proceedings of the International Congress of Photobiology, 1996.

Hawk, J.L.M., Black, A.K., Jaenicke, K.F. *et al.* (1983) Increased concentrations of arachidonic acid, prostaglandins E2, D2 and 6-oxo-F1α and histamine in skin following UVA irradiation. *Journal of Investigative Dermatology*, **80**, 496–9.

Hawk, J.L.M., Murphy, G.M. and Holden, C.A. (1988) The presence of neutrophils in human cutaneous ultraviolet-B inflammation. *British Journal of Dermatology*, **118**, 27–30.

Heckmann, M. and Pirthauer, M. (1994) Repetitive exposure to UVA reduces dermal endothelial responsiveness to pro-inflammatory stimuli. *Journal of Investigative Dermatology*, **103**, 442.

Hogan, P.A., Morelli, J.G. and Norris, D.A. (1992) Effect of ultraviolet radiation on human melanocyte and keratinocyte integrin expression. *Journal of Investigative Dermatology*, **98**, 653.

James, L.C., Moore, A.M., Wheeler, L.A. *et al.* (1991) Transforming growth factor α: *in vivo* release by normal human skin following UV irradiation and abrasion. *Skin Pharmacology*, **4** (43), 61–4.

Kirnbauer, R., Charvat, B., Schauer, E. *et al.* (1992) Modulation of intercellular adhesion molecule-1 expression on human melanocytes and melanoma cells: evidence for a regulatory role of IL-6, Il-7, TNFα and UVB light. *Journal of Investigative Dermatology*, **98**, 320–6.

Krutmann, J. (1996) UVAI radiation-induced immunomodulatory and gene regulatory effects in human keratinocytes. *European Journal of Dermatology*, **6**, 229–30.

Krutmann, J. and Grewe, M. (1995) Involvement of cytokines, DNA damage, and reactive oxygen intermediates in ultraviolet radiation-induced modulation of intercellular adhesion molecule-1 expression. *Journal of Investigative Dermatology*, **105**, 67S–70S.

Krutmann, J., Kock, A., Schauer, E. *et al.* (1990) Tumour necrosis factor beta and ultraviolet radiation are potent regulators of human keratinocyte ICAM-1 expression. *Journal of Investigative Dermatology*, **95**, 127.

Kupper, R., Kock, A., Neuner, P. *et al.* (1987) Interleukin 1 gene expression in cultured human keratinocytes is augmented by ultraviolet radiation. *Journal of Clinical Investigation*, **80**, 430–6.

Kurimoto, I. and Streilein, J.W. (1993) Studies of contact hypersensitivity induction in mice with optimal sensitising doses of hapten. *Journal of Investigative Dermatology*, **101**, 132.

Lavker, R.M., Gerberick, G.F., Veves, D., Irwin, C.J., Kaidbey, K.H. (1995) Cumulative effects from repeated exposures to subthreshold doses of UVB and UVA in human skin. *Journal of the American Academy of Dermatology*, **32**, 53–62.

Lowe, N.J., Weider, J., Bourget, T. *et al.* (1994) Small daily doses of UVA induce major changes in previously unexposed skin within several months. *Journal of Investigative Dermatology*, **102**, 649.

Margolis, R.J., Sherwood, M., Maytum, D.J. *et al.* (1989) Longwave ultraviolet radiation (UVA, 320–400 nm)-induced tan protects human skin against further UVA injury. *Journal of Investigative Dermatology*, **93**, 713–18.

McKenna, D., O'Reilly, F. and Murphy, G.M. (1996) Ultraviolet light-induced suppression of primary allergic reactions. *British Journal of Dermatology*, **135**, (Suppl 47), 65.

Morita, A., Grewe, M., Grether-Beck, S. *et al.* (1996) Induction of proinflammatory cytokines in human epidermoid carcinoma cells by *in vitro* ultraviolet A1 irradiation. *Photochemistry* and *Photobiology*, **65**, 630–5.

Murphy, G.M., Dowd, P.M., Hudspith, B.N., Brostoff, J. and Greaves, M.W. (1989) Local increase in interleukin-1-like activity following UVB irradiation of human skin *in vivo*. *Photodermatology*, **6**, 268–74.

Murphy, G.M., Norris, P.G., Young, A.R., Corbett, M.F. and Hawk, J.L. (1993) Low dose ultraviolet B irradiation depletes human epidermal Langerhans cells. *British Journal of Dermatology*, **129**, 674–7.

Murphy, G.M., Quinn, D.G., Camp, R.D.R., Hawk, J.L.M. and Greaves, M.W. (1991) *In vivo* studies of the action spectrum and time course for release of transforming growth factor by ultraviolet irradiation in man. *British Journal of Dermatology*, **125**, 566–8.

Noonan, F.P., Bucana, C., Sauder, D.N. and DeFabo, E.D. (1984) Mechanism of systemic immune suppression by UV irradiation *in vivo*. II The UV effects on number and morphology of epidermal Langerhans cells and the UV-induced suppression of contact hypersensitivity have different wavelength dependencies. *Journal of Immunology*, **132**, 2408.

Norris, D.A., Lyons, B., Middleton, M.H., Yohn, J.J. and Kashihara-Swami, M. (1990) Ultraviolet radiation can either suppress or induce expression of intercellular adhesion molecule 1 (ICAM-1) on the surface of cultured human keratinocytes. *Journal of Investigative Dermatology*, **95**, 132.

Norris, P., Poston, R.N., Sian, T.D. *et al.* (1991) The expression of endothelial adhesion molecules (ICAM-1) and vascular cell adhesion molecule-1 (VCAM-1) in experimental cutaneous inflammation: a comparison of ultraviolet B erythema and delayed hypersensitivity. *Journal of Investigative Dermatology*, **96**, 763.

Olaizola-Horn, S., Christoph, H., Budnik, A. *et al.* (1993) Ultraviolet A1 radiation-induced upregulation of keratinocyte expression of intercellular adhesion molecule-1 (ICAM-1) is mediated via the generation of free radicals. *Archives of Dermatology Research*, **286**:38

Olaizola-Horn, S., Christoph, H., Budnik, A. *et al.* (1994) Ultraviolet A1 radiation-induced immunomodulation is mediated via the generation of singlet oxygen. *Journal of Investigative Dermatology*, **103**, 429.

Parrish, J.A., Jaenicke, K.F. and Anderson R.R. (1982) Erythema and melanogenesis action spectrum of normal human skin. *Photochemistry and Photobiology*, **36** 187–91.

Powles, A.V., Murphy, G.M., Rutman, A.J. *et al.* (1989) Effect of simulated sunlight on Langerhans cells in malignant melanoma patients. *Acta Dermato-Venereologica*, **69**, 482–6.

Riemann, H., Schwarz, A., Grabbe, S. *et al.* (1996) Neutralisation of IL-12 *in vivo* prevents induction of contact hypersensitivity and induces hapten-specific tolerance. *Journal of Immunology*, **156**, 1799–803.

Rivers, J.K., Norris, P.G., Murphy, G.M. *et al.* (1989) UVA sunbeds: tanning, photoprotection, acute adverse effects and immunological changes. *British Journal of Dermatology*, **120**, 767–77.

Rosario, R., Mark, G.J., Parrish, J.A. and Mihm, M.C. Jr. (1979) Histological changes produced in skin by equally erythemogenic doses of UV-A, UV-B, UV-C and UVA with psoralens. *British Journal of Dermatology*, **101**, 299–300.

Schauer, E., Trautinger, F., Kock, A. *et al.* (1994) Propiomelanocortin-derived peptides are synthesized and released by human keratinocytes. *Journal of Clinical Investigation*, **83**, 2258–62.

Schwarz, A., Bhardwaj, R., Aragane, Y. *et al.* (1995) Ultraviolet-B-induced apoptosis of keratinocytes: evidence for partial involvement of tumor necrosis factor-alpha in the formation of sunburn cells. *Journal of Investigative Dermatology*, **104**, 922–7.

Streilein, J.W. (1993) Sunlight and the skin-associated lymphoid tissues (SALT): if UVB is the trigger and TNFα is its mediator, what is the message? *Journal of Investigative Dermatology*, **100**, 47S.

Urbanski, A., Schwarz, T., Neuner, P. *et al* (1990) Ultraviolet light induces circulating interleukin-6 in humans. *Investigative Dermatology*, **94**, 808–11.

Vermeer, M., Schneider, G.J., Yoshikawa, T. *et al.* (1991) Effects of ultraviolet B light on cutaneous immune responses of humans with deeply pigmented skin. *Journal of Investigative Dermatology*, **97**, 729.

Wintzen, M. and Gilchrest, B.A. (1996) Propiomelanocortin, its derived peptides, and the skin. *Journal of Investigative Dermatology*, **106**, 3–10.

Wintzen, M., Yaar, M., Burbach, J.P.H. and Gilchrest, B.A. (1996) Propiomelanocortin gene product regulation in keratinocytes. *Journal of Investigative Dermatology*, **106**, 673–8.

PHOTOIMMUNOLOGY

5

Gary L. Stevens and Paul R. Bergstresser

INTRODUCTION

The field of photoimmunology has developed remarkably since the 1970s, at which time ultraviolet radiation (UVR) was mostly recognized just as a cutaneous carcinogen. However, this situation changed abruptly when several investigative groups demonstrated it also to be immunosuppressive, thus providing an impetus for study of its effects on cutaneous immunity in detail. Unfortunately, the large variety of interactions between this radiation and photon-absorbing molecules in skin has tended to necessitate a reductionist approach, such that only individual molecules and limited radiation spectra are examined, often in closed experimental systems. As a result of this and of the diverse experimental methods listed, the *in vitro* approach has often produced reports not necessarily representative of the highly interactive situation in *in vivo* mammalian immune mechanisms. Nevertheless, the relevant photoreceptors, effector cells and soluble factors that play roles in UVR-induced immunosuppression are now gradually being identified, while concomitantly, experimental information from basic immunology is changing our interpretation of these data. Thus, it is becoming steadily apparent that immune recognition is a highly interactive process and one that responds to multiple signals simultaneously, rather than to the presence of foreign antigen alone. This review of UVR effects on skin now focuses on the recent findings in photoimmunology, interpreted in the context of an emerging new model of immune recognition and guided by the realization that its effects are not limited to a single molecule or event.

FEATURES OF CUTANEOUS IMMUNITY

Cellular contributions to the cutaneous microenvironment are highly interactive, with keratinocytes, endothelial cells and leucocytes all playing important signalling roles. These signals, which are mediated by soluble factors and cell surface molecules, then influence the responses of the various leucocytes that effect immunity in skin. Evidence for the complexity of this process is indicated by the following.

Lymphocyte-mediated responses in skin are determined by a balance among subpopulations of T cells, which constantly recirculate between that site and the systemic circulation. Thus, antigen-specific effector and suppressor T cells commonly co-exist, the balance between activation and tolerance depending on the relative strengths of their competing effects.

Lymphocyte trafficking, in turn, depends on integrins, selectins and soluble factors which mediate competitive homing to microenvironmental niches (Butcher and Picker, 1995).

Resident antigen-presenting cells (APC), both dendritic cells (DC) (including Langerhans cells (LC)) and macrophages, initiate and

Photodermatology. Edited by J.L.M. Hawk. Published in 1998 by Chapman & Hall, London. ISBN 0 412 72460 X.

regulate immune responses by responding to and contributing to the local environment. Ultimately, it is clear that the overall communication between this variety of effector and regulator cells establishes whether the integrated response is activating or tolerizing in nature. Further, although the stimuli determining this balance of signals are not yet fully understood, it is now also certain that UVR has the capacity to distort these effects by distorting the cutaneous microenvironment.

MODELS OF IMMUNITY

SELF/NON-SELF DISCRIMINATION

In a widely accepted model, immune reactivity defends against microbiological invasion in a process that requires discrimination between 'self' and 'non-self'. This process begins in the thymus, where T cells highly reactive against 'self' proteins are eliminated, while those capable of recognizing 'non-self' are expanded greatly in number. Unfortunately, this conventional model does not explain several well-established observations, including, for example, the presence of autoantibodies in otherwise healthy individuals and the utility of adjuvants. Recent experiments have now demonstrated that the activation or suppression of an immune response is critically dependent on the amount of antigen present (Sarzotti *et al.*, 1996), the effect of any adjuvant (Forsthuber *et al.*, 1996) and the APC type initiating the response (Ridge *et al.*, 1996). This therefore means that the conditions under which an immune response is initiated are just as important as the antigen itself and the long-standing model described above is now clearly deficient.

TWO-SIGNAL HYPOTHESIS

Although the molecular mechanisms that determine the activation or suppression of immune responses remain uncertain, they now seem more likely to be related to a 'two-signal hypothesis' of immune discrimination (Bretscher and Cohn, 1970; Lafferty and Cunningham, 1975), which has broad experimental support (Harding *et al.*, 1992; Jenkins and Schwartz, 1987; Quill and Schwartz, 1987; Schwartz, 1990) (Fig. 5.1). In the application of this hypothesis to T-cell activation, therefore, the first signal ('signal 1') is an antigen–T-cell receptor interaction mediated by an APC (a DC), while the second ('signal 2') occurs via accessory molecules or cytokines. The delivery of these signals simultaneously then activates the T cell, while the delivery of signal 1 in the absence of signal 2 leads instead to an antigen-specific state of unresponsiveness (**cellular anergy**) in association with a Th2 profile (for a further discussion of the Th1/Th2 paradigm, see p. 60).

A MODEL BASED ON DANGER

Beyond the two-signal hypothesis of ageing, an intriguing new model has now emerged that offers an alternative explanation of self/non-self discrimination. This model is based on the recognition of 'danger' and proposes that the immune system is designed not to identify non-self, but instead to protect self from the harm associated with cell stress or

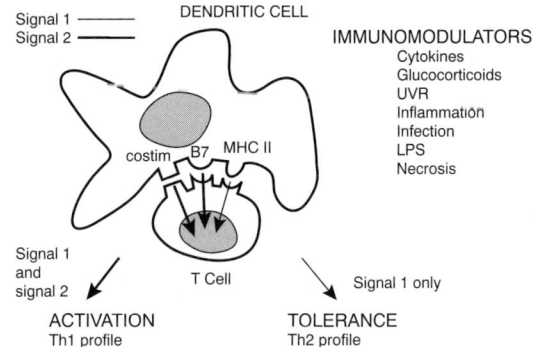

Figure 5.1 Two-signal mechanism of immune recognition ('costim' represents other, less well-defined co-stimulatory signals). UVR, ultraviolet radiation; LPS, lipopolysaccharide.

necrotic cell death (Matzinger, 1994). The distinction between dangerous or not is made by APCs, which are also responsible for both signals, namely presenting antigen to T-cell receptors (signal 1) and providing appropriate co-stimulatory signals (signal 2). It is thus the presence of local tissue injury (danger) that causes APCs to be recruited and then to upregulate such co-stimulatory signals.

Important tenets of the danger model are that:

- Effector T cells require both signal 1 and signal 2 to become activated;
- T cells become tolerant, or even die, if signal 1 is received without signal 2;
- only certain types of APC can deliver signal 2 (Table 5.1).

Thus, it is probable that only DCs (including LCs) can provide signal 2 for virgin T cells, meaning that they alone can initiate a primary response, while DCs, macrophages and B cells can all activate memory T cells. Thus, when T cells encounter new antigen (self or non-self), it is only APCs (DCs) that determine whether tolerance or activation occurs, while only danger (or signals that mimic danger) first recruits and activates such DCs.

ANTIGEN AND ANTIGEN-PRESENTING CELL CONCENTRATIONS

Contact hypersensitivity (CH) is a well-studied immune response and one that can be

examined in the context of the danger model. Thus, it includes a typical sequence of cellular events leading to a cutaneous inflammatory response (Kondo and Sauder, 1995) and has among its variables the types and amounts of inducing antigen. Not only are the chemical structure and haptenic nature of such an antigen important (Basketter *et al.*, 1995) but also its quantity, which often determines whether hypersensitivity or tolerance occurs (Macher and Chase, 1969). Low-dose tolerance to contact allergen has recently been shown to be LC independent (Steinbrink *et al.*, 1996a), whereas higher doses induce an LC-dependent response. For the integration of this phenomenon into the danger model, it is also important to remember that only certain APCs can provide an immune-enhancing signal, in this case LCs, and if for any reason a contact sensitizer bypasses LCs, for example by escape into the circulation or having too low an affinity for haptenization, alternative APCs without co-stimulatory capacity (signal 2) will instead present the antigen in a tolerogenic fashion (Fig. 5.2). Candidates for such alternative APCs include CD11b+ macrophages (Kang *et al.*, 1994) and circulating B cells and, importantly, the latter possess several characteristics making this likely. Thus, they circulate systemically and reside in the spleen, where they are certainly more

Table 5.1 Tenets of the danger model

Resting T cells require two signals to be activated:
- signal 1 – binding of T-cell receptor to MHC–peptide complex
- signal 2 – co-stimulation from molecules on surface of APC

Resting T cells receive co-stimulatory signals only from certain APCs: Langerhans cells and dendritic macrophages

T cells remain activated for finite period of time

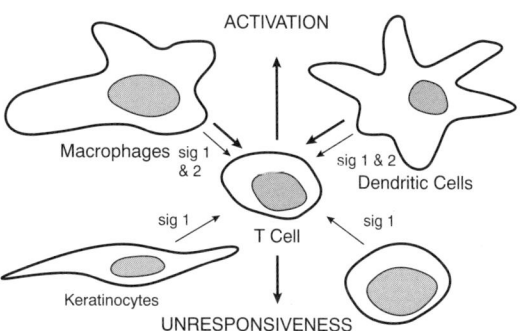

Figure 5.2 Antigen-presenting cell–T cell interactions. T cells require signal 1 and signal 2 for activation.

numerous than DCs and have a much greater affinity for capturing antigen than other cells (Lanzavecchia, 1985); indeed, they have already been demonstrated to evoke tolerance in virgin T cells (Eynon and Parker, 1992; Fuchs and Matzinger, 1992). However, normal optimal presentation of antigen by LCs will generally occur when it is present in intermediate amounts.

The danger model also predicts that large antigen concentrations, which saturate the antigen-presenting ability of APCs capable of co-stimulation, will leave additional remnants to be presented by the more numerous B cells, again resulting in tolerance. Indeed, this prediction has recently been verified in neonatal mice (Sarzotti *et al.*, 1996) which, when exposed to small doses of a leukaemia virus, mounted a Th1 response and eliminated the virus upon subsequent exposure; however, large doses instead provoked a tolerogenic Th2 response. The investigators reasoned that the large viral doses had simply overwhelmed the ability of DCs to provide co-stimulatory signals, thereby allowing the tolerogenic signals from B cells to dominate. Further, in related experiments (Ridge *et al.*, 1996), adult mice were also tolerized as easily as neonates if antigen was presented to them with a large inoculum of spleen or bone marrow cells, presumably because many such cells are again alternative APCs, such as B cells, as in the neonatal circumstance. These experiments thus lend credence to the danger model, because they suggest that the neonatal period is not an immunologically privileged one for the immune system to learn self from non-self, but rather one during which immune activation or tolerance are still options, just as in the adult; however, tolerance is generated more easily in the neonate because of a relative paucity of DCs. Thus, antigen concentration determines in part the balance between APCs providing and not providing signal 2.

LOW-DOSE/HIGH-DOSE UVR-INDUCED IMMUNOSUPPRESSION

Two models have demonstrated the capacity of animals to induce antigen-specific, T cell-mediated immune suppression in response to UVR exposure. Thus, the 'high-dose' model utilizes 5–30 kJ/m² of UVB radiation several days before the topical or subcutaneous application of hapten or antigen to irradiated or unirradiated skin. In this situation, hapten application in control mice induces the expected CH or delayed-type hypersensitivity (DTH) reaction, whereas its administration in irradiated mice results in an abrogated response, with tolerizing lymphocytes detectable in the spleen. This effect, which can occur at the site of irradiation or a distant site, is thought to involve soluble factors, namely interleukin (IL)-10 in DTH and tumour necrosis factor (TNF)-α in CH (Rivas and Ullrich, 1994).

In the 'low-dose' model, on the other hand, 1–2 kJ/m² of UVB radiation is used to irradiate the mice, again several days before the application of reactive hapten. Once again, antigen-specific immune tolerance transferable by T lymphocytes is induced, but only when the hapten is applied at the site of irradiation and only for CH, not DTH. Several mechanisms have been proposed for this, namely a direct effect on APCs, a modified elaboration of cytokines locally, an influx of CD11b+ macrophages and an immunosuppressive effect of cis-urocanic acid (UCA) (Streilein *et al.*, 1994).

In both these models, the end result is clearly downregulated hypersensitivity and a tolerizing Th2-type immune response and studies implicating DNA damage as the initiating photochemical event for this suggest two models representing local and systemic manifestations respectively of the same photobiological phenomenon. Thus, in the unifying model, DNA damage leads to the generation of local immunomodulatory factors such as IL-10 and cis-UCA, which at higher UVR doses gain access to the systemic circulation, as well as mediating distant effects (Nishigori *et al.*, 1996).

PHOTORECEPTORS

Identification of the photoreceptor responsible for initiating UVR-induced immunosuppression has been difficult, in part because of the large number of known skin chromophores with associated secondary chemical activities. Thus to date, DNA, UCA and cell membranes, all well recognized to undergo changes following UVR exposure, have been studied for their possible roles in the process (Table 5.2).

TRANS-UCA

Trans-UCA is a normal component of stratum corneum, formed from histidine during keratinization. Irradiation then causes trans to cis isomerization with subsequent diffusion of the more soluble cis form into the underlying dermis and systemic circulation. Cis-UCA has relatively recently been linked with cutaneous immune suppression because of its capacity to reduce LC numbers (Moodycliffe *et al.*, 1992; Norval *et al.*, 1990), suppress CH in mice (Ross *et al.*, 1988), stimulate TNF-α production (Streilein, 1993) and compete with histamine as an immunomodulatory factor (Norval *et al.*,

Table 5.2 Photoreceptors studied

Cis-urocanic acid
- Decreases Langerhans cell numbers
- Decreases contact hypersensitivity in mice

Cell membranes
- Adhesion molecules
- Squalenes
- Lipoperoxides

DNA
- T4N5 liposomes remove cyclobutyl pyrimidine dimers and prevent immunosuppression
- T4N5 liposomes decrease IL-10 secretion

1990). On the other hand, its relevance has also been called into question, other studies having revealed that although LCs are altered, CH is not in fact affected (El-Ghorr and Norval, 1995) while, more importantly, there appears to be a lack of correlation between the action spectra for UCA photoisomerization and for CH suppression (Reeve *et al.*, 1994). Thus, although cis-UCA does appear to enhance cutaneous immune suppression *in vivo*, the conflicts in data outlined have currently tempered enthusiasm regarding a primary role for it in the process.

CELL MEMBRANES

Cell membrane lipids are also attractive candidates as possible photoreceptors for UVR-induced immunological effects. Thus, the cell surface contains an array of regulatory molecules highly dependent upon the integrity of their local microenvironment and many of these are known to be affected by UVR. For example, the regulatory protein nuclear factor kappa B (NFκB) has been shown to be activated at the cell membrane after UVR exposure in a DNA-independent fashion (Devary *et al.*, 1993), while UVR also causes a dose-dependent decomposition of skin surface lipids, especially squalene, with the subsequent generation of active lipoperoxides (Picardo *et al.*, 1991). Further, the application of UVR-peroxidated squalene to the skin surface of mice inhibits CH induction to dinitrofluorobenzene along with decreasing with LC number. Again, UVB irradiation upregulates cytosolic phospholipase A_2, with increased prostaglandin E_2 production through free radical formation (Chen *et al.*, 1996), also most likely within membranes.

Finally, B7 adhesion molecules, important sources of the co-stimulation provided by APC, are also present on cell membranes and these are negatively affected by UVR (Fujihara *et al.*, 1996; Tesmann *et al.*, 1996; Weiss *et al.*, 1995); however, it is not certain whether this effect is direct or mediated by a soluble factor such as IL-10 (Allison and Krummel, 1995)

DNA

DNA has long been regarded as the major chromophore in UVR-induced carcinogenesis, but has only recently also been implicated in UVR-induced immunosuppression. However, both phenomena indeed appear to be mediated, at least partly, through UVR-induced DNA cyclobutyl pyrimidine dimer (CPD) formation (Sutherland *et al.*, 1980), a well-established phenomenon. Thus, when liposomes containing the excision repair enzyme T4 endonuclease V (T4N5) are used *in vivo* to increase DNA CPD removal, the UVR-induced suppression of CH and DTH (Applegate *et al.*, 1989) is simultaneously prevented. This apparent link between local cutaneous DNA damage and systemic immunosuppression may well be mediated by IL-10, recent studies having demonstrated that T4N5 also inhibits secretion of this cytokine, albeit in irradiated murine keratinocytes *in vitro* (Vink *et al.*, 1996).

THE MICROENVIRONMENT AS AN IMMUNOMODULATOR

An important current concept is that certain anatomical sites provide unique microenvironments with a capacity to regulate the immune responses emerging therefrom and the cutaneous microenvironment is one of these which has been studied in considerable detail. As a result, it is now known that multiple factors contribute to the immunomodulating properties of this milieu and in the following sections, cutaneous factors signalling the presence of 'danger' to DCs will in particular be examined. These will include a well-recognized potential threat to the organism, namely bacterial lipopolysaccharide (LPS), and one that prevents the signalling of 'danger', namely topically applied glucocorticoids, the latter instead

mediating a tolerizing response, for example to contact sensitizers (Amkraut *et al.*, 1996; Burrows and Stoughton, 1976). Following this, the direct and indirect effects of UVR on the cutaneous microenvironment will also be examined in more detail.

BACTERIAL CELL WALL CONSTITUENTS AS USEFUL ADJUVANTS

As noted previously, an appropriate activation signal ('danger') within a microenvironment facilitates the initiation of an immune response. In this model, danger is identified as 'anything that causes or resembles cell stress or necrotic cell death' (Fuchs and Matzinger, 1996) and one reproducible such danger is bacterial cell wall constituents, as at sites of infection. LPS, part of the outer membrane of gram-negative bacterial cell walls, thus exerts a powerful immunostimulatory effect in mammals, which has long been exploited in the immunization process (Fig. 5.3).

The enhancement of co-stimulation by the use of LPS has also been emphasized recently in studies with mice. Thus, neonatal or adult mice were injected with a 'foreign' protein, namely egg lysozyme, in either Freund's complete adjuvant, containing killed mycobacteria, or in incomplete adjuvant, lacking mycobacterial products (Forsthuber *et al.*, 1996). Immunization with both antigen and

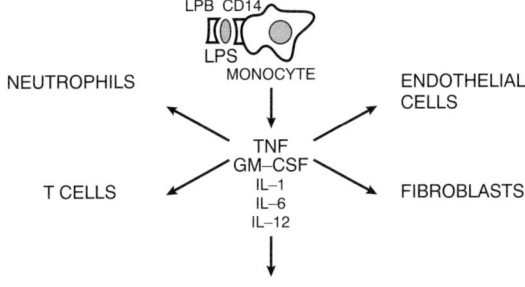

Figure 5.3 Lipopolysaccharide as danger signal. LPS, lipopolysaccharide; LPB, lipopolysaccharide-binding protein.

mycobacterial adjuvant together evoked a Th1 response, whereas exposure to the antigen alone evoked Th2 activity. Thus, it was the adjuvant, not the antigen or age of the mice, that determined the response. Besides supporting the idea that the neonatal period is not necessarily immunologically privileged, this work again indicates that the local cutaneous milieu is of great immunological importance. In addition, the immune upregulation described above was also associated with the release from APC of important soluble factors such as thromboxane, reduced oxygen species, IL-1, IL-6 and TNF-α (Schletter *et al.*, 1995).

An analogous situation occurs in the presence of a tolerizing microenvironment, but with opposite results. Thus, the co-administration of a contact sensitizer with topical glucocorticoids is known to inhibit the induction of sensitization (Burrows and Stoughton, 1976) and this observation is now used to evoke tolerance to topical therapies known to be contact sensitizers (Amkraut *et al.*, 1996). Therefore, it seems possible that UVR may mediate its effects in similar fashion, also providing a tolerizing microenvironment for co-administered antigens. Hence, the immune response appears to be adjustable so as to generate either tolerizing or activating responses according to the nature of the cutaneous microenvironment and in fact, this may be the means by which contact sensitizers representing only a minimal threat to the organism are able to induce strong local reactions.

UVR AS AN IMMUNOMODULATOR OF THE CUTANEOUS MICROENVIRONMENT

This review of the effects of UVR on cutaneous immunity has been organized around the 'danger' model of immune recognition as described above, in which counter to the activities of environmental danger signals such as LPS which upregulate immune responses, we now propose that UVR acts to distort the cutaneous microenvironment by causing inappropriate signalling through a variety of mechanisms. Thus, the radiation profoundly affects the APC types available in skin, produces a cytokine and adhesion molecule milieu causing the remaining APCs to express tolerizing signals and distorts adhesion molecule expression such that T-cell migration to lymph nodes and recirculation is adversely affected (Fig. 5.4).

CELLULAR IMMUNITY

During CH, APCs process antigen, migrate to regional lymph nodes and present antigen-specific stimulatory signals to T cells (Kripke *et al.*, 1990). However, UVR decreases epidermal LC numbers, destroys their dendricity, alters their expression of major histocompatibility complex (MHC) class II molecules, decreases their adenosine triphosphatase activity (Toews *et al.*, 1980) and, perhaps most importantly, alters the activation signals between these cells and the various T-cell subsets; the CH response is clearly likely to be altered thereby.

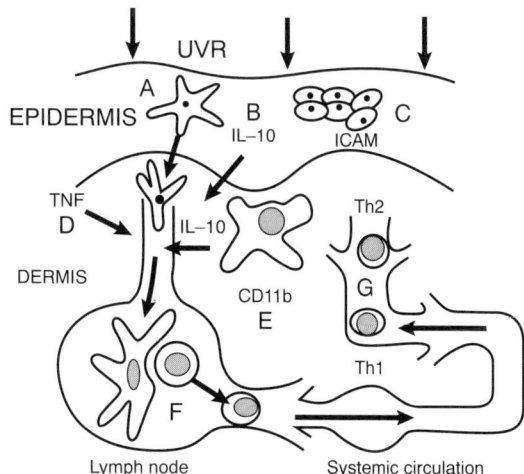

Figure 5.4 Features of UVR effects on cutaneous immunity. A. Langerhans cells; B. IL-10; C. ICAM; D. TNF; E. macrophages; F. APC–T cell interaction; G. Th1–Th2 cell balance.

Thus, there is now good evidence for the existence of distinct helper T-cell subsets, distinguished mainly by their cytokine production profile and the consequent immune responses induced. Of these, T helper 1 cells (Th1) secrete IL-2 and gamma interferon (IFN-γ), thereby mediating proinflammatory immune responses such as CH and DTH, natural killer (NK) cell activation and the stimulated production of complement fixing antibodies, while T helper 2 (Th2) cells instead produce ILs-4, 5, 6 and 10, inhibiting cellular responses but facilitating those associated with IgE. On the other hand, this duality is unfortunately not absolute, some human T cells deemed Th0 producing both IL-4 and IFN-γ, while IL-10, a cytokine with potent downregulating properties, is now known to be secreted by Th1 as well as Th2 cells. Nevertheless, through its effects on LCs, UVR also exerts important indirect effects on the activation of Th cells, in particular preventing LCs from activating Th1 cells in an antigen-specific fashion, thus creating a state of functional inactivation (Simon *et al.*, 1991); however, their capacity to evoke a Th2 pattern is retained (Simon *et al.*, 1990). Thus, UVR exposure appears to shift the cutaneous microenvironment overall towards a suppressive state by the preferential activation of Th2 cells.

However, LCs are not the only APCs affected by UVR in the CH model. Thus, although no response develops when dinitrochlorobenzene (DNCB) is applied to a skin site immediately after UVB exposure, the development of tolerance to a second application as well requires an interval of 48 hours between exposure and the first application (Hammerberg *et al.*, 1994); this delay is now known to enable a population of CD11b+ macrophages, distinct from LCs to migrate into skin and provide immune suppression through the production of IL-10 (Kang *et al.*, 1994). Indeed, a variety of APC populations reach the draining lymph nodes after UVR exposure (Bucana *et al.*, 1994) and it appears that the dose of a contact sensitizer, even in the absence of UVR, is important, LC activation being bypassed at subsensitizing doses and tolerance induced (Steinbrink *et al.*, 1996b), perhaps through the other APCs. Interestingly, higher, sensitizing doses of contact allergen generate Th2-like cells as well, but these are apparently non-functional in the fact of another, effector T-cell subset generated by LC stimulation (Steinbrink *et al.*, 1996b). The 'effector' and 'suppressor' cells are present together, the final outcome thus depending on the balance of signals received from the APCs and environment. Thus, UVR may abrogate the effector function of one APC, the LC, and allow the activity of another to promote tolerizing effects, ultimately mediated by the balance of T-cell subpopulations. However, in the danger model of immunity, a contact sensitizer bypassing the initial cutaneous sentry, namely LC processing and local inflammation, may not represent a systemic threat and therefore, tolerance is likely to be appropriate.

CYTOKINES

UVR-mediated immune suppression has been associated with the effects of a number of cytokines, acting both locally and systemically; these include IL-1 (Gahring *et al.*, 1984), an IL-1 inhibitor (Sutherland *et al.*, 1980), TNF-α (Kock *et al.*, 1990), IL-10 (Rivas and Ullrich, 1992) and IL-12 (Bradley *et al.*, 1995). Of these, the last three have generated the greatest interest.

TNF is a proinflammatory cytokine with a broad spectrum of activities. Secreted by a variety of cells, particularly macrophages and keratinocytes, its effects include the upregulation of intercellular adhesion molecule (ICAM) and MHC class I and II molecule expression and the co-stimulation of lymphocytes. UVR stimulates its release in humans after a single total body exposure (Kock *et al.*, 1990), while its intradermal injection into mice mimics the immunosuppressive effects of

UVR on CH. This latter observation also corresponds with the finding that CH impairment by UVR is a polymorphic trait determined by alleles at two different loci, namely the TNF and LPS sites (Yoshikawa and Streilein, 1990), the associated genetic variability being thought to determine UVB-induced TNF production and thus CH suppressibility in mice. Moreover, intracutaneously injected TNF has been shown to cause the loss of epidermal LC dendricity within 1–2 minutes, correlating with a delayed ability to migrate to regional lymph nodes (Vermeer and Streilein, 1990). On the other hand, some work suggests that TNF enhances CH (Polla *et al.*, 1986) and that the accumulation of DCs in draining lymph nodes during the process may be abrogated by preirradiation TNF antibody treatment (Moodycliffe *et al.*, 1994). These discrepancies have still to be resolved but in spite of this, a role for TNF in UVR-induced immunosuppression seems probable, very likely acting through its effects on the cutaneous microenvironment.

IL-10 is a cytokine associated with downregulated immune responses in a variety of models, often appearing late and therefore particularly thought to function as a natural dampener. It is secreted by a variety of cells, particularly T cells, B cells, monocytes, macrophages and keratinocytes (DeVries, 1995), and its production by the latter in culture following UVB or UVAI (340–400 nm) irradiation (Grewe *et al.*, 1995) has led to its being proposed as an important mediator of UVR-induced immunosuppression. It affects T-cell responsiveness by inhibiting APC antigen presentation and accessory cell function, including the downregulation of APC class II MHC and B7 (CD80 and CD86) molecule expression, the latter important in co-stimulation. In addition, it inhibits IL-2 gene expression in responding T cells and is particularly intriguing because of its role in the differential regulation of Th1 and Th2 responses, thought to be critical in the systemic modulation of immunity. Further, it suppresses T cell cytokine production by blocking the ability of APC to present antigen to the Th1 subset (Enk *et al.*, 1993; Fiorentino *et al.*, 1991; Moore *et al.*, 1993), while T cells cultured with IL-10-treated LCs do not respond to subsequent antigen restimulation, although still proliferating in response to IL-2, thus suggesting that IL-10 may induce a state of clonal anergy. Systemic impairment of APC function by IL-10 also occurs, spleen cells from UVR-irradiated mice demonstrating enhanced antigen presentation to Th2 cells (Ullrich, 1994), while IL-10 antibodies importantly interrupt this effect. Likewise, murine contact photosensitivity may be mediated by an antigen-specific T cell subpopulation releasing IL-10 (Bitto *et al.*, 1995; Burrows and Stoughton, 1976), a suppressive activity which is transferable and again inhibited by IL-10 antibodies. Thus, keratinocyte-, macrophage- and lymphocyte-derived IL-10 may modulate immunity by causing a shift towards a tolerizing T-cell response, the strength of which is clearly demonstrated by its ability to protect mice from LPS-induced shock (DeVries, 1995). In man, this natural downregulator of the immune response may have been similarly incorporated into a protective response, this time against the potentially damaging effects of UVR, although other antigens present during exposure are of necessity tolerated as well.

IL-12 is a cytokine secreted by polymorphonuclear leucocytes, keratinocytes and APC, being important in the activation of Th1 cells (Hsieh *et al.*, 1993) and having been shown to interfere with Th2 cell differentiation and IL-10 production (Bradley *et al.*, 1995); in addition, prostaglandin E_2, the production of which is upregulated by UVR, is a potent inhibitor of the substance (Van Der Pouw Krann *et al.*, 1995). Recently, IL-12 has been demonstrated to prevent both systemic (Schmitt *et al.*, 1995) and local (Schwarz *et al.*, 1996) UVR-induced immunosuppression.

ADHESION MOLECULES AND CO-STIMULATION

B7 MOLECULE INTERACTIONS

Although the exact mechanisms of IL-10-induced immunosuppression are not yet clear, they may be related to its effects on the antigen-independent accessory signals involved in APC co-stimulation, which are in turn mediated by engagement of the T-cell surface molecules CD28 and CTLA-4 with members of the B7 family of APC surface receptors (B7-1 or CD80, and B7-2 or CD86) (Allison and Krummel, 1995). Thus CD28 ligation promotes T-cell stimulation and the secretion of IL-2, whereas CTLA-4 induces inhibition, the resulting T-cell activity then depending on the balance of signals between the two. Importantly, it has also been demonstrated that B7-1 and B7-2 differentially activate the commitment of T-cell precursors to a Th1 or Th2 lineage, again acting through their interactions with CD28 and CTLA-4 (Kuchroo *et al.*, 1995), this cellular interaction thus representing a source of signal 2 in the danger model. Its relevance to the field of photoimmunology, however, lies in the fact that IL-10 interferes with both B7-1 (Ding *et al.*, 1993) and B7-2 (Buelens *et al.*, 1994) upregulation on APCs and the cutaneous immunosuppressive effects of UVR may thus be mediated through the effects of this cytokine on these surface receptor molecules, thereby providing a tolerizing co-stimulation signal.

ICAM

ICAM-1 is a keratinocyte surface molecule providing adhesion to infiltrating leucocytes, thereby making an important contribution to the cutaneous immunological process. UVR may paradoxically exert both pro- and anti-inflammatory effects through ICAM, a situation similar to that in skin as a whole. Thus, it has been shown that the TNF receptor (TNFR), which mediates TNF-induced keratinocyte ICAM expression, is downregulated within 0–12 hours of UVB irradiation (Trefzer *et al.*, 1993), although such exposure also upregulates constitutive expression of the molecule beyond this time. In the same setting, however, UVB upregulates keratinocyte IL-1α sensitivity, thus also upregulating both ICAM-1 messenger RNA and cell surface expression (Krutmann and Grewe, 1995). Additionally, it now appears that UVAI irradiation can also increase keratinocyte expression of this molecule, although apparently by a different mechanism (Krutmann and Grewe, 1995), namely through the generation of reactive oxygen intermediates and lipid peroxides, while by contrast the UVB induction of keratinocyte DNA damage prevents IFN-γ-mediated upregulation of ICAM (Krutmann *et al.*, 1994). This further corroborates the relevance of DNA as a chromophore for UVR-induced immunosuppression but, more importantly, helps reflect the diversity of regulatory and counterregulatory signals affecting just one immunomodulatory facet of the cutaneous microenvironment.

UVR-INDUCED SKIN CANCER

It is now well established that UVR is not only the carcinogen, but also the immunosuppressive agent promoting continuing skin tumour growth in irradiated laboratory animals. The evidence for such immunosuppression has been strongly supported by the finding that it can be transferred in T lymphocytes (Fisher and Kripke, 1982) and the data from several studies have now suggested that this is because of a shift to a Th2-like response, perhaps mediated by IL-10 (Ullrich, 1996). Such a response then permits tumour spread in an environment poorly equipped to mount the necessary cell-mediated immune response against it.

Although the mechanism linking UVR-induced immunosuppression and cutaneous malignancy remains uncertain, there is still compelling evidence that the susceptibility to such suppression in humans correlates with a susceptibility to carcinogenesis. Thus, it has been demonstrated convincingly that the acute, low-dose exposure of Caucasian skin to UVB impairs CH induction to DNCB in approximately 40% of normal individuals, but virtually 100% of patients with a previous biopsy-proven skin cancer, a trait termed **UVB susceptibility** (Yoshikawa *et al.*, 1990); this therefore provides strong evidence that a tendency to immunosuppression is also a risk factor for skin cancer. Importantly, it has further been found that this UVB suscepti-bility exists as a polymorphic trait of equal incidence in both highly pigmented and Caucasian skin (Vermeer *et al.*, 1991), thus suggesting that cutaneous melanin does not protect against the immunosuppressive effects of acute, low-dose UVB irradiation, regardless of skin type. Other studies, however, suggest that UVR-induced immuno-suppression may not always be required for the development and progression of some skin cancers (Menzies *et al.*, 1991).

The danger model provides a useful perspective from which tumour immunity and immunotherapy can be approached. Thus, the model suggests that a neoantigen on a developing tumour cell would not be sufficient to induce an immune response in the absence of co-stimulation. Therefore, an immune system responding to danger in the microenvironment would have difficulty in responding to tumours and, without co-stim-ulation in the form of adhesion molecules or local immunomodulatory signals, would actually delete tumour-specific T cells or produce a state of clonal anergy; in addition, the presence of IL-10 after cutaneous irradia-tion would further reduce the response. Hence, tumour-specific T cells such as lymphokine-activated killer cells (Rosenberg and Lotze, 1986) may ultimately fail, because although signal 1 is provided in the form of T-cell specificity, there is no additional co-stimulatory signal from APC adhesion mole-cules or cytokines in the microenvironment.

Therefore, effective immunotherapy might theoretically use both tumour-specific lymphocytes and a source of co-stimulation or else of inhibition of the negative regulators of co-stimulation. Indeed, blocking of the inhibitory signals of CTLA-4, which normally functions as such an inhibitor, has already been shown to enhance antitumour immunity in mice (Leach *et al.*, 1996), while B7-trans-fected tumour cells have likewise shown early potential in immunotherapy and are now being studied in clinical trials (Williams, 1996). However, the phenotypes of experi-mental animals with adhesion molecule dysfunction have revealed that there may also be other co-stimulatory molecules functioning independently of the B7-CD28/CTLA-4 inter-action (Kuiper *et al.*, 1995) and these may also be worthy of study in due course as potential therapeutic agents.

CONCLUSION

It is now clear that the regulation of cutaneous immunity after UVR exposure is both dynamic and redundant. Thus, rather than being a series of unilateral pathways set irrevocably in motion by antigen activation, it is instead, a highly interactive balance of multiple simultaneous signals based on infor-mation obtained from the local cutaneous environment. In this system, the early effects of UVR exposure, which are very probably initiated by DNA as a photoreceptor, involve APCs, namely LCs, which are altered both structurally and functionally, culminating in their inability to activate lymphocyte subsets in an antigen-specific fashion; a state of func-tional anergy is thereby created for all anti-gens presented during exposure. In addition, a subset of dermal macrophages induced by the exposure appears to be a major source of IL-10, which also has a suppressive effect on the immunological microenvironment, down-regulating adhesion molecule expression, inhibiting antigen presentation and the co-stimulatory functions of APCs and shifting

cutaneous immune activity from a Th1-
toward a Th2-like pattern of response.
Although other cytokines such as TNF also
appear to be involved, many of the changes
can be created by IL-10 alone, thus suggesting
a critical role for this cytokine. Hence, in
summary, by its alteration of the co-stimulatory function of APCs, UVR exposure induces
a shift in the balance of cytokine production,
adhesion molecule expression and T cell
subpopulations toward a tolerance of any
antigens presented at that time. In addition,
these responses are overlapping, perhaps
reflecting a need for the prevention of deleterious immune activation. However, as the
co-stimulatory pathways and regulatory
signals become better understood, progress
will steadily be made towards our complete
understanding of the heterogeneous cutaneous disorders induced by UVR exposure
and their treatment.

REFERENCES

Allison, J.P. and Krummel, M.F. (1995) The Yin and Yang of T cell costimulation [see comments]. *Science*, **270**, 932–3.

Amkraut, A.A., Jordan, W.P. and Taskovich, L. (1996) Effect of coadministration of corticos-teroids on the development of contact sensitiza-tion. *Journal of the American Academy of Dermatology*, **35**, 27–31.

Applegate, L.A., Ley, R.D., Alcalay, J. and Kripke, M.L. (1989) Identification of the molecular target for the suppression of contact hypersensitivity by ultraviolet radiation. *Journal of Experimental Medicine*, **170**, 1117–31.

Basketter, D., Dooms-Goossens, A., Karlberg, A.T. and Leopittevin, J.P. (1995) The chemistry of contact allergy: why is a molecule allergenic? [review]. *Contact Dermatitis*, **32**, 65–73.

Bitto, T., Ueda, M., Nagano, T., Fujii, S. and Ichihashi, M. (1995) Reduction of ultraviolet-induced skin cancer in mice by topical application of DNA excision repair enzymes. *Photodermatol-ogy, Photoimmunology and Photomedicine*, **11**, 9–13.

Bradley, L.M., Yoshimoto, K. and Swain, S.L. (1995) The cytokines IL-4, IFN-gamma, and IL-12 regu-late the development of subsets of memory effector helper T cells *in vitro*. *Journal of Immunology*, **155**, 1713–24.

Bretscher, P. and Cohn, M. (1970) A theory of self-nonself discrimination. *Science*, **169**, 1042–9.

Bucana, C.D., Tang, J.M., Dunner, K. Jr., Stickland, F.M. and Kripke, M.L. (1994) Phenotypic and ultrastructural properties of antigen-presenting cells involved in contact sensitization of normal and UV-irradiated mice. *Journal of Investigative Dermatology*, **102**, 928–33.

Buelens, C., Willems, F., Delvaux, A. *et al.* (1994) Interleukin-10 differentially regulates B7-1 (CD80) and B7-2 (CD86) expression on human peripheral blood dendritic cells. *European Journal of Immunology*, **25**, 2668–72.

Burrows, W.M. and Stoughton, R.B. (1976) Inhibition of induction of human contact sensi-tization by topical glucocorticosteroids. *Archives of Dermatology*, **112**, 175–8.

Butcher, E.C. and Picker, L.J. (1995) Lymphocyte homing and homeostasis [review]. *Science*, **272**, 60–6.

Chen, X., Gresham, A., Morrison, A. and Pentland, A.P. (1996) Oxidative stress mediates synthesis of cytosolic phospholipase A2 after UVB injury. *Biochimica et Biophysica Acta*, **1299**, 23–33.

Devary, Y., Rosette, C., Didonato, J.A. and Karin, M. (1993) NF-kappa B activation by ultraviolet light not dependent on a nuclear signal. *Science*, **261**, 1442–5.

DeVries, J.E. (1995) Immunosuppressive and anti-inflammatory properties of interleukin 10 [review]. *Annals of Medicine*, **27**, 537–41.

Ding, L., Linsley, P.S., Huang, L.Y., Germain, R.N. and Shevach, E.M. (1993) IL-10 inhibits macrophage costimulatory activity by selectively inhibiting the up-regulation of B7 expression. *Journal of Immunology*, **151**, 1224–34.

El-Ghorr, A.A., and Norval, M. (1995) A mono-clonal antibody to cis-urocanic acid prevents the ultraviolet-induced changes in Langerhans cells and delayed hypersensitivity responses in mice, although not preventing dendritic cell accumulation in lymph nodes draining the site of irradiation and contact hypersensitivity responses. *Journal of Investigative Dermatology*, **105**, 264–8.

Enk, A.H., Angeloni, V.L., Udey, M.C. and Katz, S.I. (1993) Inhibition of Langerhans cell antigen-presenting function by IL-10. A role for IL-10 in induction of tolerance. *Journal of Immunology*, **151**, 2390–8.

Eynon, E.E. and Parker, D.C. (1992) Small B cells as antigen-presenting cells in the induction of tolerance to soluble protein antigens. *Journal of Experimental Medicine*, **175**, 131–8.

Fiorentino, D.F., Zlotnik, A., Vieira, P. *et al.* (1991) IL-10 acts on the antigen-presenting cell to inhibit cytokine production by Th1 cells. *Journal of Immunology*, **146**, 3444–51.

Fisher, M.S. and Kripke, M.L. (1982) Suppressor T lymphocytes control the development of primary skin cancer in ultraviolet-irradiated mice. *Science*, **216**, 1133–4.

Forsthuber, T., Yip, H.C. and Lehmann, P.V. (1996) Induction of T sub H 1 and T sub H 2 immunity in neonatal mice. *Science*, **271**, 1728–30.

Fuchs, E. and Matzinger, P. (1992) B cells turn off virgin, but not memory T cells. *Science*, **258**, 1156–9.

Fuchs, E. and Matziner, P. (1996) Beyond 'self' and 'nonself': immunity is a conversation, not a war. *Journal of NIH Research*, **8**, 35–9.

Fijihara, M., Takahashi, T.A., Axuma, M. *et al.* (1996) Decreased inducible expression of CD80 and CD86 in human monocytes after ultraviolet-B irradiation: its involvement in inactivation of allogenecity. *Blood*, **87**, 2386–93.

Gahring, L., Baltz, M., Pepys, M.B. and Daynes, R. (1984) The effect of ultraviolet radiation on production of epidermal cell thymocyte-activating factor/interleukin 1 *in vivo* and *in vitro*. *Proceedings of the National Academy of Sciences of the USA*, **81**, 1198.

Grewe, M., Gyufko, K. and Krutmann, J. (1995) Interleukin-10 production by cultured human keratinocytes: regulation by ultraviolet B and ultraviolet A1 radiation. *Journal of Investigative Dermatology*, **104**, 3–6.

Hammerberg, C., Duraiswamy, N. and Cooper, K.D. (1994) Active induction of unresponsiveness (tolerance) to DNFB by *in vivo* ultraviolet-exposed epidermal cells is dependent upon infiltrating class I MHC + CD11b bright (superscript) monocyte/macrophagic cells. *Journal of Immunology*, **153**, 4915–24.

Harding, F.A., McArthur, J.G., Gross, J.A., Raulet, D.H. and Allison, J.P. (1992) CD28-mediated signalling co-stimulates murine T cells and prevents induction of anergy in T-cell clones. *Nature*, **356**, 607–9.

Hsieh, C.-S., Macatonia, S.E., Tripps, C.S. *et al.* (1993) Development of Th1 CD4+ T cells through IL-12 produced by Listeria-induced macrophages. *Science*, **260**, 547–9.

Jenkins, M.K. and Schwartz, R.H. (1987) Antigen presentation by chemically modified splenocytes induces antigen-specific T cells unresponsiveness *in vitro* and *in vivo*. *Journal of Experimental Medicine*, **165**, 302–19.

Kang, K., Hammerberg, C., Meunier, L. and Cooper, K.D. (1994) CD11b+ macrophages that infiltrate human epidermis after *in vivo* ultraviolet exposure potently produce IL-10 and represent the major secretory source of epidermal IL-10 protein. *Journal of Immunology*, **153**, 5256–64.

Kock, A., Schwartz, T., Kirnbauer, R. *et al.* (1990) Human keratinocytes are a source for tumor necrosis factor alpha: evidence for synthesis and release upon stimulation with endotoxin or ultraviolet light, *Journal of Experimental Medicine*, **172**, 1609–14.

Kondo, S. and Sauder, D.N. (1995) Epidermal cytokines in allergic contact dermatitis [review]. *Journal of the American Academy of Dermatology*, **33**, 786–800.

Kripke, M.L., Munn, C.G., Jeevan, A., Tang, J.M and Bucana, C. (1990) Evidence that cutaneous antigen-presenting cells migrate to regional lymph nodes during contact sensitization. *Journal of Immunology*, **145**, 2833–8.

Krutmann, J. and Grewe, M. (1995) Involvement of cytokines, DNA damage and reactive oxygen intermediates in ultraviolet radiation-induced modulation of intercellular adhesion molecule-1 expression [review]. *Journal of Investigative Dermatology*, **105**, 67S–70S.

Krutmann, J., Bohnert, E. and Jung, E.G. (1994) Evidence that DNA damage is a mediate in ultraviolet B radiation-induced inhibition of human gene expression: ultraviolet B radiation effects on intercellular adhesion molecule-1 (ICAM-1) expression. *Journal of Investigative Dermatology*, **102**, 428–32.

Kuchroo, V.K., Das, M.P., Brown, J.A. *et al.* (1995) B7-1 and B7-2 costimulatory molecules activate differentially the Th1/Th2 developmental pathways: application to autoimmune disease therapy. *Cell*, **80**, 707–18.

Kuiper, H.M., Lens, S.M., Hintzen, R.Q. and Van Lier, R.A. (1995) Lymphocyte costimulation: multiple pathways, multiple functions? [review]. *Research in Immunology*, **146**, 180–3.

Lafferty, K.J. and Cunningham, A.J. (1975) A new analysis of allogenic interactions. *Australian Journal of Experimental Biology and Medical Science*, **53**, 1734–6.

Lanzavecchia, A. (1985) Antigen-specific interaction between T and B cells. *Nature*, **314**, 537–9.

Leach, D.R., Krummel, M.F. and Allison, J.P. (1996) Enhancement of antitumor immunity by CTLA-4 blockade [see comments]. *Science*, **271**, 1734–6.

Macher, E. and Chase, M.W. (1969) Studies on the sensitization of animals with simple chemical compounds. XI. The fate of labeled picryl chloride and dinitrochlorobenzene after sensitizing injections. *Journal of Experimental Medicine*, **129**, 81–102.

Matzinger, P. (1994) Tolerance, danger, and the extended family [review]. *Annual Review of Immunology*, **12**, 991–1045.

Menzies, S.W., Greenoak, G.E., Reeve, V.E. and Gallagher, C.H. (1991) Ultraviolet radiation-induced murine tumors produced in the absence of ultraviolet radiation-induced systemic tumor immunosuppression. *Cancer Research*, **51**, 2772–9.

Moodycliffe, A.M., Kimber, I. and Norval, M. (1992) The effect of ultraviolet B irradiation and urocanic acid isomers on dendritic cell migration. *Immunology*, **77**, 394–9.

Moodycliffe, A.M., Kimber, I. and Norval, M. (1994) Role of tumor necrosis factor-alpha in ultraviolet B light-induced dendritic cell migration and suppression of contact hypersensitivity. *Immunology*, **81**, 79–84.

Moore, K., O'Garra, A., De Waal Malefyt, R., Vieira, P. and Mosmann, T. (1993) Interleukin-10. *Annual Review of Immunology*, **11**, 165–90.

Nishigori, C., Yarosh, D.B., Donawho, C. and Kripke, M.L. (1996) The immune system in ultraviolet carcinogenesis. *Journal of Investigative Dermatology*, **1**, 143–6.

Norval, M., Gilmour, J.W. and Simpson, T.J. (1990) The effect of histamine receptor antagonists on immunosuppression induced by the cis-isomer of urocanic acid. *Photodermatology, Photoimmunology and Photomedicine*, **7**, 243–8.

Picardo, M., Zompetta, C., De Luca, C. *et al.* (1991) Squalene peroxides may contribute to ultraviolet light-induced immunological effects. *Photodermatology, Photoimmunology and Photomedicine*, **8**, 105–10.

Polla, L., Margolis, R., Goulston, C., Parish, J.A. and Granstein, R.D. (1986) Enhancement of the elicitation phase of the murine contact hypersensitivity response by prior exposure to local ultraviolet radiation. *Journal of Investigative Dermatology*, **86**, 13–17.

Quill, H. and Schwartz, R.H. (19987) Stimulation of normal inducer T cell clones with antigen presented by purified Ia molecules in planar lipid membranes: specific induction of a long-lived state of proliferative nonresponsiveness. *Journal of Immunology*, **138**, 3704–12.

Reeve, V.E., Boehm-Wilcox, C., Bosnic, M., Cope, R. and Ley, R.D. (1994) Lack of correlation between suppression of contact hypersensitivity by UV radiation and photoisomerization of epidermal urocanic acid in the hairless mouse. *Photochemistry and Photobiology*, **60**, 268–73.

Ridge, J.P., Fuchs, E.J. and Matzinger, P. (1996) Neonatal tolerance revisited: turning on newborn T cells with dendritic cells. *Science*, **271**, 1723–6.

Rivas, J.M. and Ullrich, S.E. (1992) Systemic suppression of delayed-type hypersensitivity by supernatants from UV-irradiated keratinocytes. *Journal of Immunology*, **149**, 3865–71.

Rivas, J.M. and Ullrich, S.E. (1994) The role of IL-4, IL-10 and TNF-α in the immune suppression induced by ultraviolet radiation. *Journal of Leukocyte Biology*, **56**, 769–75.

Rosenberg, S.A. and Lotze, M.T. (1986) Cancer immunotherapy using interleukin-2 and interleukin-2-activated lymphocytes [review]. *Annual Review of Immunology*, **4**, 681–709.

Ross, J.A., Howie, S.E.M., Norval, M. and Maingay, J. (1988) Systemic administration of urocanic acid generates suppression of the delayed type hypersensitivity response to herpes simplex virus in a murine model of infection. *Photodermatology*, **5**, 9–14.

Sarzotti, M., Robbins, D.S. and Hoffman, P.M. (1996) Induction of protective CTL responses in newborn mice by a murine retrovirus. *Science*, **271**, 1726–8.

Schletter, J., Heine, H., Ulmer, A.J. and Riteschel, E.T. (1995) Molecular mechanisms of endotoxin activity [review] *Archives of Microbiology*, **164**, 383–9.

Schmitt, D.A., Owen-Schaub, L. and Ullrich, S.E. (1995) Effect of IL-12 on immune suppression and suppressor cell induction by ultraviolet radiation. *Journal of Immunology*, **154**, 5114–20.

Schwartz, R.H. (1990) A cell culture model for T lymphocyte clonal anergy. *Science*, **248**, 1349–56.

Schwartz, A., Grabbe, S., Aragane, Y. *et al.* (1966) Interleukin-12 prevents ultraviolet B-induced local immunosuppression and overcomes UVB-induced tolerance. *Journal of Investigative Dermatology*, **106**, 1187–91.

Simon, J.C., Cruz, P.D., Bergstresser, P.R. and Tigelaar, R.E. (1990) Low-dose UVB-irradiated Langerhans cells preferentially activate CD4 cells of the Th1 subset. *Journal of Immunology*, **145**, 2087–91.

Simon, J.C., Tigelaar, R.E., Bergstresser, P.R., Edelbaum, D. and Cruz, P.D. (1991) UVB radiation converts Langerhans cells from immunogenic to tolerogenic antigen presenting cells. Induction of specific clonal anergy in CD4+ T helper 1 cells. *Journal of Immunology*, **146**, 485–91.

Steinbrink, K., Kolde, G., Sorg, C. and Macher, E. (1996a) Induction of low zone tolerance to contact allergens in mice does not require functional Langerhans cells. *Journal of Investigative Dermatology*, **10**, 243–7.

Steinbrink, K., Sorg, C. and Macher, E. (1996b) Low zone tolerance to contact allergens in mice: a functional role for CD8+ helper type 2 cells. *Journal of Experimental Medicine*, **183**, 243–7.

Streilein, J.W. (1993) Sunlight and skin-associated lymphoid tissues (SALT): if UVB is the trigger and TNFα is its mediator, what is the message? *Journal of Investigative Dermatology*, **100**, 47s–52s.

Streilein, J.W., Taylor, J.R., Vincek, V. *et al.* (1994) Immune surveillance and sunlight-induced skin cancer [review]. *Immunology Today*, **15**, 174–9.

Sutherland, B.M., Harber, L.C. and Kochevar, I. (1980) Pyrimidine dimer formation and repair in human skin. *Cancer Research*, **40**, 3181–5.

Tesmann, L.P., Denfeld, R.W., Weiss, J.M., Schopf, E. and Simon, J.C. (1996) Effects of UVB-radiation (UVBR) on the functional expression of B7-1 and B7-1 by murine Langerhans cells (LC). *Journal of Investigative Dermatology*, **106**, 824.

Toews, G.B., Bergstresser, P.R. and Streilein, J.W. (1980) Epidermal Langerhans cell density determines whether contact hypersensitivity or unresponsiveness follows painting with DNFB. *Journal of Immunology*, **134**, 445–53.

Trefzer, U., Brockhaus, M., Lotscher, H. *et al.* (1993) The 44kD tumor necrosis factor receptor on human keratinocytes is regulated by tumor necrosis factor-alpha and by ultraviolet B radiation. *Journal of Clinical Investigation*, **92**, 462–70.

Ullrich, S.E. (1994) Mechanism involved in the systemic suppression of antigen-presenting cell function by UV irradiation. *Journal of Immunology*, **152**, 3410–16.

Ullrich, S.E. (1996) Does exposure to UV radiation induce a shift to a Th-1-like immune reaction? *Photochemistry and Photobiology*, **64**, 254–8.

Van Der Pouw Krann, T.C., Boeije, L.C., Smeenk, R.J., Wijdenes, J. and Aarden, L.A. (1995) Prostaglandin-E2 is a potent inhibitor of human interleukin 12 production. *Journal of Experimental Medicine*, **181**, 775–9.

Vermeer, M. and Streilein, J.W. (1990) Ultraviolet B light-induced alterations in epidermal Langerhans cells are mediated in part by tumor necrosis factor-alpha. *Photodermatology, Photoimmunology and Photomedicine*, **7**, 258–65.

Vermeer, M., Schmieder, G.J., Yoshikawa, T. *et al.* (1991) Effects of ultraviolet B light on cutaneous immune responses of humans with deeply pigmented skin. *Journal of Investigative Dermatology*, **97**, 729–34.

Vink, A.A., Yarosh, D.B. and Kripke, M.L. (1996) Chromophore for UV-induced immunosuppression: DNA. *Photochemistry and Photobiology*, **63**, 383–6.

Weiss, J.M., Renkl, A.C., Denfeld, R.W. *et al.* (1995) Low-dose UVB radiation perturbs the functional expression of B7.1 and B7.2 co-stimulatory molecules on human Langerhans cells. *European Journal of Immunology*, **25**, 2858–62.

Williams, N. (1996) An immune boost to the war on cancer [news]. *Science*, **272**, 28–30.

Yoshikawa, T. and Streilein, J.W. (1990) Tumor necrosis factor-alpha and ultraviolet light have similar effects on contact hypersensitivity in mice. *Regional Immunology*, **3**, 139–44.

Yoshikawa, T., Rae, V., Bruins-Slot, W. *et al.* (1990) Susceptibility to effects of UVB radiation on induction of contact hypersensitivity as a risk factor for skin cancer in humans. *Journal of Investigative Dermatology*, **95**, 530–6.

6

THE CUMULATIVE EFFECTS OF ULTRAVIOLET RADIATION ON THE SKIN: PHOTOAGEING

Rachel E. Herschenfeld and Barbara A. Gilchrest

Photoageing refers to the cumulative changes that occur in the ageing skin as a consequence of repeated exposure to sunlight. These changes are distinct from those due to chronological ageing alone, both clinically and histologically, with epidemiological and direct experimental evidence supporting this concept. Photodamage is a more general term that refers to the deleterious effects of chronic sun exposure on skin overall, to encompass both photoageing and photocarcinogenesis. Recent research has provided insight into the possible mechanisms of these processes and identified potential treatment and prevention strategies.

This chapter describes the clinical and histopathological features of photoageing, then considers its epidemiology, aetiology, pathogenesis and prevention.

CLINICAL MANIFESTATIONS

The clinical manifestations of photoageing depend on an individual's burning and tanning skin type (Table 6.1). In fair-skinned individuals an atrophic pattern predominates, fine wrinkling, freckles and telangiectasia developing initially, with the subsequent appearance of lentigines, guttate hypomelanosis

Photodermatology. Edited by J.L.M. Hawk. Published in 1998 by Chapman & Hall, London. ISBN 0 412 72460 X.

and amelanotic pseudoscars as the damage becomes more severe (Plates 1–3). In darker skinned individuals, there is a hypertrophic pattern, lentigines and diffuse hyperpigmentation developing, followed by the thickened pebbly skin texture often referred to as elastosis (Gilchrest, 1992, 1994) (Plate 4), a word also used to describe the histopathological changes seen in sun-exposed skin and discussed further below. Persistent erythema, dryness, roughness, purpura, premalignant neoplasia and malignancies may also develop as a result of photodamage (Calderone and Fenske, 1995).

Other characteristic clinical hallmarks of photoageing can be observed in some exposed individuals. Delicate parallel lines along the sides of the neck and upper chest, referred to as striated beaded lines, may be formed by hypertrophic sebaceous glands surrounded by variable degrees of elastotic material. The skin of the posterolateral neck may become thickened, leathery and yellow with deep criss-crossing furrows, a condition referred to as cutis rhomboidalis nuchae. Elastotic plaques studded with comedones and keratinous cysts characterize the Favre–Racouchot syndrome and tend to develop over the malar skin or temples; they may also occur on the upper extremities but are referred to there as actinic comedonal plaques. In addition, elastotic nodules consisting of pale 4–6 mm

Table 6.1 Classification of photoageing by type and severity (from Gilchrest, 1992)

Type A*		Type B**	
I	Freckling	I	Diffuse hyperpigmentation
II	Telangiectasia and/or fine wrinkling	II	Lentigines
III	Actinic keratoses and/or irregular pigmentation	III	Thickened, pebbly skin (elastosis) and/or sallowness
IV	Focal or diffuse atrophy with irregular depigmentation	IV	Severe elastosis with deep furrows

* Usually seen in skin types I and II
** Usually seen in skin types III, IV and V

papules may develop on the ear (Calderone and Fenske, 1995), while bullous solar elastosis, demonstrating extensive dermal elastosis and intradermal vesicle formation, has also been reported (Gilchrest, 1993).

HISTOPATHOLOGY

Photoaged skin has distinct histopathological characteristics which differentiate it from intrinsically aged skin (Table 6.2). The latter typically demonstrates flattening of the dermoepidermal junction with a decrease in the number of rete ridges and dermal papillae per unit surface area of skin, variability in epidermal thickness and keratinocyte size and dermal atrophy with decreased collagen content, the appearance of disorganized and granular appearing collagen fibrils, decreased proteoglycan concentration, elastic fibre diminution and disintegration and decreased vascularity (Gilchrest, 1993; Montagna and Carlisle, 1990; West, 1994). Overall, therefore, it is a picture of atrophy and cell loss.

On the other hand, the most marked changes in photoaged skin are found in the dermis, although some of the changes are epidermal. Thus, the papillary and reticular zones contain accumulations of basophilic, thickened and hyperplastic connective tissue

Table 6.2 Histopathological features of intrinsically aged and photoaged skin

	Intrinsically aged skin	Photoaged skin
Epidermal changes	Flattened dermoepidermal junction	Flattened dermoepidermal junction
	Variable epidermal thickness	Early: epidermal thickening Late: epidermal atrophy
	Variable keratinocyte size	Variable keratinocyte size
	Decreased number of melanocytes	Increased number of melanocytes, melanin content and melanocyte atypia
Dermal changes	Atrophy	Collagen degeneration
	Decreased collagen	Increased proteoglycans
	Decreased proteoglycans	Increased elastin, elastic fibre fragmentation
	Decreased elastic fibres	Thickening of vessel walls
	Decreased vascularity	Low-grade perivascular inflammation

fibres which curl, branch and tangle to form the amorphous masses referred to as solar elastosis (Braverman and Fonferko, 1982a; Kligman, 1969). This material stains as for elastic tissue and immunohistochemical studies reveal it to be composed mainly of elastin mixed with smaller amounts of microfibrillar proteins, fibrillin and versican (Bernstein *et al.*, 1994; Chen *et al.*, 1986; Dahlback *et al.*, 1990; Mera *et al.*, 1987). Electron microscopy further reveals swollen, degenerate elastic fibres containing irregular masses of electron-dense material (Lavker, 1995) and a grenz border zone of eosinophilic material separates these masses from the epidermis (Plate 5). Histological evidence of elastosis can predate any clinical signs of photodamage and has regularly been observed in the skin of subjects in the second and third decades of life (Kligman, 1969). Additional dermal features are the accumulation of glycosaminoglycans (GAGs) and the degeneration of collagen, immunohistochemical staining revealing decreases of 20–30% in types I and III collagen in the sun-exposed skin of the posterior neck as compared to the protected skin of the buttock (Bernstein *et al.*, 1996). Microvascular changes have also been found in photoaged skin, particularly thickening of vessel walls, most marked in post-capillary venules, and low-grade perivascular inflammation consisting of lymphocytes, histiocytes and mast cells (Braverman and Fonferko, 1982b; Lavker, 1995).

Epidermal changes in photoageing affect keratinocytes, melanocytes and the dermoepidermal junction, epidermal thickening being present early on, while atrophy is seen in the later stages. Basal keratinocytes vary in size and shape to a greater degree in photoaged than intrinsically aged skin, while the melanosome distribution amongst keratinocytes is also more irregular (Lavker, 1995). A twofold increase in melanocyte number per unit area, an increase in melanin content and increased melanocytic atypia are also found in chronically sun-exposed facial skin (crow's

feet area) as compared with protected postauricular skin (Bhawan *et al.*, 1995). Finally, in both intrinsically and photoaged skin, there is flattening of the dermoepidermal junction.

There are regional variations in these histopathological changes of photoageing. In a study comparing the facial and arm skin of patients with mild to moderate photoageing, for example, Bhawan *et al.* (1992) noted an increase in stratum corneum compaction and keratinocyte atypia, increased number of granular cell layers, the presence of melanophages and an increased degree and prevalence of perivascular inflammation in the facial skin. Whether these differences were due to local skin characteristics or to the relatively greater or more continuous sun exposure of the face as compared with the arm of the same patients could not be deduced from the available biopsies.

The histological changes of photoageing in humans have also been reproduced by the chronic exposure of animals to ultraviolet light (UV). Elastosis, for example, was first induced on the shaved backs of albino mice by Sams in 1964 and later in irradiated hairless mice by others (Young, 1990). Since then, studies in these animals have provided excellent experimental models with which to examine the contribution of the various UV wavelengths to photodamage, as discussed below.

EPIDEMIOLOGY OF PHOTOAGEING

Epidemiological assessment of photoageing is complicated by a lack of widely employed objective criteria for its diagnosis and grading and for the accurate measurement of prior solar exposure, as well as by the absence of any centralized recording of the incidence or prevalence of the disorder. Therefore, it is useful to examine the data concerning other more easily quantified chronic effects of sunlight on human skin, such as photocarcinogenesis, and those following quantified UV exposures of PUVA therapy.

PHOTOAGEING

There are small studies which suggest a strong role for sunlight in the photoageing of human skin. Asymmetrical facial photo-damage, with a small but significant increase in left-sided as compared with right-sided changes, was associated with a high per-centage of time spent driving a car among 120 American subjects (Singer *et al.*, 1994). Accentuation of age-induced alterations at sun-exposed relative to non-sun exposed adjacent skin sites has also been demonstrated by non-invasive measurements of cutaneous properties such as electrical conductance, colour, microrelief and thickness (Richard *et al.*, 1994). Thickening of the subepidermal non-echogenic band, as assessed by ultra-sound and corresponding to the presence of actinic elastosis, was also found. Higher levels of self-reported sun exposure have also been associated with greater perceived age, more wrinkles and histological changes demon-strating increased elastosis and decreased collagen in a group of 41 Caucasian women (Warren *et al.*, 1991).

The National Health and Nutrition Examination Survey is the only major popu-lation-based survey which has included a full skin examination and questions about sunlight exposure. Examinees were classified into groups having had low, moderate or high sunlight exposure according to occupation and reported time spent out of doors. They were also examined for the presence of actinic keratoses, telangiectasia and elastosis as markers of actinic damage. In both white males and females, the prevalence of actinic damage and its components increased with increasing levels of reported sun exposure (Engel *et al.*, 1988).

PHOTOCARCINOGENESIS

Epidemiological evidence concerning the carcinogenic effects of sunlight is abundant, the incidence of squamous cell carcinoma (SCC) and basal cell carcinoma (BCC), as well as of actinic keratoses (AK), being strongly linked to sun exposure.

In a group of Maryland watermen, the risk of AK was increased 1.5 times for those with a cumulative UVB exposure above the median level (Vitasa *et al.*, 1990). AKs were also more prevalent among US white men and women with increasing levels of sunlight exposure (Engel *et al.*, 1988), while other studies have also found AKs to be a sensitive indicator of cumulative exposure (Marks and Selwood, 1985; Marks *et al.*, 1988; Preston and Stern, 1992). Furthermore, sun protection with a sunscreen in Australia over one summer season was found to decrease the develop-ment of new AKs and increase the regression of such lesions in adults (Thompson *et al.*, 1993), while sun protection over two years decreased the development of new AKs in adults in Texas (Naylor *et al.*, 1995).

Skin cancer development is strongly asso-ciated with sunlight exposure and Australia, with its strong insolation and largely fair-skinned Celtic population, has the highest incidence of skin cancers in the world (Giles *et al.*, 1988). In 1985, an Australia-wide survey revealed age-standardized rates of 823 per 100 000 person years for non-melanoma skin cancer (NMSC), with rates for BCC and SCC of 657 and 166 per 100 000 person years respectively (Giles *et al.*, 1988; Marks *et al.*, 1993). In contrast, the SCC rate in the United States in 1983 was only 41.4 cases (Kwa *et al.*, 1992), a difference presumably related to lower UV exposure and a darker skinned population.

A second Australian survey in 1990 reported an NMSC rate of 977 per 100 000 person-years and documented an inverse association between latitude and the risk of the condition. Furthermore, incidence was highest among men over 70 years of age, the subgroup with the highest cumulative UV exposure (Marks *et al.*, 1993). The amount of occupational and non-occupational sun expo-sure also correlates with the development of

SCC (Kwa *et al.*, 1992; Vitasa *et al.*, 1990), most cutaneous SCC in Caucasians being found on sun-exposed areas, and in the United States, 86.7% of cutaneous SCCs in Caucasian men and 76.5% in Caucasian women are found on the head, neck or hands (Kwa *et al.*, 1992), less than 10% of the total body surface.

The incidence of BCC is also strongly correlated with cumulative sunlight exposure, again showing a latitudinal correlation in Australia, although the gradient is not as steep as for SCC (Marks *et al.*, 1993). In the United States, approximately 80% of such lesions occur on the head and neck, areas maximally exposed to sunlight (Preston and Stern, 1992). Incidence rates around the world strongly parallel regional insolation. Thus in Iceland, it is ten per 100 000 person years, while in Rochester, Minnesota, it was 146 from 1976 to 1984 and in Hawaii in 1983, it was 692 (Chuang *et al.*, 1990; Kaminer, 1995).

PUVA AND PHOTODAMAGE

PUVA photochemotherapy involves the administration of oral psoralen, a photosensitizing medication, followed by controlled cutaneous exposures to UVA irradiation. Histopathological and clinical evidence suggests that such therapy leads to photodamage, long-term treatment producing lentigines differing from solar lentigines by the presence in the former of large melanocytes with aberrant and giant melanosomes (Wolff, 1990), as well as leading to mottled hyper- and hypopigmentation with atrophy, usually restricted to areas of overdosage (Wolff, 1990). Stern and colleagues (1985) studied these changes in the skin of psoriatic patients, noting an increased incidence and severity of fine wrinkling, telangiectasia, diffuse hyperkeratosis and freckling on both buttock and dorsal hand skin with increasing numbers of PUVA treatments. Non-invasive measurement of cutaneous microrelief by means of surface replicas also revealed a significant increase in both the number and

depth of wrinkles on the buttock skin after long-term PUVA (cumulative UVA dose > 1000 J/cm^2) as compared with psoriatic patients not receiving the treatment. The response was dose dependent, no significant differences being found between controls and patients who were undergoing PUVA therapy for the first time (Brazzelli *et al.*, 1994).

PUVA therapy also increases the risk of skin cancer (SCC more than BCC), particularly in PUVA-treated, non-sun exposed areas, the risk of such cancer being related to the total cumulative UVA dose, any history of prior carcinogen exposure, the patient's burning and tanning skin type and the intensity of the PUVA treatment (Lerman and Van Voorhees, 1992; Roenigk and Caro, 1981; Stern and Lange, 1988; Stern *et al.*, 1979).

Histological studies reveal both dermal and epidermal changes in PUVA-treated skin. Dermal changes include elastic fibre fragmentation and reduction, basement membrane thickening, eosinophilic homogenization of the dermis, the accumulation of eosinophilic material around blood vessels and the formation of colloid-amyloid bodies (Stern *et al.*, 1985; Wolff, 1990). The degeneration of elastic fibres may be seen as early as two weeks into PUVA therapy in superficial, smaller fibres, progressing thereafter in both severity and depth with continued PUVA treatment (Zelickson *et al.*, 1980). Epidermal changes include the clustering of melanocytes, increases in melanocyte size and the increased melanization of keratinocytes. Focal epidermal dystrophy, consisting of single or clustered keratinocytes with large hyperchromatic nuclei, focal keratinocyte disorientation and atypical cells with multiple or lobulated nuclei, has also been reported inconsistently, but only in patients who have received very high radiation doses (Naylor *et al.*, 1995; Wolff, 1990). Similar changes have also been produced in mice and are clearly dose dependent, while after 20 weeks of PUVA, albino mice also develop basement membrane thickening and the dermal deposition of acid mucopolysaccharides and, after 30 or 40 weeks, hyperkeratosis, acanthosis and dyskeratotic epidermal cells, along with progressive elastotic change in both albino and pigmented mice (Pfau *et al.*, 1986).

AETIOLOGY OF PHOTOAGEING

Photoageing results, by definition, from exposure of the skin to solar radiation over the lifetime of an individual. Certain parts of the solar energy spectrum contribute more to the disorder than others, while its severity in any individual depends in turn upon the amount of sunlight absorbed by the skin, a process influenced by both environmental and behavioural factors.

ACTION SPECTRUM

The action spectrum for photoageing, unlike those for sunburn and tanning, has never been and presumably will not be determined experimentally in humans. Hence, the relative contributions of the different UV wavelengths to the observed epidermal and dermal sequelae of lifelong sun exposure must be extrapolated from the available animal studies and our understanding of skin optics and photochemistry.

UVB irradiation of hairless mice produces epidermal hyperplasia and the proliferation, thickening and curling of dermal elastic fibres, increased dermal GAG deposition, an increase in thin argyrophilic dermal collagen bundles and the thickening of the dermoepidermal basement membrane, all changes similar to those observed in photoaged human skin (Kligman, 1995; Margelia *et al.*, 1993). UVA exposure, on the other hand, produces less dense elastic fibre hyperplasia extending more deeply into the dermis, GAG deposition at the dermoepidermal junction and the reduplication of vascular basement membrane with endothelial cell damage; however, there is no collagen damage or dermal inflammatory infiltrate (Kligman,

1995; Kligman *et al.*, 1985; Zheng and Kligman, 1993). UVA also produces mitochondrial damage in vascular endothelial and dermal cells (Zheng and Kligman, 1993), while both UVB and UVA exposure increase wrinkles and change surface microtopography in hairless mice. Ultrastructural studies also reveal elastic fibre hyperplasia, epidermal basement membrane duplication and an increased variability of collagen fibre diameter in response to UVB, while UVA exposure produces elastic fibre hyperplasia and duplication of the vascular basement membrane (Kligman, 1995). These studies suggest that the changes in sun-exposed human skin result from the combined effects of UVB and UVA in sunlight.

In humans, a single exposure to high-dose UVA (86 J/cm^2 or 173 J/cm^2) leads to minimal epidermal change but to striking dermal vascular alterations, including the opening of endothelial junctions, platelet aggregation and red blood cell extravasation. Repeated exposure, however, results in epidermal changes as well as the deposition of thick amorphous masses around blood and lymphatic vessels (Kumakiri *et al.*, 1977). Twice-weekly exposure of human buttock skin to suberythemal doses of UVA ($3–5 \text{ J/cm}^2$), on the other hand, produced epidermal changes consisting of increased stratum corneum thickness and an increased number of granular and stratified cell layers, along with vascular dilatation and inflammation and decreased elastic tissue content (Lowe *et al.*, 1995); these doses are similar to those expected during cutaneous sun exposure through window glass or through UVB-filtering sunscreens.

EXPOSURE

Levels of sunlight exposure correlate with severity of actinic damage. As described above, higher reported levels of sun exposure have been associated with an increasing prevalence of clinical actinic damage and persons who live in areas with greater sunlight exposure have had higher numbers of actinic keratoses and skin cancers (Engel *et al.*, 1988; Marks and Selwood, 1985; Marks *et al.*, 1988; Preston and Stern, 1992; Vitasa *et al.*, 1990).

RISK FACTORS

Risk factors for photoageing include environmental and behavioural factors which influence exposure to solar radiation, as well as individual characteristics such as burning and tanning skin type (reflecting inducible skin colour) and pigmentation (or constitutive skin colour), which determine an individual's response to solar exposure (Table 6.3).

Skin pigmentation plays a key role in determining an individual's susceptibility to photoageing, melanin being the most important endogenous factor protecting the skin from UV radiation and acting by scattering and absorbing the radiation and by quenching any free radicals generated in spite of this (Pathak and Fitzpatrick, 1993). Dark black skin has a minimal erythemogenic dose (MED) 33 times as great as white skin, while in white skin the stratum corneum, as opposed to the melanin-poor epidermis, is instead the main but relatively ineffective site of UV filtration (Pathak and Fitzpatrick, 1993).

The National Health and Nutrition Survey found an incidence of clinical actinic damage (senile elastosis, AKs and fine telangiectasia) among black Americans of 3–4%, compared with an incidence of approximately 20–30% for white Americans (Engel *et al.*, 1988).

Actinic damage was also found to be significantly higher among whites with lighter coloured eyes as compared to those with brown eyes. A study of 164 albino patients (of whom 52% were under 16 years old) enrolled in an outreach skin care programme in Northern Tanzania revealed actinic changes in almost 90% of patients (wrinkling of the dorsal hand in 89%, solar elastosis in 85% and actinic cheilitis in 77%). The oldest patient without wrinkling or elastosis was 13 and the oldest without actinic cheilitis was 24 (Lookingbill *et al.*, 1995), while a history of sunburns after the age of 20 and of a tendency to freckling in adolescence were also significantly related to the presence of actinic lentigines (Garbe *et al.*, 1994).

This protective effect of pigmentation on photodamage can be more precisely quantified in mice exposed to UV radiation. Compared to pigmented mice, albino mice display more marked acanthosis, dyskeratosis, basement membrane thickening, dermal inflammation, acid mucopolysaccharide deposition and elastic fibre degeneration after 20–30 weeks of UVB irradiation; in addition, they display more marked elastotic changes in response to PUVA exposure (Pfau *et al.*, 1986). Further, black and other dark-skinned people have a much lower incidence of skin cancer than whites, the greater abundance and different distribution of melanin and the increased number and density of stratum corneum layers in black skin having been proposed as major contributors to these differences (Taylor *et al.*, 1990). Skin type, as assessed by an individual's judgement of his or her own response to sunlight exposure,

Table 6.3 Risk factors for photoageing

Individual characteristics	Behavioural and environment factors
Light skin pigmentation	Residence in area of high insolation
Light-coloured eyes (blue, green)	Outdoor occupation or avocation
Skin type	History of sunburns
Tendency to freckling	Sunscreen and sun-protective clothing use
	Exposure to PUVA or UVB phototherapy or to tanning bed

also inversely correlates with skin cancer risk (Taylor *et al.*, 1990) and directly with MED as measured by exposure to a solar simulator, although not with minimal phytotoxic dose after psoralen sensitization or with MED as measured by exposure to UVB (Fitpatrick, 1988; Sayre *et al.*, 1981; Stern and Momtaz, 1984; Taylor *et al.*, 1990).

Acclimatization is the decreased sensitivity to acute sun exposure noted after repeated exposures to sunlight, both pigmentation and epidermal thickening contributing to this process; it is not, however, known whether acclimatization decreases the risk of photoageing due to continued sunlight exposure.

Behavioural factors which contribute to the development of photoageing include the failure to use sunscreens and wear sun-protective clothing such as long-sleeved shirts and hats, factors which will be discussed further in due course along with preventive measures.

PATHOGENESIS

Normal human cells in tissue culture have a finite lifespan, as first demonstrated by Hayflick in the 1960s; intrinsic ageing is reflected in the inverse relationship between cell donor age and this lifespan (Gilchrest and Yaar, 1992). The impact of photoageing at the cellular level is, however, demonstrated by comparison of keratinocytes and fibroblasts derived from sun-exposed sites (lateral upper arm or preauricular region) with controls derived from sun-protected sites (medial upper arm or postauricular region). Such studies reveal that cells from chronically sun-exposed areas have a shorter *in vitro* lifespan (fewer population doublings) and that the lifespan varies inversely with donor age and the severity of clinical photoageing (Gilchrest and Yaar, 1992; Gilchrest *et al.*, 1983). *In vitro* dermal fibroblast growth rate and confluent density at early passage, as well as their response to retinoic acid, are similarly reduced in cultures derived from sun-exposed sites (Gilchrest and Yaar, 1992).

Recent research has further examined the changes produced by photoageing at the cellular and molecular levels and now suggests several mechanisms which may contribute to this process. Specifically, changes in gene expression, cytokine production and oxidative status have been implicated in the process.

GENETIC ALTERATIONS

Many changes in gene expression have been found in photoaged skin and skin-derived cells. Whether these are attributable to UV-induced mutations in the genes or their regulatory elements or to less direct UV effects mediated by such stimuli as altered cytokine release or a changed character of the extracellular matrix is presently unknown. Of particular interest, however, are increases in elastin mRNA in the photoaged skin of the neck and in elastin and fibrillin mRNA in fibroblast explants from photoaged skin, as compared with the levels in the sun-protected skin of the buttocks from the same individuals. This increased mRNA expression correlated wtih enhanced elastin promoter activity in the fibroblast explants and with immunohistochemical evidence of elastosis as demonstrated by antibody staining of both elastin and fibrillin (Bernstein *et al.*, 1994). These findings thus suggest a possible mechanism for the characteristic accumulation of elastotic material in photoaged skin, the role of UV light in activation of the human elastin promoter having been further clarified by experiments in transgenic mice expressing this promoter linked to a chloramphenicol acetyl transferase (CAT) reporter gene. In these studies UVB exposure induced a 4.6-fold increase in elastin promoter activity as compared with controls, which persisted for more than 72 hours, while exposure of fibroblast cultures derived from transgenic mouse skin explants to as little as 0.07 MED also increased this activity, demonstrating that inflammatory cells are not necessary for UVB-induced elastin promoter activation. In addition, exposure of mice to approximately 0.25 MED of UVA produced a 60% increase in CAT activity (Bernstein *et al.*, 1995).

Other genes whose baseline expression and UV inducibility are affected by photoageing include the c-fos proto-oncogene, a 'master switch' involved in signal transduction, whose induction by solar-simulated radiation declines with chronological ageing but is greater in skin cells derived from the photoaged skin of the outer upper arm than in those from the sun-protected skin of the inner upper arm from the same donors (Garmyn *et al.*, 1995; Gilchrest *et al.*, 1994). Conversely, baseline mRNA levels of SPR2 and interleukin-1-receptor antagonist (IL-1ra), two differentiation-associated genes encoding a cornified envelope protein and immunomodulatory protein respectively, are lower in skin cells derived from photoaged rather than photoprotected areas of the same donor (Garmyn *et al.*, 1995; Gilchrest *et al.*, 1994). This combination of a greater reactivity to UVR with an apparently decreased differentiation state may thus perhaps contribute to photocarcinogenesis risk in habitually sun-exposed skin.

Genetic changes in mitochondrial DNA also have been shown to be associated with sunlight exposure, sun-exposed skin having been found to harbour higher levels of such DNA deletions than non-sun exposed skin (Pang *et al.*, 1994), a finding also observed in tissues from animals and humans with increasing chronological age (Melor *et al.*, 1995a, b). Scant data also suggest that aberrations in the expression of cell cycle regulatory proteins may appear early in the process of photodamage, perhaps being associated with excessive atrophy or apoptotic cell death, thus leading to tissue damage or malignant behaviour. Thus, acute exposure to broad-spectrum UV radiation induces epidermal p53, also overexpressed in AKs and SCCs, as well as both epidermal and papillary dermal p21 expression (Paten *et al.*, 1995).

Recently, Fisher *et al.* (1996) further demonstrated an increase in the mRNA and protein levels, as well as enzyme activity, of three matrix-degrading metalloproteinase proteins (MMP) (interstitial collagenase, stromelysin 1 and 92K-gelatinase) following UVB irradiation of human buttock skin *in vivo* with doses as low as 0.1 MED, equivalent to just 1–3 minutes of solar irradiation on a sunny day. This exposure also induced half-maximal binding of the nuclear transcription factors AP-1 (composed of jun and fos proteins and known to stimulate gene transcription for the MMPs mentioned) and NF-kappa-KB (composed of Rel family members and positively regulating 92K-gelatinase gene transcription) to their DNA response elements while pretreatment of the skin with glucocorticoids or all-transretinoic acid (t-RA), both of which have receptors capable of trans-repressing AP-1, reduced the AP-1 binding by approximately 70% (Fisher *et al.*, 1996). These data thus suggest that repeated modest sun exposures over many years may lead to the loss of normal collagen and elastin in photoaged skin by chronic upregulation of their respective degradative enzymes and, further, that this presumably pathological process may be blocked by topical tretinoin therapy and probably also by sunscreen use.

UVA is also reported to induce proteases collagenase mRNA and protein in cultured human fibroblasts, as well as tissue inhibitor of metalloproteinases (TIMP) to a lesser extent, possibly through activation of protein kinase C (Petersen *et al.*, 1992), while Wlaschek and colleagues (1994) demonstrated both *in vivo* and *in vitro* UVA induction of fibroblast-derived collagenase/MMP-1. The increases in collagenase mRNA (maximal at 24 hours) were preceded by increases in interleukin-1 (IL-1) and interleukin-6 (IL-6) mRNA levels (maximal at 12 and 3–6 hours, respectively) and by an early rise in IL-1 activity at three hours. Moreover, antibodies to IL-1α and IL-1β decreased the steady-state levels of IL-6 and abrogated the increases in IL-6 activity and collagenase mRNA, while antisense oligonucleotides to IL-1α and IL-1β mRNA decreased these responses (Wlaschek *et al.*, 1994). These data thus suggest that interleukins may in part mediate UVA-induced increases in collagenase mRNA.

ROLE OF CYTOKINES

UVB irradiation of human keratinocytes *in vitro* leads to the release of numerous cytokines such as tumour necrosis factor α (TNF-α), IL-1α and IL-6, all of which have proinflammatory and proliferative effects on numerous cell types such as fibroblasts, endothelial cells and Langerhans cells (Chung *et al.*, 1996; Grewe *et al.*, 1995). In mice, UVB irradiation also induces IL-1 and TNF-α and causes an increase in myeloperoxidase (MPO), a marker for polymorphonuclear infiltration (Griswold and Tzimas, 1995). Oral administration of a phosphodiesterase inhibitor, rolipram, known to block cAMP production, however, inhibited both release of TNF-α and MPO accumulation, thus implicating cAMP in the regulation of UVB-induced inflammation (Griswold and Tzimas, 1995).

Ultraviolet radiation can also promote anti-inflammatory cascades in human keratinocytes, some studies having demonstrated increased IL-10 mRNA and protein in response to UVA and UVB irradiation, with a twofold greater response to UVA, although others have failed to confirm these results (Grewe *et al.*, 1995; Jackson *et al.*, 1996). UVB and UVA also transiently inhibit interferon gamma (IFN-γ) and TNF-α-induced intercellular adhesion molecule-1 (ICAM-1) expression by human keratinocytes while upregulating constitutive ICAM-1 expression (Krutmann and Grewe, 1995). UVB can downregulate keratinocyte expression of IL-15 (a cytokine which enhances the proliferation and activity of activated T cells, B cells, lymphocyte-activated killer cells and natural killer cells), thereby contributing to UV-induced immunosuppression (Blauvelt *et al.*, 1996). The effect of ageing and photoageing on these UV-induced cytokine modulations is virtually unexamined, although donor age-associated reductions in keratinocyte production of IL-1 (then termed epidermal cell-derived thymocyte activating factor or ETAF) have been reported (Sander *et al.*, 1988). In addition, stratum corneum from sun-exposed human facial skin was found to have higher levels of activity of IL-1ra, a competitive inhibitor of IL-1, than sun-protected inner upper arm skin and these IL-1ra levels increased with UVB irradiation, perhaps also contributing to UV-induced immunosuppression (Hirao *et al.*, 1996).

FREE RADICALS AND PHOTOAGEING

Substantial evidence implicates free radical damage, incurred during the course of normal cellular metabolism, in the intrinsic ageing processes, while it is also hypothesized that such damage plays an important additional role in skin photoageing. The free radical theory proposes that:

1. UV irradiation produces free radicals in the skin;
2. sufficiently high UV doses produce enough free radicals to overwhelm antioxidant defences;
3. these excessive free radicals then damage proteins, lipids and DNA;
4. this damage finally leads to the observed chronic changes in skin.

Generation of free radicals by UV irradiation is well established *in vitro*, although difficult to demonstrate *in vivo*; such irradiation, however, enhances the electron spin resonance signals of eumelanins and phaeomelanins, thus indirectly indicating an increase in radical generation (Emerit, 1992). Exposure of compounds present in all cells, for example riboflavin and other endogenous photosensitizers such as NADP, NADPH, porphyrins and quinones, to UVA and UVB also produces free radicals (Dalle Carbonare and Pathak, 1992; Emerit, 1992) and *in vitro* experiments have demonstrated that exposure of riboflavin-containing solutions under aerobic conditions to UVA or UVB produces singlet oxygen which can then crosslink and inactivate the antioxidant enzyme catalase, at least in solution. UVA irradiation of collagen solutions in the presence of riboflavin (but not UVA irradiation alone) also produced crosslinking which was then minimized by the addition of specific oxygen radical quenchers (Dalle Carbonare and Pathak, 1992). Further UVA irradiation of cultured human fibroblasts increases lipid hydroperoxides, indicators of oxygen-associated photodynamic reactions, and decreases levels of reduced glutathione (Schmitz *et al.*, 1995), presumably because this antioxidant species is consumed during repair of the oxidative damage.

UVB and UVA have also been shown to decrease antioxidant defences in the skin of hairless mice (Darr *et al.*, 1992; Fuchs and Packer, 1990; Fuchs *et al.*, 1990; Punnonen *et al.*, 1991), solar-simulating radiation (containing a mixture of UVA and UVB) decreasing the levels of enzymic antioxidants, such as glutathione peroxidase (GSH-Px), glutathione reductase, superoxide dismutase (SOD) and catalase, and of non-enzymic antioxidants such as α-tocopherol, ubiquinone 9, ubiquinol 9, ascorbate and glutathione in murine epidermis *in vivo* (Shindo *et al.*, 1993). In addition, a dose–response relationship between total UVB and UVA exposure and the degree of antioxidant reduction has been demonstrated, as well as a dramatic reduction in epidermal versus dermal antioxidant defences after exposure (Shindo *et al.*, 1994a, b). In addition, UVA exposure increases lipid peroxidation in cultured human keratinocytes and reduces the activity of both SOD and catalase, while psoralen pretreatment causes a significant further reduction in SOD but not catalase activity (Punnonen *et al.*, 1991).

Maeda *et al.* (1991) further studied photoageing-related changes in collagen and elastin solubility, lipid-soluble antioxidants and SOD and GSH-Px activity in the skin of hairless mice irradiated with UVA and 2% UVB. SOD and GSH-Px activities increased during a six-week period of irradiation, at which point GSH-Px activity stabilized but SOD declined. Lipid-soluble antioxidants, however, decreased dramatically with irradiation, while the insoluble, crosslinked fraction of collagen increased significantly as compared to that in age-matched controls.

Preliminary evidence also suggests that free radicals may mediate a UV radiation-associated induction of enzymes important in photoageing, UVB-mediated induction of MMP1 mRNA, for example inhibited by iron chelators, scavengers of hydroxyl radicals and a vitamin E derivative that inhibited lipid peroxidation (Brenneisen *et al.*, 1996). These results thus suggest a role for ferrous/ferric ion in catalysing UVB-mediated hydroxyl radical and lipid peroxide formation, which may ultimately lead to the induction of MMP1 mRNA.

SUMMARY

Taken together, the available research provides several insights into the possible mechanisms of photoageing. Exposure of human skin to sunlight activates multiple processes simultaneously via different pathways, UVB and UVA irradiation through fibroblast elastin promoter activation perhaps contributing to the accumulation of elastic fibres, while a simultaneous increase in binding of AP-1 and NFκB to promoters of metalloproteinase genes may upregulate expression of these proteins with the consequent degradation of stromal elements such as elastin and collagen. UVA might also produce additional activation of the metalloproteinases through increases in the production of mediators such as IL-1 and IL-6. Recruitment of inflammatory cells through UVA- and UVB-induced production of pro-inflammatory cytokines such as TNF-α may further increase the production and release of proteolytic enzymes and the finding that collagen levels are decreased in the papillary dermis of sun-exposed skin, but that collagen mRNA levels from fibroblasts derived from such skin are not, supports the idea that the decreased collagen is due to degradation and not altered production (Bernstein *et al.*, 1996).

Generation of reactive oxygen species mediated by endogenous chromophores such as melanin, flavins, quinones and NADH may produce direct oxidative damage to DNA, proteins and lipid membranes, while such damage may also occur in the extracellular space, which has relatively few antioxidant defences (Maeda *et al.*, 1991). This and directly UV-mediated DNA damage could further influence gene expression, while protein damage such as collagen crosslinking could again contribute to the development of elastosis. Finally, membrane lipid peroxidation may enhance the release of soluble mediators into the dermis, further amplifying the inflammatory process and its associated cellular responses.

PREVENTION OF PHOTOAGEING

A significant proportion of age-associated cosmetic skin defects are caused by photodamage and it is estimated that 80% of this damage may take place by the age of 20 (Leyden, 1990). Therefore, any prevention of photoageing must be promoted at an early age and there is evidence that sunscreens, physical barriers, antioxidants and other pharmacological agents are likely to be useful.

SUNSCREENS

Sunscreens decrease exposure to UV radiation by absorbing, reflecting or scattering it before it reaches the skin. In mice, application of a sunscreen with protection factor 15 prevented elastosis, neutral and acid mucopolysaccharide deposition and melanin production in response to exposure to UVA and UVB (Kligman *et al.*, 1982), while even application of a sunscreen protection factor 2 prevented

some photodamage in these animals (Young, 1990; Young *et al.*, 1988). In humans, application of such screens can also slow the development of actinic keratoses (Thompson *et al.*, 1993), while application of a sunscreen of protection factor 29, blocking both UVB and short wavelength UVA, decreased solar elastosis over two years as assessed by computer enhancement of histological specimens, but did not decrease epithelial thickness, keratinocyte atypia or dermal inflammation (Boyd *et al.*, 1995). Furthermore, application of a sunscreen containing cinnamate to block UVB and benzophenone to block UVA also inhibited the induction of p53 and p21 nuclear protein expression in human skin exposed to broad-spectrum UV radiation (Ponten *et al.*, 1995).

CLOTHING AND OTHER FORMS OF PHYSICAL PROTECTION

Appropriate clothing is a simple and effective means of protecting against sun exposure and its use is recommended wherever possible.

ANTIOXIDANTS

Antioxidants such as α-tocopherol and vitamin C have been shown to reduce UV-induced damage *in vitro* and in animal models (Summers and Summers, 1993), in particular, decreased sunburn cell formation and erythema in response to UVB and decreased sunburn cell formation and blistering in response to PUVA being found in pigs treated with topical vitamin C (Darvr *et al.*, 1992). These results were not due to sunscreening properties, however, as the absorption peak of vitamin C is below 300 nm. In albino hairless mice, topical α-tocopherol and ascorbic acid also reduced UVB- but not UVA-induced skin wrinkling, tumour formation and histopathological changes (though a protection factor 4 sunscreen was more effective for the latter), and since a common feature among these antioxidants was the ability to scavenge superoxide *in vitro*, thus suggests a role for this radical in UV-induced skin damage (Bissett *et al.*, 1990). In a human study of ten people, application of 10% L-ascorbic acid solution to the volar forearm also reduced UVB erythema significantly as compared to vehicle control (Murray *et al.*, 1996), while preincubation of mouse keratinocytes with vitamin C, Trolox (a water-soluble vitamin E analogue) or selenite (a nutrient required for glutathione peroxidase activity) again significantly reduced UVB-induced DNA damage (Stewart *et al.*, 1996). Finally, human fibroblasts cultured with α-tocopherol were protected from UVB-induced cytotoxicity as reflected by a lack of increase in levels of malondialdehyde, an endproduct of lipid peroxidation (Kondo *et al.*, 1990).

PHARMACOLOGICAL APPROACHES

Topical retinoids and corticosteroids may help to prevent photoageing by blocking some of the harmful effects of UV radiation that reaches the dermis because, as discussed above, these compounds have receptors which transrepress AP-1, a transcription factor which may mediate the UVB induction of matrix-degrading metalloproteinases (Fisher *et al.*, 1996). An additional anti-inflammatory property of 13-cis retinoic acid was also recently described, namely its ability to decrease nitrite and thereby TNF-α production by activated cultured human keratinocytes (Becherel *et al.*, 1996). Whether this mechanism may play a role in the prevention of UV-induced inflammation and photoageing, however, is not known.

EDUCATION

The success of any of these measures is dependent upon its utilization by individuals at risk and therefore information about the dangers of sun exposure must accompany recommendations for the use of sun protection. Unfortunately, some studies have failed to find a significant correlation between aware-ness of the risks of sun exposure and the use of sunscreens or avoidance of tanning bed use (Mawn and Fleischer, 1993; Ross and Sanchez, 1990). Intensive education of 9–11-year-olds as part of their school curriculum, however, was shown to increase their use of sun-protective measures, while one study of adults attending a skin cancer screening clinic did find a positive correlation between knowledge of the risks of sun exposure and sunscreen use (Berwick *et al.*, 1992; Girgis *et al.*, 1993). In addition, sunscreen use in children correlates strongly with parental sunscreen use and, therefore, parental education is particularly important in the photoprotection of children (Zinman *et al.*, 1995).

TREATMENT OF ESTABLISHED PHOTOAGEING

Established photoageing is at least partially reversible, the dermal changes of elastosis and mucopolysaccharide deposition produced by 20 weeks of UVB in mice becoming less pronounced if the animals were allowed to spend 20 weeks without further exposure (Pfau *et al.*, 1986) and, even with continued exposure, a factor 15 sunscreen was shown to allow dermal repair of collagen and elastic fibres (Kligman *et al.*, 1983). In large multicentre trials of photoageing therapy, control groups using a so-called placebo regimen consisting of regular use of a factor 15 sunscreen and a moisturizer experienced subtle but statistically significant improvement clinically and histologically, as compared with their own baseline status (Bhawan *et al.*, 1991; Olsen *et al.*, 1992; Weinstein *et al.*, 1991). In another study, however, use of a sunscreen blocking UVB and short wavelength UVA diminished the progression of solar elastosis in preauricular skin over 24 months but did not decrease dermal inflammation, epidermal thickening or keratinocyte atypia (Boyd *et al.*, 1995).

Topical tretinoin is very effective at reversing the wrinkling and pigmentary changes associated with photoageing, enhancing the intrinsic repair of UV-damaged skin in mice (Kligman *et al.*, 1984). In humans, 0.05% and 0.1% topical tretinoin creams have also been found to improve the appearance of photoaged skin, as judged by its texture, wrinkling, pigmentation (solar lentigines and mottled hyperpigmentation) and sallowness (Futoryan and Gilchrest, 1994; Griffiths *et al.*, 1995; Olsen *et al.*, 1992; Rafal *et al.*, 1992; Weiss *et al.*, 1988). Although the histological changes in the epidermis, including the increased epidermal thickness, increased granular layer thickness and stratum corneum compaction, then return to baseline after 48 weeks of therapy, the clinical improvement still persists (Bhawan *et al.*, 1991; Futoryan and Gilchrest, 1994). In the dermis, on the other hand, topical tretinoin increases type I collagen synthesis, reduced in photoaged as compared to sun-protected skin, and this may partially account for the wrinkle effacement (Chen *et al.*, 1992; Griffiths *et al.*, 1993; Kligman *et al.*, 1986).

α-hydroxy acids also seem effective in the treatment of photodamage, producing epidermal thickening and increased GAG deposition in the dermis. Glycolic acid 70% peels, for example, can produce improvement in mild photoageing (Roenigk, 1995), while 12% lactic acid produced mild improvement in periorbital wrinkling and skin texture after eight weeks in one uncontrolled trial of 21 patients (Ridge *et al.*, 1990). α-hydroxy acid (25% lactic acid, glycolic acid or citric acid lotion pH 3.5) treatment of forearm skin for six months was also reported to produce increased epidermal thickness, a more undulating rete ridge pattern, decreased basal cell atypia, less melanin clumping and longer, thicker elastic fibres with less clumping as compared to placebo-treated sites on the other forearm (Ditre *et al.*, 1996); the increased skin thickness seemed to be caused by increased synthesis of GAGs, collagen and possibly elastic fibres. Another study demonstrated significant improvement in the severity of photodamage (as graded by the assessment of mottled pigmentation, wrinkling, laxity, telangiectasia, sallowness and tactile roughness) on the face and arm after 22 weeks of topical 8% glycolic acid or 8% lactic acid creams, as compared with vehicle cream (Stiller *et al.*, 1996).

Additional, more invasive options are also available for the improvement of photoaged skin, namely soft tissue augmentation with collagen, gelatin matrix implants, autologous fat transplantations, chemical peels, CO_2 laser resurfacing, dermabrasion and rhytidectomy.

CONCLUSION

Photoageing is the result of cumulative exposure to sunlight over the lifetime of an individual and is characterized by specific clinical and histopathological changes in the skin. The cellular and molecular events that produce these changes include alterations in gene expression, changes in cytokine levels and the production of free radicals and while our understanding of these mechanisms has progressed, it is still incomplete. The ageing of populations in developed countries, the lengthening of the average lifespan, individuals' continued habit of sun exposure and the continuation of ozone depletion all ensure that photoageing and photodamage will remain important clinical problems well into the future. Studies further characterizing the molecular changes involved in the process will probably steadily provide improvements in its treatment.

REFERENCES

Becherel, P.A., LeGoff, I., Ktorza, S. *et al.* (1996) CD-23 mediated nitric oxide synthase pathway induction in human keratinocytes is inhibited by retinoic acid derivatives. *Journal of Investigative Dermatology*, **106**, 1182–6.

Bernstein, E.F., Brown, D.B., Urbach F. *et al.* (1995) Ultraviolet radiation activates the human elastin promoter in transgenic mice: a novel *in vivo* and *in vitro* model of cutaneous photoageing. *Journal of Investigative Dermatology*, **105**, 269–73.

Bernstein, E.F., Chen, Y.Q., Tamai, K. *et al.* (1994) Enhanced elastin and fibrillin gene expression in chronically photodamaged skin. *Journal of Investigative Dermatology*, **103**, 182–6.

Bernstein, E.F., Chen, Y.Q., Kopp, J.B. *et al.* (1996) Long-term sun exposure alters the collagen of the papillary dermis. *Journal of the American Academy of Dermatology*, **34**, 209–18.

Berwick, M., Fine, J.A. and Bolognia, J.L. (1992) Sun exposure and sunscreen use following a community skin cancer screening. *Preventive Medicine*, **21**, 302–10.

Bhawan, J., Gonzalez-Serva, A., Nehal, K. *et al.* (1991) Effects of tretinoin on photodamaged skin: a histological study. *Archives of Dermatology*, **127**, 666–72.

Bhawan, J., Oh, C., Lew, R. *et al.* (1992) Histopathologic differences in the photoageing process in facial versus arm skin. *American Journal of Dermatopathology*, **14**, 224–30.

Bhawan, J., Andersen, W., Lee, J., Labadie, R. and Solares, G. (1995) Photoageing versus intrinsic ageing: a morphologic assessment of facial skin. *Journal of Cutaneous Pathology*, 154–9.

Bissett, D.L., Chatterjee, R. and Hannon, D.P. (1990) Photoprotective effect of superoxide scavenging antioxidants against ultraviolet radiation-induced chronic skin damage in the hairless mouse. *Photodermatology, Photoimmunology and Photomedicine*, **7**, 56–62.

Blauvelt, A., Asada, H., Klaus-Kotvun, V. *et al.* (1996) Interleukin-15 mRNA is expressed by human keratinocytes, Langerhans cells, and blood-derived dendritic cells and is downregulated by ultraviolet B radiation. *Journal of Investigative Dermatology*, **106**, 1047–52.

Boyd, A.S., Naylor, M., Cameron, G.S. *et al.* (1995) The effects of chronic sunscreen use on the histological changes of dermatoheliosis. *Journal of the American Academy of Dermatology*, **33**, 941–6.

Braverman, I.M. and Fonferko, B.A. (1982a) Studies in cutaneous ageing: I. The elastic fibre network. *Journal of Investigative Dermatology*, **78**, 434–43.

Braverman, I.M. and Fonferko, E. (1982b) Studies in cutaneous ageing: II. The microvasculature. *Journal of Investigative Dermatology*, **78**, 444–8.

Brazzelli, V., Borroni, G., Berardesca, E. *et al.* (1994) PUVA-treated psoriatic skin as a model for cutaneous wrinkling assessed by skin replicas. *Acta Dermato-Venereologica*, **74** (suppl 186), 162–3.

Brenneisen, P., Brivibka, K., Wlaschek, M. *et al.* (1996) Involvement of ferrous/ferric iron in the UVB mediated induction of interstitial collagenase (MMP1) mRNA. *Journal of Investigative Dermatology*, **107**, 515.

Calderone, D.C. and Fenske, N.A. (1995) The clinical spectrum of actinic elastosis. *Journal of the American Academy of Dermatology*, **32**, 1016–24.

Chen, V.L., Fleischmajer, R. and Schwartz, E. (1986) Immunochemistry of elastotic material in sun-damaged skin. *Journal of Investigative Dermatology*, **87**, 334–7.

Chen, S., Kiss, I. and Tramposch, K.M. (1992) Effects of all-trans RA on UVB irradiated and non-irradiated hairless mouse skin. *Journal of Investigative Dermatology*, **98**, 248–54.

Chuang, T.Y., Popescu, A., Su, W.P. *et al.* (1990) Basal cell carcinoma. A population based incidence study in Rochester, Minnesota. *Journal of the American Academy of Dermatology*, **22**, 413–17.

Chung, J.H., Youn, S.H., Koh, W.S. *et al.* (1996) Ultraviolet B irradiation-enhanced Il-6 production and mRNA expression are mediated by IL-1a in cultured human keratinocytes. *Journal of Investigative Dermatology*, **106**, 715–20.

Dahlback, K., Ljungquist, A., Lofberg, H. *et al.* (1990) Fibrillin immunoreactive fibres constitute a unique network in the human dermis: immuno-histochemical comparison of the distribution of fibrillin, vitronectin, amyloid p component, and orcein stainable structures in normal skin and elastosis. *Journal of Investigative Dermatology*, **94**, 284–91.

Dalle Carbonare, M. and Pathak, M.A. (1992) Skin photosensitizing agents and the role of reactive oxygen species in photoageing. *Journal of Photochemistry and Photobiology*, **14**, 105–24.

Darr, D., Combs, S., Dunston, S., Manning, T. and Pinnell, S. (1992) Topical vitamin C protects porcine skin from ultraviolet radiation-induced damage. *British Journal of Dermatology*, **127**, 247–53.

Ditre, C.M., Griffin, J.D., Murphy, G.F. *et al.* (1996) Effects of α-hydroxy acids on photoaged skin: a pilot clinical, histological, and ultrastructural study. *Journal of the American Academy of Dermatology*, **34**, 187–95.

Emerit, I. (1992) Free radicals and ageing of the skin, in *Free Radicals and Ageing*, (eds I. Emerit and B. Chence), Birkhauser Verlag, Basel, pp. 328–41.

Engel, A., Johnson, M. and Haynes, S.G. (1988) Health effects of sunlight exposure in the United States. *Archives of Dermatology*, **124**, 72–9.

Fisher, G.J., Datta, S.C., Talwar, H.S. *et al.* (1996) Molecular basis of sun induced premature skin ageing and retinoid antagonism. *Nature*, **379**, 335–9.

Fitzpatrick, T.B. (1988) The validity and practicality of sun-reactive skin types I through VI. *Archives of Dermatology*, **124**, 869–71.

Fuchs, J. and Packer, L. (1990) Ultraviolet irradiation and the skin antioxidant system. *Photodermatology, Photoimmunology and Photomedicine*, **7**, 90–2.

Fuchs, J., Huflejt, M., Rothfuss, L. *et al.* (1990) Dermatologic antioxidant therapy may be warranted to prevent ultraviolet induced skin damage, in *Antioxidants in Therapy and Preventive Medicine*, (ed. I. Emerit) Plenum Press, New York, pp. 533–6.

Futoryan, T. and Gilchrest, B.A. (1994) Retinoids and the skin. *Nutrition Reviews*, **52**, 299–310.

Garbe, C., Buttner, P., Weiss, J. *et al.* (1994) Associated factors in the prevalence of more than 50 common melanocytic nevi, atypical melanocytic nevi, and actinic lentigines: multicenter case-control study of the central malignant melanoma registry of the German dermatological society. *Journal of Investigative Dermatology*, **102**, 700–5.

Garmyn, M., Degreef, H. and Gilchrest, B.A. (1995) The effect of acute and chronic photodamage on gene expression in human keratinocytes. *Dermatology*, **190**, 305–8.

Gilchrest, B.A. (1992) The variable face of photoageing: influence of skin type. *Cosmetics and Toiletries*, **107**, 41–2.

Gilchrest, B.A. (1993) Ageing of the skin, *Dermatology in General Medicine*, (eds T.B. Fitzpatrick *et al.*), McGraw-Hill, New York, 150–8.

Gilchrest, B.A. (1994) Ultraviolet damage to the skin: a strategy for August, a month of sun days. *Modern Medicine*, **62**, 43–6.

Gilchrest, B.A. and Yaar, M. (1992) Ageing and photoageing of the skin: observations at the cellular and molecular level. *British Journal of Dermatology*, **127** (suppl 41), 25–30.

Gilchrest, B.A., Szabo, G., Flynn, E. and Goldwyn, R. (1983) Chronologic and actinically induced ageing in human facial skin. *Journal of Investigative Dermatology*, **80**, 81s–85s.

Gilchrest, B.A., Garmyn, M. and Yaar, M. (1994) Ageing and photoageing affect gene expression in cultured human keratinocytes. *Archives of Dermatology*, **130**, 82–6.

Giles, G.G., Marks, R. and Foley, P. (1988) The incidence of non-melanocytic skin cancer treated in Australia. *British Medical Journal*, **296**, 13–17.

Girgis, A., Sanson-Fisher, R.W., Tripodi, D.A. and Golding, T. (1993) Evaluation of interventions to improve solar protection in primary schools. *Health Education Quarterly*, **20**, 275–87.

Grewe, M., Gyufko, K. and Krutmann, J. (1995) Interleukin-10 production by cultured human keratinocytes: regulation by ultraviolet B and ultraviolet A1 radiation. *Journal of Investigative Dermatology*, **104**, 3–6.

Griffiths, C.E.M., Russman, A.N., Majmudar, G. *et al.* (1993) Restoration of collagen formation in photodamaged human skin by tretinoin (retinoic acid). *New England Journal of Medicine*, **329**, 530–5.

Griffiths, C.E.M., Kang, S., Ellis, C.N. *et al.* (1995) Two concentrations of topical tretinoin (retinoic acid) cause similar improvement of photoageing but different degrees of irritation. *Archives of Dermatology*, **131**, 1037–44.

Griswold, D.E. and Tzimas, M.N. (1995) Ultraviolet B-induced inflammatory cytokine production, *in vivo*: initial pharmacological characterization. *Inflammation Research*, **44** (suppl 2), s209–s210.

Hirao, T., Aoki, H., Yoshida, T., Sato, Y. and Kamoda, H. (1996) Elevation of interleukin-1 receptor antagonist in the stratum coreneum of sun-exposed and ultraviolet B-irradiated human skin. *Journal of Investigative Dermatology*, **106**, 1102–7.

Jackson, M., Thomson, K.E., Laker, R. and Norval, M. (1996) Lack of induction of IL-10 expression in human keratinocytes (letter). *Journal of Investigative Dermatology*, **106**, 1329.

Kaminer, M.S. (1995) Photodamage: magnitude of the problem, in *Photodamage*, (ed. B.A. Gilchrest), Blackwell Science, Oxford, pp. 1–11.

Kligman, A.M. (1969) Early destructive effect of sunlight on human skin. *Journal of the American Medical Association*, **210**, 2377–80.

Kligman, A.M., Grove, G.L., Hirose, R.H. and Leyden, J.J. (1986) Topical tretinoin for photoaged skin. *Journal of the American Academy of Dermatology*, **15**, 536–59.

Kligman, L.H. (1995) Animal models of photodamage and its treatment, *Photodamage*, (ed. B.A. Gilchrest), Blackwell Science, Oxford, pp. 136–56.

Kligman, L.H., Akin, F.J. and Kligman, A.M. (1982) Prevention of ultraviolet damage to the dermis of hairless mice by sunscreens. *Journal of Investigative Dermatology*, **78**, 181–9.

Kligman, L.H., Akin, F.J. and Kligman, A.M. (1983) Sunscreens promote repair of ultraviolet radiation-induced dermal damage. *Journal of Investigative Dermatology*, **81**, 98–102.

Kligman, L.H., Duo, C.H. and Kligman, A.M. (1984) Topical retinoic acid enhances the repair of ultraviolet damaged dermal connective tissue. *Connective Tissue Research*, **12**, 139–50.

Kligman, L.H., Akin, F.J. and Kligman, A.M. (1985) The contributions of UVA and UVB to connective tissue damage in hairless mice. *Journal of Investigative Dermatology*, **84**, 272–6.

Kondo, S., Mamada, A., Yamaguchi, J. and Fukuro, S. (1990) Protective effect of di-tocopherol on the cytotoxicity of ultraviolet B against human skin fibroblasts *in vitro*. *Photodermatology, Photoimmunology and Photomedicine*, **7**, 173–7.

Krutmann, J. and Grewe, M. (1995) Involvement of cytokines, DNA damage, and reactive oxygen intermediates in ultraviolet radiation-induced modulation of intercellular adhesion molecule-1 expression. *Journal of Investigative Dermatology*, **105**, 67s–70s.

Kumakiri, M., Hashimoto, K. and Willis, I. (1977) Biologic changes due to long-wave ultraviolet irradiation on human skin: ultrastructural study. *Journal of Investigative Dermatology*, **69**, 392–400.

Kwa, R.E., Campana, K. and Moy, R.L. (1992) Biology of cutaneous squamous cell carcinoma. *Journal of the American Academy of Dermatology*, **26**, 1–26.

Lavker, R.M. (1995) Cutaneous ageing: chronologic versus photoageing, in *Photodamage*, (ed. B.A. Gilchrest), Blackwell Science, Oxford, pp. 123–35.

Lerman, S. and Van Voorhees, A. (1992) Cutaneous and ocular ramification of ultraviolet radiation. *Dermatologic Clinics*, **10**, 483–504.

Leyden, J.J. (1990) Clinical features of ageing skin. *British Journal of Dermatology*, **122** (suppl 35), 1–3.

Lookingbill, D.P. Lookingbill, G.L. and Leppard, B. (1995) Actinic damage and skin cancer in albinos on northern Tanzania: findings in 164 patients enrolled in an outreach skin care program. *Journal of the American Academy of Dermatology*, **32**, 653–8.

Lowe, N.J., Meyers, D.P., Wieder, J.M. *et al.* (1995) Low doses of repetitive ultraviolet A induce morphologic changes in human skin. *Journal of Investigative Dermatology*, **105**, 739–43.

Maeda, K., Naganuma, M. and Fukuda, M. (1991) Effects of chronic exposure ultraviolet-A including 2% ultraviolet-B on free radical reduction systems in hairless mice. *Photochemistry and Photobiology*, **54**, 737–40.

Margelin, D., Fourtanier, A., Thevenin, T. *et al.* (1993) Alterations of proteoglycans in ultraviolet-irradiated skin. *Photochemistry and Photobiology*, **58**, 211–18.

Marks, R. and Selwood, T.S. (1985) Solar keratoses: the association with erythemal ultraviolet radiation in Australia. *Cancer*, **56**, 2332–6.

Marks, R., Rennie, G. and Selwood, T. (1988) The relationship of basal cell carcinomas and squamous cell carcinomas to solar keratoses. *Archives of Dermatology*, **124**, 1039–42.

Marks, R., Staples, M. and Giles, G.G. (1993) Trends in non-melanocytic skin cancer treated in Australia: the second national survey. *International Journal of Cancer*, **53**, 585–90.

Mawn, V.B. and Fleischer, A.B. (1993) A survey of attitudes, beliefs and behavior regarding tanning bed use, sunbathing and sunscreen use. *Journal of the American Academy of Dermatology*, **29**, 959–62.

Melov, S., Lithgow, G.J., Fischer, D.R., Tedesco, P.M. and Johnson, T.E. (1995a) Increased frequency of deletions in the mitochondrial genome with age of *Caenorhabditis elegans*. *Nucleic Acids Research*, **23**, 1419–25.

Melov, S., Shoffner, J.M., Kaufman, A. and Wallace, D.C. (1995b) Marked increase in the number and variety of mitochondrial DNA rearrangements in ageing human skeletal muscle. *Nucleic Acids Research*, **23**, 4122–6.

Mera, S.L., Lovell, C.R., Jones, R.R. and Davies, J.D. (1987) Elastic fibres in normal and sun-damaged skin: an immunohistochemical study. *British Journal of Dermatology*, **117**, 21–7.

Montagna, W. and Carlisle, K. (1990) Structural changes in ageing skin. *British Journal of Dermatology*, **122** (suppl 35), 61–70.

Murray, J., Darr, D., Reich, J. and Pinnell, S. (1991) Topical vitamin C treatment reduces ultraviolet B radiation-induced erythema in human skin. *Journal of Investigative Dermatology*, **96**, 587.

Naylor, M.F., Boyd, A., Smith, D.W. *et al.* (1995) High sun protection factor sunscreens in the suppression of actinic neoplasia. *Archives of Dermatology*, **131**, 170–5.

Olsen, E.A., Katz, H.I., Levine, N. *et al.* (1992) Tretinoin emollient cream: a new therapy for photodamaged skin. *Journal of the American Academy of Dermatology*, **26**, 215–24.

Pang, C., Lee, H., Yang, J. and Wei, Y. (1994) Human skin mitochondrial DNA deletions associated with light exposure. *Archives of Biochemistry and Biophysics*, **312**, 534–8.

Pathak, M.A. and Fitzpatrick, T.B. (1993) Preventive treatment of sunburn, dermatoheliosis and skin cancer with sun-protective agents, in *Dermatology in General Medicine*, (eds T.B. Fitzpatrick *et al.*), McGraw-Hill, New York, pp. 1689–716.

Petersen, M.J., Hansen, C. and Craig, S. (1992) Ultraviolet A irradiation stimulates collagenase production in cultured human fibroblasts. *Journal of Investigative Dermatology*, **99** (4), 440–4.

Pfau, R.G., Hood, A.F. and Morison, W.L. (1986) Photoageing: the role of UVB, solar-simulated UVB, visible and psoralen UVA radiation. *British Journal of Dermatology*, **114**, 319–27.

Ponten, F., Berne, B., Ren, Z., Nister, M. and Ponten, J. (1995) Ultraviolet light induces expression of p53 and p21 in human skin: effect of sunscreen and constitutive p21 expression in skin appendages. *Journal of Investigative Dermatology*, **105**, 402–6.

Preston, D.S. and Stern, R.S. (1992) Nonmelanoma cancers of the skin. *New England Journal of Medicine*, **327**, 1649–62.

Punnonen, K., Jansen, C.T., Puntala, A. and Ahotupa, M. (1991) Effects of *in vitro* irradiation and PUVA treatment on membrane fatty acids and activities of antioxidant enzymes in human keratinocytes. *Journal of Investigative Dermatology*, **96**, 255–9.

Rafal, E.S., Griffiths, C.E.M., Ditre, C.M. *et al.* (1992) Topical tretinoin (retinoic acid) treatment for liver spots associated with photodamage. *New England Journal of Medicine*, **326**, 368–74.

Richard, S., De Rigal, J., De Lacharriere, O. *et al.* (1994) Noninvasive measurement of the effect of lifetime exposure to the sun on the aged skin. *Photodermatology, Photoimmunology and Photomedicine*, **10**, 164–9.

Ridge, J.M., Siegle, R.J. and Zuckermann, J. (1990) Use of α-hydroxy acids in the therapy for 'photoaged' skin (letter). *Journal of the American Academy of Dermatology*, **23**, 932.

Roenigk, H.H. (1995) Treatment of the ageing face. *Cosmetic Dermatology*, **13** (2), 245–61.

Roenigk, H.H. Jr. and Caro, W.A. (1981) Skin cancer in the PUVA-48 cooperative study. *Journal of the American Academy of Dermatology*, **4**, 319–24.

Ross, S.A. and Sanchez, J.L. (1990) Recreational sun exposure in Puerto Rico: trends and cancer risk awareness. *Journal of the American Academy of Dermatology*, **23**, 1090–2.

Sauder, D.N., Stanulis-Prager, B.M. and Gilchrest, B.A. (1988) Autocrine growth stimulation of human keratinocytes by epidermal cell-derived thymocyte activating factor: implications for skin ageing. *Archives of Dermatology Research*, **280**, 71–6.

Sayre, R.M., Desrochers, D.L., Wilson, C.J. and Marlowe, E. (1981) Skin type, minimal erythema dose (MED), and sunlight acclimatization. *Journal of the American Academy of Dermatology*, **5**, 439–43.

Schmitz, S., Garbe, C., Jimbow, K. *et al.* (1995) Photodynamic action of ultraviolet A: induction of cellular hydroperoxides. *Recent Results in Cancer Research*, **139**, 43–5.

Shindo, Y., Witt, E. and Packer, L. (1993) Antioxidant defense mechanisms in murine epidermis and dermis and their responses to ultraviolet light. *Journal of Investigative Dermatology*, **100**, 260–5.

Shindo, Y., Witt, E., Han, D. and Packer, L. (1994a) Dose–response effects of acute ultraviolet irradiation on antioxidants and molecular markers of oxidation in murine epidermis and dermis. *Journal of Investigative Dermatology*, **102**, 470–5.

Shindo, Y., Witt, E., Han, D. *et al.* (1994b) Recovery of antioxidants and reduction in lipid lhydroperoxides in murine epidermis and dermis after acute ultraviolet radiation exposure. *Photodermatology, Photoimmunology and Photomedicine*, **10**, 183–91.

Singer, R.S., Hamilton, T.A., Voorhees, J.J. *et al.* (1994) Association with asymmetrical facial photodamage with automobile driving. *Archives of Dermatology*, **130**, 121–3.

Stern, R.S. and Lange, R. (1988) Non-melanoma skin cancer occurring in patients treated with PUVA five to ten years after first treatment. *Journal of Investigative Dermatology*, **91** (2), 120–4.

Stern, R.S. and Momtaz, T.K. (1984) Skin typing for assessment of skin cancer risk and acute response to UV-B and oral methoxsalen photochemotherapy. *Archives of Dermatology*, **120**, 869–73.

Stern, R.S., Thibodeau, L.A., Kleinerman, R. *et al.* (1979) Risk of cutaneous carcinoma in patients treated with oral methoxsalen photochemotherapy for psoriasis. *New England Journal of Medicine*, **300**, 809–13.

Stern, R.S., Parrish, J., Fitzpatrick, T.B. and Bleich, H.L. (1985) Actinic degeneration in association with long-term use of PUVA. *Journal of Investigative Dermatology*, **84**, 135–8.

Stewart, M.S., Cameron, G.S. and Pence, B.C. (1996) Antioxidant nutrients protect against UVB-induced damage to DNA of mouse keratinocytes in culture. *Journal of Investigative Dermatology*, **106**, 1086–9.

Stiller, M.J., Bartolone, J., Stern, R. *et al.* (1996) Topical 8% glycolic acid and 8% L-lactic acid creams for the treatment of photodamaged skin. *Archives of Dermatology*, **132**, 631–36.

Summers, R.S. and Summers, B. (1993) Update – skin photodamage protection. *South African Medical Journal*, **83**, 242–3.

Taylor, C.R., Stern, R.S., Leyden, J.J. and Gilchrest, B.A. (1990) Photoageing/photodamage and photoprotection. *Journal of the American Academy of Dermatology*, **22**, 1–15.

Thompson, S.C., Jolley, D. and Marks, R. (1993) Reduction of solar keratoses by regular sunscreen use. *New England Journal of Medicine*, **329**, 1147–51.

Vitasa, B.C., Taylor, H.R., Strickland, P.T. *et al.* (1990) Association of nonmelanoma skin cancer and actinic keratosis with cumulative solar ultraviolet exposure in Maryland watermen. *Cancer*, **65**, 2811–17.

Warren, R., Gartstein, V., Kligman, A. *et al.* (1991) Age, sunlight and facial skin: a histological and quantitative study. *Journal of the American Academy of Dermatology*, **25**, 751–60.

Weinstein, G.D., Nigra, T.P., Pochi, P. *et al.* (1991) Topical tretinoin for treatment of photodamaged skin: a multicenter study. *Archives of Dermatology*, **127**, 659–65.

Weiss, J.S., Ellis, C., Headington, J.T. *et al.* (1988) Topical tretinoin improves photoaged skin: a double-blind, vehicle-controlled study. *Journal of the American Medical Association*, **259**, 527–32.

West, M.D. (1994) The cellular and molecular biology of skin ageing. *Archives of Dermatology*, **130**, 87–95.

Williams, B.T. (1996) Bullous solar elastosis. *Journal of the American Academy of Dermatology*, **34**, 856–8.

Wlaschek, M., Heinen, G., Poswig, A. *et al.* (1994) UVA-induced autocrine stimulation of fibroblast derived collagenase/MMP-1 by interrelated loops of interleukin-1 and interleukin-6. *Photochemistry and Photobiology*, **59**, 550–6.

Wolff, K. (1990) Side-effects of psoralen photochemotherapy. *British Journal of Dermatology*, **122** (suppl 36), 117–25.

Young, A.R. (1990) Senescence and sunscreens. *British Journal of Dermatology*, **122** (suppl 35), 111–14.

Young, A.R., Harrison, J.A. and Walker, S.L. (1988) Low SPF sunscreens reduce photoageing in mice. *Cosmetics and Toiletries*, **103**, 49–51.

Zelickson, A.S., Mottaz, J.H., Zelickson, B.D. and Muller, M.D. (1980) Elastic tissue changes in skin following PUVA therapy. *Journal of the American Academy of Dermatology*, **3**, 186–92.

Zheng, P. and Kligman, I.H. (1993) UVA-induced ultrastructural changes in hairless mouse skin: a comparison to UVB-induced damage. *Journal of Investigative Dermatology*, **100**, 194–9.

Zinman, R., Schwartz, S., Gordon, K., Fitzpatrick, E. and Camfield, C. (1995) Predictors of sunscreen use in childhood. *Archives of Pediatric and Adolescent Medicine*, **149**, 804–7.

THE CUMULATIVE EFFECTS OF ULTRAVIOLET RADIATION ON THE SKIN: PHOTOCARCINOGENESIS

7

Frederick Urbach

Repeated ultraviolet (UV)-B exposure, prolonged over years, is known to result in chronic degenerative changes of the skin, namely characteristic ageing effects and the development of premalignant and malignant tumours. Major interest in this topic, and in photocarcinogenesis in particular, however, has been stimulated by the relatively recent appearance in the scientific literature of three different concepts. One has been the concern that human activities might adversely affect the ability of the earth's atmosphere to remove harmful solar UV radiation by optical filtration (Van Der Leun *et al.*, 1995), a second the realization that photocarcinogenesis could be greatly enhanced by a variety of chemicals (Urbach *et al.*, 1982) and the third the discovery that UV radiation could affect photocarcinogenesis via the immune system (Kripke, 1990). In each case, the concept enriched the field of photobiology while also contributing to the understanding of immediately relevant problems.

THE ROLE OF LIGHT IN THE PATHOGENESIS OF SKIN CANCER

In 1858 Charcot determined that UV radiation caused acute erythema and Unna (1894)

Photodermatology. Edited by J.L.M. Hawk. Published in 1998 by Chapman & Hall, London. ISBN 0 412 72460 X.

proved that it may also cause pigmentation. It soon became apparent that the capability of the skin to react to light by pigmenting was most variable and that this variability pertained not only to different races, but also to individuals of apparently similar ancestry. Hausser and Vahle (1927) next showed that the longer UV wavelengths were more effective in producing pigmentation than the more erythemogenic shorter ones.

Changes in the stratum corneum, epidermis and dermis due to chronic light exposure had first been associated with exposure by Unna (1894), while Miescher (1930) documented in detail that thickening of the stratum corneum provided some measure of protection against further UV injury, but noted also that an eventual marked degeneration of the elastica and collagen of the skin develops virtually only on the most exposed areas of very heavily subexposed persons.

The first intimation that skin cancer might also be due to prolonged and repeated exposure to light came almost simultaneously from two sources, namely Unna again (1894), who associated the severe degenerative changes of the exposed areas of the skin of sailors with the development of the skin cancer, and Dubreuilh (1896) who, during a study of skin diseases in the Bordeaux region of France, observed the frequent incidence of keratoses and skin cancer in vineyard workers, but only occasionally in the city dwellers nearby. These observations were then confirmed by Hyde (1906), Paul (1918) and others, who also observed a high incidence of skin cancer among country people in the USA and Australia, where sun exposure is much more intense than in Central Europe.

In 1928, Findlay discovered that daily irradiation of mice with UV radiation from a mercury arc induced skin cancer and also that when they were treated with coal tar before irradiation, the time to induction of the cancer was reduced. Following this, the person most responsible for calling attention to the causal relation between solar and artificial UV radiation and skin cancer in man and animals was Roffo (1939), who showed that skin cancer could be induced in rats with natural sunlight as well as mercury arc radiation and was the first to carry out a real epidemiological study in man. He also undertook the first action spectrum study by showing that clear window glass was sufficient to prevent the development of skin cancer by both natural sunlight and mercury arc radiation and thus set an approximate limit of less than 320 nm for carcinogenically effective UV radiation.

Between 1941 and 1944, Blum, Grady and Kirby-Smith at the US National Cancer Institute then performed a comprehensive series of experiments on UV carcinogenesis in mice, for details of which, Blum's classic work *Carcinogenesis by Ultraviolet Light* (1959) should be consulted. As a result, Blum reported several important observations on tumour induction.

1. A single dose of UV radiation did not induce tumours in the lifetime of the animals.
2. A useful measure for tumour induction was the 'development time', i.e. the time lapse between the first UV dose and the appearance of a tumour of certain volume. Within an identically treated population of animals, this was distributed in a consistently regular fashion.

3. Differences in dose, intensity or interval between doses did not alter the shape or the slope of the dose–time relation, but only moved their relative position along the dose axis.
4. The incidence of tumours was widely distributed in the mouse population when plotted against the log of the square of the number of doses.
5. Time–dose reciprocity held until the doses became too small to produce tumours in the lifetime of the animals.

CELLULAR AND MOLECULAR PHOTOBIOLOGY

Widely varied effects of UV radiation on many cell types and organisms have been reported over the past 100 years, but the early work failed to appreciate both the need to control the wavelength of the radiation and the importance of the physiological state of the biological system before, during and after the irradiation. In 1929, however, it was discovered by Gates that the relative effectiveness of different wavelengths for killing bacteria paralleled the absorption spectrum of nucleic acid. In fact, we now know that many types of photoproducts are formed in the nucleic acid of cells, some of which were early isolated and characterized (Smith and Hanawalt, 1969). In several, their relative biological importance has also been determined. The molecular mechanism for UV carcinogenesis was, however, poorly understood until results of the effects of UV radiation on DNA structure and replication became available and it is now established that UV radiation results in pyrimidine dimer formation in DNA and that both excision repair and photoreactivation repair may occur in mammalian cells (Hart and Setlow, 1975). The observation that cells from a cancer–prone skin disease (xeroderma pigmentosum) are unable to repair DNA damage also resulted in a flurry of activity (Cleaver, 1968), although xeroderma variants were soon discovered in which excision repair systems were apparently normal, while patients remained cancer prone.

In addition to the well-documented capability of UV radiation to induce cancer of the skin in man and mice, Hart and Setlow (1975) further showed that fish liver cells, UV irradiated *in vitro* and reinjected into isogeneic recipients, give rise to tumours. This tumour induction was UV dose dependent, while illumination of the irradiated cells before reinjection with visible light markedly reduced tumour production. Since fish cells possess the photoreactivating enzyme, these data strongly suggested that pyrimidine dimers, induced by UV radiation in DNA, were related to the development of the tumours. Ley *et al.* (1988) have also shown that the induction of skin cancer in a South American opossum by UV irradiation can also be prevented by photoreactivating light.

More recent work has gone on to show that gene expression as well as mutation can be induced by UV irradiation and such changes are found in experimental and human skin cancer (Peak and Peak, 1983). Furthermore, UV-induced tumours display mutations preferentially in the N-ras oncogene, suggesting that these sites may be targets for UV-induced mutation and transformation (Kanjilal *et al.*, 1993). Also, loss of a putative suppressor function associated with an epidermal differentiation phenotype (p53) may lead to tumours, progressing to highly anaplastic lesions, and in human lesions, heterozygous mutations in the p53 gene have been found in basal cell and invasive squamous cell cancers, either CC-TT double base changes or mutations exclusively at the dipyridine sites (Pierceall *et al.*, 1991). Consequently it appears that in all phases of photocarcinogenesis, genomic changes attributable to UV exposure can be found.

ACTION SPECTRA FOR PHOTOCARCINOGENESIS

In the period of about 40 years after the early experiments noted above, there was little advance in knowledge of the wavelength dependency of photocarcinogenesis. This began to change, however, when in the 1960s a hairless mouse became available for experimental studies (Forbes and Urbach, 1969). The change in carcinogenicity with UV wavelength has long been a topical question, but has assumed even greater importance with the threat of depletion of the earth's protective stratospheric ozone. Skin cancer has been known for many years to be induced by UVB and UVC (Blum, 1959) while Roffo (1939) apparently showed that wavelengths longer than 320 nm did not produce such cancer in rats. However, more recently, evidence has shown that UVA can indeed induce skin cancer, at least in animals, although 1000 times less effectively than UVB (Sterenborg and Van Der Leun, 1992). In fact, the latest skin carcinogenesis action spectrum shows a rapid drop in effectiveness from 295 to 330 nm (by about four orders of magnitude) and then a fairly flat response out to 390 nm. These latest animal photocarcinogenesis action spectra thus parallel the human skin erythema action spectrum in the UVB and the short UVA wavelengths, but are well below the human erythema action spectrum in efficacy in the long UVA region (De Gruijl and Van Der Leun, 1994) (Fig. 7.1).

INTERACTION OF UVR AND CHEMICALS IN PHOTOCARCINOGENESIS

Evidence is long-standing and compelling that chemical agents can modify the carcinogenic effects of radiation (Urbach *et al.*, 1982) and there are several possibilities for such an interaction.

1. Chemical carcinogenesis may be modified by UV irradiation (Findlay, 1928).
2. Chemically enhanced photocarcinogenesis follows the topical or systemic administration of phototoxic agents not in themselves carcinogenic, in association with irradiation by UV doses not primarily carcinogenic under the conditions of the experiment.

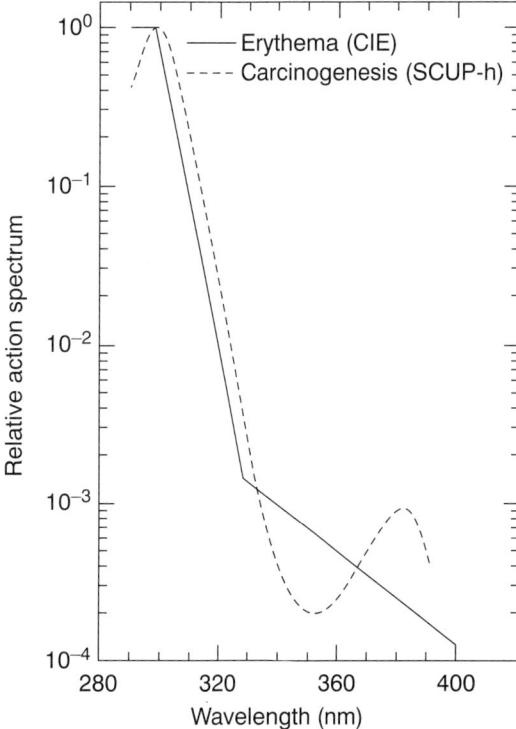

Figure 7.1 (——) Action spectrum for minimal erythema (24 hours after irradiation). (- - -) Action spectrum for human photocarcinogenesis (calculated from animal data and estimated human skin transmission). Based on data from De Gruijl and Van Der Leun (1994).

Chemical promotion of photocarcinogenesis consists of the enhancement of minimal UV irradiation-induced carcinogenesis by the application of a non-carcinogenic compound, such as croton oil or all-transretinoic acid (Forbes *et al.*, 1979), the classic example being that induced by psoralen medication and UVA irradiation (psoralen photochemotherapy, PUVA). That psoralens can enhance photocarcinogenesis has been known since 1959 (Urbach) and since 1974, PUVA therapy has been extensively used worldwide for the treatment of psoriasis and other skin diseases. The first report indicating an increased risk for skin cancer following such treatment was

published by Stern *et al.* in 1979 and since then, it has been confirmed that there is a small but dose-related increasing risk of SCC in patients treated in this way. Important co-factors in increasing risk are a history of arsenic exposure, ionizing radiation therapy or severe sunlight-induced skin damage (Studniberg and Weller, 1995).

PHOTOIMMUNOLOGY

It has long been known that skin cancers induced in mice by UV radiation are highly antigenic (Kripke, 1990), a finding which raised the question of how such tumours were able to survive in the original host without being destroyed by the immune system. The answer turned out to be that UV irradiation (particularly UVB) alters host immunity against UVB-induced cancers, leading to the production of suppressor lymphocytes that prevent the immunological destruction of the developing primary skin cancers. Thus, UV irradiation may induce new antigens in the skin, cause the transformation of normal cells into cancer cells and also block the immune response against these cancers. In addition, UV radiation also induces antigen-specific suppression of contact dermatitis and of delayed-type hypersensitivity, a process perhaps important for protection against some infectious diseases (Kripke, 1990). That immunosuppression can also increase the risk of skin cancer in humans has been demonstrated by the observation that renal transplant patients may develop SCCs in large numbers, mostly on previously sun-exposed sites (Glover *et al.*, 1993).

SKIN CANCER IN HUMANS

Repeated sunlight exposure prolonged over many years can result in chronic degenerative changes in human skin, characterized by the features of skin ageing and the development of premalignant and malignant skin lesions. Human skin cancers can be divided into two types: non-melanoma skin cancers ((NMSC; BCCs and SCCs) and malignant melanoma (MM). There is excellent although circumstantial evidence that at least NMSC are primarily due to repeated exposure of the skin to UV irradiation. The major arguments in favour of such a causal role for UVR exposure are:

- the most frequent location of NMSC is on the exposed sites (head, neck, arms);
- pigmented races, who sunburn much less readily than people with white skin, have much less NMSC and when it does occur, it does not preferentially affect exposed areas;
- among white-skinned people, those who spend more time outdoors and who live in areas of greater UV exposure (such as tropical and semitropical areas) have a much greater risk of developing NMSC;
- genetic diseases resulting in greater sensitivity to solar UV radiation (such as albinism) are associated with premature NMSC;
- skin cancers of the NMSC type can be readily induced in the skin of experimental animals and the wavelength distribution is similar to that causing sunburn in man.

Together, BCCs and SCCs add up to the most frequently detected cancers in man and have increased in frequency over the past decades (Glass and Hoover, 1989; Marks *et al.*, 1993). However, they are also the most easily and successfully treated of human cancers. The quantitative extent to which agents other than UV exposure cause NMSC in the white population has not been established, but is believed to be small. Some NMSCs are caused by exposure to arsenic, pitch and X-rays, usually during the course of work and sometimes following treatment for skin disorders, while in some less developed countries, many NMSCs may arise in neglected wounds (Davies *et al.*, 1968; Foster and Webb, 1988). NMSC at present remains a serious problem because of its potential for disfigurement, particularly in Australia, the United States, in Europe and in emigrants from these regions to other parts of the world.

ANATOMICAL DISTRIBUTION OF BASAL CELL AND SQUAMOUS CELL CANCER

Numerous studies have shown that NMSCs arise (in those most susceptible, namely white-skinned people) primarily on sun-exposed sites. From these studies, it is demonstrable that 75–85% of BCCs (Kricker *et al.*, 1990; Scotto and Fears, 1981; Serrano *et al.*, 1991) and more than 70% of SCCs (Czarnecki *et al.*, 1992; Glass and Hoover, 1989; Kricker *et al.*, 1990) occur on the head and neck, while the majority of SCCs not occurring on the head are found on the hands and forearms; the ears of females are relatively spared, apparently being protected by hair.

Comparing the sites of NMSC with major sites of insolation of the head and neck areas, as determined by geometric studies, it becomes clear that two thirds of all BCCs occur on those areas receiving the highest UV doses and that virtually all SCCs occur at these sites (Urbach, 1969). Furthermore, the histological changes due to chronic solar exposure (namely epithelial dysplasia and connective tissue damage) are also most severe there (Marks *et al.*, 1989).

RACE AND ETHNIC EXTRACTION

It has long been known that whites have a much higher incidence of skin cancer than pigmented races (Davies *et al.*, 1968), BCC in particular being very rare in dark skin (Matsuoka *et al.*, 1981; Foster and Webb, 1988). Further, in contrast to the anatomical distribution of SCCs in white subjects (70% on the head and neck), Isaacson (1979) found only one third of these tumours in urban blacks in South Africa to be at these sites. In addition, the male–female ratio was 60:40, as compared to 85:15 in whites. Age of onset was also much earlier in blacks than whites, 50% of SCCs occurring before age 50.

In several carefully controlled studies, comparing white patients with NMSC to age- and sex-matched controls from the same populations, it has been shown that the patients with skin cancer have a much greater frequency of certain genetically transmitted traits than those without cancer (Marks *et al.*, 1993; O'Beirn *et al.*, 1970). These patients as a group also have a greater frequency of light-coloured eyes, complexion and hair than the controls. They also sunburn more frequently and tan less easily than the controls, though the degree of tan achieved was only marginally less. Male cancer patients also experience a greater cumulative outdoor exposure than male controls, while the proportion of Irish, English, Scots and Welsh ancestry was greater in the cancer patients, the Slavic and 'other' categories of national origin being smaller (O'Beirn *et al.*, 1970; Urbach *et al.*, 1972).

GEOGRAPHICAL DISTRIBUTION

Incidence data for skin cancer other than MM must be treated with considerable reserve, most national cancer registries not registering NMSC at all, and those which do so incompletely, because most of these tumours are treated in physicians' offices and thus are either not reported or reported without histological verification.

Europe

The data available for incidence and prevalence of NMSC in Europe are fragmentary and extremely difficult to interpret, since surveys, such as they are, have been performed by variably rigorous methods and over several decades, during which the incidence of NMSC has greatly increased (Glass and Hoover, 1989). However, it is clear, just as in the US and Australia, that a marked North–South gradient exists, incidences in 1987 being reported as follows per 100 000 person-years (Muir *et al.*, 1987): Finland – male/female 5.1/3.3; Norway –

8.2/4.7; Germany – 35/27; Denmark – 38/27; Hungary – 32/33; France – 35/27. In addition, unusually high incidences have been reported from The Netherlands (60/35), Ireland (63/48), Switzerland (53/36) and the UK (c. 65 male and female).

Africa

Information relating to skin cancer in Africa, gathered from various sources (mainly the reports of Oettle (1963), Davies *et al.* (1968) and Isaacson (1979)) shows that native Africans have very low rates of NMSC as well as MM, incidence rates in Johannesburg Bantus and in Uganda being of the order of 1–2 per 100 000 person-years for NMSC, almost all SCCs of the lower extremities. Exceptions, however, are albino natives, who are extremely prone to skin cancer and in South Africa, where they are quite common among the Bantu, Oettle estimated a crude annual incidence rate for SCC of 579/100 000 for males and 408 for females, while for BCC, it was 36/100 000 for both sexes combined, although only one lesion was actually found.

India

Realistic data for NMSC in India are not available, but incidence rates seem to be less than 1/100 000, except in whites. Among native Indians, however, special types of SCC are found, apparently due to extreme heat, combustion products or chronic friction (Mulay, 1963).

Japan and Taiwan

While again incidence figures are not reliable, it is clear that NMSC is uncommon in Japan and Taiwan, rates being about 1/100 000 person-years. SCC is two to three times more common than BCC, again frequently arising at sites of premalignant skin change such as burns and chronic trauma or after arsenic ingestion (Kikuchi *et al.*, 1996).

Australia

Probably the best skin cancer surveys in recent years have been carried out in Australia (Kricker *et al.*, 1990, 1991; Marks *et al.*, 1993), overall incidence being the highest in the world, namely 977/100 000 person-years (Marks *et al.*, 1993), having increased by 19% in the five-year period between 1985 and 1990. There is also a distinct latitude gradient, the incidence for SCC having been estimated as 201/100 000 in the temperate South (Marks *et al.*, 1989), 585/100 000 in subtropical, more Northern regions (Kricker *et al.*, 1990) and 774/100 000 in the Northern tropics (Stenbeck *et al.*, 1990). From such information, one may plot the global distribution of annual solar radiation against the incidence of NMSC on a global basis, this suggesting a doubling of the incidence for every 10° in latitude (Fig. 7.2).

USA

While NMSC data are not routinely collected by tumour registries in the US, data do exist from special surveys, namely the Texas Tumour Registry (MacDonald and Bubendorf, 1964), a survey of NMSC in four areas of the US (Scotto and Fears, 1981, 1987), a special survey by the National Cancer Institute (Scotto *et al.*, 1981) and a recent report of 25 years' SCC incidence data from the West Coast (Glass and Hoover, 1989). Thus, the total NMSC incidence reported in 1981 was 312/100 000 for males and 174/100 000 for females, while the SCC incidence in 1986 on the West Coast was 106/100 000 in males and 30/100 000 in females. These incidence figures had increased by a factor of 3.5 over a 25-year period.

RELATIONSHIP TO ENVIRONMENTAL EXPOSURE

Recent epidemiological research has resulted in the development of preliminary dose–response relationships for NMSC following UVR exposure, reasonable hypotheses having

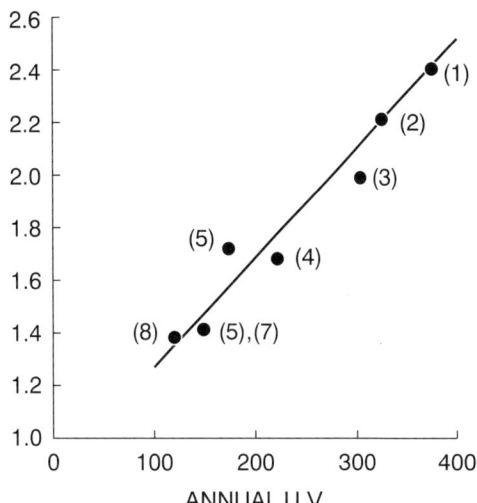

LOG (INCIDENCE)

ANNUAL U.V.

(1) Queensland
(2) Texas
(3) South Africa (Cape Province/Whites)
(4) Nevada
(5) Canada (6 Provinces)
(6) England (5 Regions)
(7) German Democratic Republic
(8) Scotland

Figure 7.2 Incidence of NMSC compared with amounts of biologically effective UV radiation (arbitrary units). The amount of UV radiation is linearly related to latitude. Note power relationship of NMSC incidence to UV radiation. It can be estimated that NMSC doubles for each 10° of latitude.

been proposed based on tissue culture and animal experiments for the relevant wavelengths. Thus, while uncertainty remains regarding the exact relationships of the various UVR spectral segments to carcinogenesis, models predicting probable NMSC incidence increases with increasing UVR exposure now seem possible. For instance, an increase of 50% in solar exposure every year for the 30-year period from the ages of 15 to 45 could be expected to increase BCC by 500% and SCC by 700% in the remaining lifetime of the individual (Van Der Leun *et al.*, 1995). There is also evidence that BCC incidence has been increasing by 3% each year (Scotto and Fears, 1981), while SCCs rose threefold in females and 2.6-fold in males between 1960 and 1986 in the USA. From the most recent calculations based on the actual decreases of stratopheric ozone over the Northern hemisphere, however, one would have expected an increase per decade of 11.6% for BCC and 21.6% for SCC (Fears and Scotto, 1982), while from the data of Glass and Hoover (1989), the actual increases have been 82% for BCC and 76% for SCC. Thus, it seems likely that most of the recent skin cancer increases are not due to stratospheric ozone decrease but rather to greater exposure of the population to solar radiation for social and cosmetic reasons. Although skin cancer is most often found among people with fair or lightly pigmented skin, not all people with similar skin colour, even when equally exposed, develop skin cancer. Thus, recent studies of the susceptibility of patients to develop contact sensitivity after UVR exposure have shown that skin cancer develops in those with impaired immune function. Therefore, genetic differences other than just UVR sensitivity appear also to play a role in photocarcinogenesis in humans (Yoshikawa *et al.*, 1990).

EPIDEMIOLOGY OF MALIGNANT MELANOMA

The incidence of MM varies over 100-fold around the world, from a low of 0.2/100 000 person-years in parts of Japan to nearly 50 in Queensland, Australia (Stenbeck *et al.*, 1990). However, although five-year survival after diagnosis is of the order of 85%, MM has shown a remarkable and consistent increase in incidence, varying by only about 5% per year, beginning at least in 1930 (Glass and Hoover, 1989; Muir *et al.*, 1987).

ANATOMICAL DISTRIBUTION

In contrast to NMSC, the anatomical distribution of MM is not associated with the most UVR-exposed sites (Osterlind *et al.*, 1985), only about 1% being on the head and neck. Further, these lesions are most often lentigo maligna melanomas, which basically have the same characteristics as SCCs, namely location on the most exposed sites of the head and neck, low incidence before age 50 with a progressive rise in frequency with advancing age, almost uniform presence of solar elastosis in the adjacent skin and low aggressiveness (Osterlind *et al.*, 1985). In addition, while NMSC is extremely uncommon in pigmented races, MM has an incidence in such people as high as a tenth of that of white-skinned races. Lesions are frequently acral and found in 75–85% of cases on the foot and the lower leg (Davies *et al.*, 1968; Halder and Bang, 1985; Oettle, 1963), while 6–11% appear to be of genetic origin, as evidenced by familial and multiple lesions and unusual precursors (dysplastic naevi), present from early in life (Albert *et al.*, 1990).

The remaining approximately 75% of MM in white persons are mostly superficial spreading melanomas, which also have interesting attributes (Green, 1982), their incidence rising sharply between adolescence and early adult life, stabilizing during middle age before rising again in old age because of the appearance of lentigo maligna melanoma. The disorder occurs in a preponderance of females less than 40 years old and the sites of greatest incidence differ between the sexes, more often affecting the trunk in males and the lower leg in females (Dennis *et al.*, 1993). It is also of interest that although the various populations studied live in such disparate areas as Finland (60°N latitude) and Queensland (25–15°S latitude) and are thus exposed to hugely different amounts of solar UV, the relative proportion of MM affecting the various body sites has remained quite stable in all these areas until recently. In two areas, however, Norway and Hawaii, the differences in incidence of MM between males and females on the most affected sites seem to have been decreasing over the past decade (Hinds and Kolonel, 1980).

Latitude gradients for MM incidence and mortality exist in some countries but not others. For example, there are real latitude gradients for MM in Norway, Sweden, Great Britain and the USA, but less striking or even reversed gradients in Western Australia and across Central Europe and only a partial latitude gradient in Eastern Australia, the incidence in Queensland being less in the tropical than the subtropical areas (Armstrong, 1984).

In contrast to NMSC, again, the individuals most affected are not outdoor workers but rather white-collar, more educated, affluent subjects (Cooke *et al.*, 1984). As a result the demonstrable concentration of MM in large cities almost cancels out any latitude gradient in such places as Finland and Western Australia where this matter has been investigated.

The worldwide rapid increase in the incidence of MM (but interestingly, much slower increase in mortality rates, as if MM were perhaps becoming less aggressive) has been attributed to changes in lifestyle, with apparently greater exposure to solar UV radiation during leisure activities and vacations (Armstrong, 1984; Giles, 1996). Since the more affluent might be considered more likely to partake in such activities, the reasoning therefore goes that men removing their shirts outdoors and women wearing shorter skirts or shorts might account for the unusual anatomical distribution of MM (Cooke *et al.*, 1984).

GEOGRAPHICAL DISTRIBUTION

In contrast to the regularly increasing incidence with decreasing latitude seen in NMSC, such a relationship is by no means so obvious for MM.

Europe

The data for incidence of MM tend to be reliable, most tumour registries having collected such information since at least 1954. The details below come primarily from Muir *et al.* (1987) and are for each 100 000 person-years, males first, then females. In Europe, the Middle European countries have low incidences, namely Hungary 1.6/2.7, United Kingdom 2.8/5.1, Czechoslovakia 3.2/4.0, Poland 2.6/3.1 and Spain 2.8/3.0. Somewhat higher, although not further south are France 3.4/6.0, Italy 4.5/5.1, Netherlands 4.3/6.8 and Germany 5.4/7.1. The Nordic countries, however, have the highest incidence, Sweden having 10.0/11.6, Norway 13.0/15.8 and, unaccountably, Switzerland 11.8/12.4.

Japan and Far East

Since most of the population of these areas is constitutionally pigmented, the incidence of MM is very low and mostly involves the lower extremity. The following data have been reported: Singapore 0.9/0.4, Shanghai 0.4/0.4, Bombay 0.12/0.09, Japan 0.21, 50% on acral areas (Elwood, 1989).

Africa

As expected, incidence figures are very low: Nigeria 0.2/0.7 (Davies *et al.*, 1968), South African Bantu 0.4/1.7 and South African whites, in contrast, 5.3/7.0 (Isaacson, 1979).

Australia and New Zealand

The incidence of MM in Australia is the highest in the world, probable factors accounting for this being the relative nearness to the equator, the relative preponderance of genetically UV-sensitive skin and frequent tendency to work outdoors.

Incidences are as follows: for all Australian males 30.2, females 23.9 (Marks *et al.*, 1989); for Queensland males 50.9, females 42.3 (Stenbeck *et al.*, 1990); for New South Wales males 19.4, females 21.0 (Stenbeck *et al.*, 1990); and for New Zealand, constitutionally pigmented Maoris 2.9 (males and females), whites 16.1.

United States

The incidence rates for MM in the United States have also risen spectacularly, going up in males in the 25-year period from 1960 to 1986 from 4.4/100 000 to 20.1/100 000 and in females from 4.9 to 17.0/100 000 (Glass and Hoover, 1989). In 1991, Scotto *et al.* reported a more recent incidence of 20.6 for males and 15.9 for females. However, in Hispanics it was only 2.4 and in blacks only 0.8, while in Hawaii it ranged in non-white males from 0.67 to 3.3 and in non-white females from 0.33 to 2.9, depending on skin colour.

RELATIONSHIP TO ENVIRONMENTAL FACTORS

Anatomically, MM are frequently associated with melanocytic naevi and the number of naevi present in a given subject is a good indicator of his MM risk (Swerdlow and Green, 1987). In addition, families exist with a very high likelihood of developing MM and it was in these that dysplastic naevi were first described (Albert *et al.*, 1990). However, the relationship of such naevi to common acquired and sporadic MM is not clear (Cooke *et al.*, 1984), although the development of naevi is clearly influenced by environmental factors, mainly solar exposure (Green *et al.*, 1995).

In contrast to the case for NMSC, where the causal association with solar UV exposure is very strong, there are clearly inconsistencies in assuming that sun exposure is the major risk factor for the causation of MM (Armstrong, 1984), which include the following.

- Inconsistency in patterns of MM incidence by latitude (e.g. the incidence in populations in the far North of Europe and the Scandinavian states is often higher than those further South).
- Inconsistency in skin areas affected as compared with those receiving the greatest solar exposure (in men, highest incidence on the back, in women, on the leg, less than 20% incidence on head and neck).
- Inconsistency in terms of cumulative lifetime UV exposure (risk greater for indoor than outdoor workers).
- Inconsistency in that experimental production of MM is very difficult in animal models in comparison with NMSC, which can rapidly be induced by UV irradiation in mice (Klein-Szanto *et al.*, 1994).

Nevertheless, the epidemiological features of cutaneous MM point to complex relationships with sunlight, some consistent with a positive association, some not. For example, the genetically determined presence of sensitive skin, freckles and an inability to tan are well-established risk factors, as are proximity to the equator for non-pigmented people and the number of melanocytic naevi, associated with a history of sun exposure in childhood.

Based on the foregoing inconsistencies and positive associations, a new hypothesis has therefore been formed, namely that intermittent and intense sun exposure of untanned skin is a strong risk factor, particularly for superficial spreading melanoma (Katsambos and Nicolaidu, 1996).

RISK FACTORS FOR CUTANEOUS CARCINOGENESIS

The two most important risk factors are an individual's genetic constitution and amount of exposure to solar UV radiation, the highest risk skin type being characterized by pale, freckled skin which does not tan at all or only very slowly. Such a skin type is most often accompanied by blue, green or grey eyes, light or red hair and Celtic (Irish, Scots, Welsh) family background and while it may only occasionally lead to a slight tan, the overall skin appearance may be quite dark because of almost confluent freckles.

An equally important risk factor is the amount and type of exposure to solar UV radiation, the most carcinogenic component of sunlight, UVB, peaking in the middle hours of the day and increasing with the height of the sun in the sky and thus its decreasing distance from the equator. Populations living at low latitudes are therefore much more affected, chronic, repeated exposure over decades being the determining factor for NMSC (Urbach, 1969), and intermittent sunburning exposure and severe sunburns in childhood seeming to be more important for MM (Armstrong, 1984). In addition, while there are not yet any absolutely firm data, exposure of predisposed persons to artificial UV radiation such as in solaria and tanning salons should be strongly discouraged.

PREVENTIVE MEASURES

The most useful preventive measures against the development of skin cancer are sun avoidance, sunscreen application and the wearing of protective clothing.

SUN AVOIDANCE

While remaining indoors to avoid solar radiation is intuitively the best protection, this is frequently neither practicable nor desirable. However, it is usually entirely practical to minimize solar exposure by taking advantage of the great differences in biologically effective UV intensity at varying times of the day (i.e. according to the height of the sun in the sky). Thus, two thirds of all UVB and half of the UVA reach the ground in the two hours on either side of the solar zenith at around noon. Furthermore, the skin surface area irradiated is much less in the middle of the day than in the morning or evening (Fig. 7.3). Thus, arranging one's time out of doors so as to perform work or play early in the morning or later in the afternoon can significantly reduce skin damage, while another useful strategy is to take advantage of shade, including one's own. However, about half the incidence of UVB will still reach shaded areas.

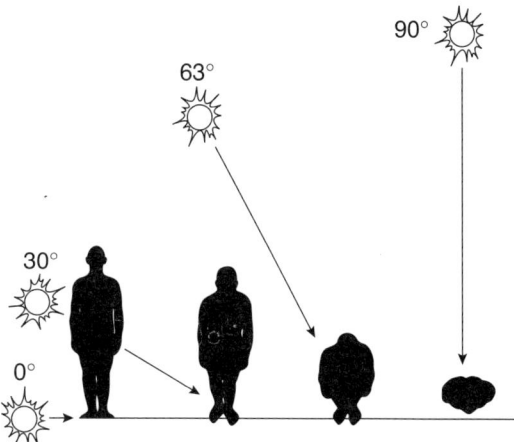

Figure 7.3 Direct sunlight-exposed surface area of a standing person facing the sun at different solar elevations. By the time solar elevation is reduced to 30°, there is insufficient UVB to cause injury.

SUNSCREENS

Sunscreens are topically applied creams or lotions containing chemicals that absorb UVR or reflect or scatter it. Since these materials basically act as filters, the concentration of the active agents and the thickness of the application are of major importance. Calculations concerning their potential efficiency have been performed, estimating that regular use of a product with a protective factor of 15 for the first 18 years of life might reduce lifetime NMSC incidence by 78% (Stern *et al.*, 1986). Animal experiments have also directly shown that sunscreens may prevent experimental photocarcinogenesis (Kligman *et al.*, 1980), while Naylor *et al.* (1995) have also shown significant reduction in the development of precancerous skin lesions by the regular use over two years of a sunscreen of protection factor 29. It would therefore appear likely that sunscreen use might also prevent photocarcinogenesis in man.

PROTECTIVE CLOTHING

Since most exposure occurs in the upright position, the skin areas at greatest risk are the top of the head (particularly in bald subjects), the ears, nose, forehead, cheeks, upper back, forearms and hands (Fig. 7.3). Thus, the wearing of a hat with a brim, a neckerchief over the neck and anterior chest and a long-sleeved shirt will help to protect the areas most at risk. The colour of such clothing is not of importance although a tight weave is, T-shirts allowing 50% of incident UV radiation to pass if wet. Small children should, however, always wear a T-shirt and a cotton hat when in the sun, even in a swimming pool or the sea.

REFERENCES

Albert, L.S., Rhodes, A.R. and Sober, A.J. (1990) Dysplastic melanocytic nevi and cutaneous melanoma. *Journal of the American Academy of Dermatology*, **22**, 69–75.

Armstrong, B.K. (1984) Melanoma of the skin. *British Medical Bulletin*, **40**, 246–350.

Blum, H.F. (1959) *Carcinogenesis by Ultraviolet Light*, Princeton University Press, Princeton, NJ.

Cleaver, J.E. (1968) Defective repair replication of DNA in xeroderma pigmentosum. *Nature*, **218**, 652–8.

Cooke, K.R., Skegg, D.G. and Fraser, J. (1984) Socioeconomic status, indoor and outdoor work and malignant melanoma. *International Journal of Cancer*, **34**, 57–62.

Czarnecki, D., Collins, N., Keehan, C. *et al.* (1992) Squamous cell carcinoma in Southern and Northern Australia. *International Journal of Dermatology*, **31**, 492–7.

Davies, N.P., Tank, R. Meyer, R. *et al.* (1968) Skin cancer in Nigeria. *Journal of the National Cancer Institute*, **41**, 31–51.

De Gruijl, F.R. and Van Der Leun, J.C. (1994) Estimate of the wavelength dependency of ultraviolet carcinogenesis in humans and its relevance of the risk assessment of a stratospheric ozone depletion. *Health Physics*, **67**, 319–25.

Dennis, L.K., White, E. and Lee, J.A.H. (1993) Recent cohort trends in malignant melanoma by anatomic site in the United States. *Cancer Causes and Control*, **4**, 93–100.

Dubreuilh, W. (1896) Des hyperkératoses circonscrites. *Annales de Dermatologie et Syphilis* (series 3), **7**, 1158–204.

Elwood, J.M. (1989) The epidemiology and control of melanoma in the white population of Japan. *Journal of Investigative Dermatology*, **92**, 214S–221S.

Fears, T.R. and Scotto, J. (1982) Changes in skin cancer morbidity between 1971–72 and 1977–78. *Journal of the National Cancer Institute*, **69**, 365–70.

Findlay, G.M. (1928) Ultraviolet light and skin cancer. *Lancet*, **2**, 1070–3.

Forbes, P.D. and Urbach, F. (1969) Vascular and neoplastic changes in mice following ultraviolet radiation, in *The Biologic Effects of Ultraviolet Radiation*, (ed. F. Urbach), Pergamon Press, Oxford, pp. 279–90.

Forbes, P.D., Urbach, F. and Davies, R.E. (1979) Enhancement of experimental photocarcinogenesis by topical retinoic acid. *Cancer Letters*, **7**, 85–90.

Foster, H.M. and Webb, S.J. (1988) Skin cancer in the North Solomons. *Australian and New Zealand Journal of Surgery*, **58**, 397–401.

Gates, F.L. (1929) A study of the bactericidal action of ultraviolet light. *Journal of General Physiology*, **13**, 231–49.

Giles, G.G. (1996) Has mortality from melanoma stopped rising in Australia? *British Medical Journal*, **312**, 1121–5.

Glass, A.G. and Hoover, R.N. (1989) The emerging epidemic of melanoma and squamous cell skin cancer. *Journal of the American Medical Association*, **262**, 2097–100.

Glover, M.T., Proby, C.R. and Leigh, I.M. (1993) Skin cancer in renal transplant patients. *Cancer Bulletin*, **45**, 220–4.

Green, A. (1982) Incidence and reporting of cutaneous melanoma in Queensland. *Australian Journal of Dermatology*, **23**, 105–9.

Green, A., Siskind, V. and Green, L. (1995) The incidence of melanocytic nevi in adolescent children in Queensland, Australia. *Melanoma Research*, **5**, 155–60.

Halder, R.M. and Bang, K.M. (1985) Skin cancer in blacks in the United States. *Dermatology Clinics*, **6**, 397–405.

Hart, R.W. and Setlow, R.B. (1975) Direct evidence that pyrimidine dimers in DNA result in neoplastic transformation, in *Molecular Mechanisms for Repair of DNA*, (eds P.C. Hanawalt and R.B. Setlow), Plenum Press, New York, pp. 719–24.

Hausser, K.W. and Vahle, W. (1927) Sonnenbrand und Sonnenbräunung, *Wissenschaftliche Veröffnungen Siemens Konzern* **6**, 101–20.

Hinds, M.W. and Kolonel, L.N. (1980) Malignant melanoma of the skin in Hawaii. *Cancer*, **45**, 811–17.

Hyde, J. (1906) On the influence of light on the production of cancer of the skin. *American Journal of Medical Science*, **31**, 1–22.

Isaacson, C. (1979) Cancer of the skin in urban blacks in South Africa. *British Journal of Dermatology*, **100**, 347–50.

Kanjilal, S., Pierceall, W.E. and Ananthaswamy, H.N. (1993) Ultraviolet radiation in the pathogenesis of skin cancers: involvement of ras and p53 genes. *Cancer Bulletin*, **45**, 205–11.

Katsambos, A. and Nicolaidu, E. (1996) Cutaneous melanoma and sun exposure. *British Medical Journal*, **312**, 1121–5.

Kikuchi, A., Shimizo, H. and Nishikawa, T. (1996) Clinical and histopathological characteristics of basal cell carcinoma in Japanese patients. *Archives of Dermatology*, **132**, 320–4.

Klein-Szanto, A.J.P., Sivers, W.K. and Mintz, B. (1994) Ultraviolet radiation induced malignant skin melanoma in melanoma susceptible transgenic mice. *Cancer Research*, **54**, 4569–72.

Kligman, L.M., Akin, F.J. and Kligman, A.M. (1980) Sunscreens prevent ultraviolet carcinogenesis. *Journal of the American Academy of Dermatology*, **3**, 30–5.

Kricker, A., English, D.R., Randell, P.L. *et al.* (1990) Skin cancer in Geraldton, Western Australia: a survey of incidence and prevalence. *Medical Journal of Australia*, **152**, 399–407.

Kricker, A., Armstrong, B.K., English, D.R. and Heenan, P.J. (1991) Pigmentary and cutaneous risk factors for non-melanocytic skin cancer – a case-control study. *International Journal of Cancer*, **46**, 650–62.

Kripke, M.L. (1990) Ultraviolet radiation and tumour immunity. *Journal of the National Cancer Institute*, **82**, 1392–6.

Ley, R.D., Applegate, L.A., Stuart, T.D. *et al.* (1988) UVA/visible light suppression of ultraviolet radiation induced skin and eye tumours of the marsupial *Monodelphis domestica*. *Photochemistry and Photobiology*, **47**, 45S.

MacDonald, E. and Bubendorf, E. (1964) Some epidemiologic aspects of skin cancer, in *Tumors of the Skin*, Yearbook Medical Publishers, Chicago, 23–66.

Marks, R., Jolley, D., Dorewitch, A.P. *et al.* (1989) The incidence of non-melanocytic skin cancers in an Australian population: results of a five year prospective study. *Medical Journal of Australia*, **150**, 475–8.

Marks, R., Staples, M. and Giles, G.G. (1993) Trends in non-melanocytic skin cancer treated in Australia: the second national survey. *International Journal of Cancer*, **53**, 585–90.

Matsuoka, L.Y., Schauer, P.K. and Sardillo, P.D. (1981) Basal cell carcinoma in black patients. *Journal of the American Academy of Dermatology*, **4**, 670.

Miescher, G. (1930) Das Problem der Lichtgewöhnung. *Strahlentherapie*, **35**, 403–43.

Muir, C., Waterhouse, J., Mack, T. *et al.* (1987) *Cancer Incidence in Five Continents, Vol. 5*, IARC Scientific Publication No. 88, International Agency for Research on Cancer, Lyon.

Mulay, D.M. (1963) Skin cancer in India, in *First International Conference on the Biology of Cutaneous Cancer*, (ed. F. Urbach), Government Printing Office, Washington DC, 215–224.

Naylor, M.F., Boyd, A., Smith, D.W. *et al.* (1995) High sunprotection factor sunscreens in the suppression of actinic neoplasia. *Archives of Dermatology*, **131**, 170–5.

O'Beirn, S.F., Judge, P., Urbach, F. *et al.* (1970) *Skin Cancer in County Galway, Ireland*. Proceedings of the 6th National Cancer Congress. J.B. Lippincott, Philadelphia, pp. 489–500.

Oettle, A.G. (1963) Skin cancer in Africa, in *The Biology of Cutaneous Cancer*, (ed. F. Urbach), US Government Printing Office, Washington DC, pp. 197–214.

Osterlind, A., Han-Jensen, K. and Jensen, O.M. (1985) Incidence of cutaneous malignant melanoma in Denmark 1978–1982. Anatomic site distribution, histologic type and comparison with non-melanoma skin cancer. *British Journal of Cancer*, **58**, 385–91.

Paul, N. (1918) The influence of sunlight in the production of cancer of the skin. H.K. Lewis, London.

Peak, M.J. and Peak, J.G. (1983) Use of action spectra for identifying molecular targets and mechanisms of action of solar ultraviolet light. *Physiologica Plantarum*, **58**, 367–72.

Pierceall, W.E., Mukhopadhyay, T., Goldberg, K.H. and Ananthaswamy, H.N. (1991) Mutations in the p53 tumour suppressor gene in human squamous cell carcinomas. *Molecular Carcinogenesis*, **4**, 445–9.

Roffo, A.H. (1939) Über die physikalische Aetiologie der Krebskrankheit. *Strahlentherapie*, **66**, 328–50.

Scotto, J. and Fears, T.R. (1981) *Incidence of non-melanoma skin cancer in the United States*. US Department of Health and Health Services, Washington DC.

Scotto, J. and Fears, T.R. (1987) The association of solar ultraviolet and skin melanoma incidence among Caucasians in the United States. *Cancer Investigations*, **5**, 275–83.

Scotto, J., Kopf, A.W. and Urbach, F. (1974) Non-melanoma skin cancer among Caucasians in four areas of the United States. *Cancer*, **34**, 1333–8.

Scotto, J., Pitcher, H. and Lee, J.A.H. (1991) Indications of future decreasing trends in skin melanoma mortality among whites in the United States. *International Journal of Cancer*, **49**, 490–7.

Serrano, H., Scotto, J., Sharnick, G. *et al.* (1991) Incidence of non-melanoma skin cancer in New Hampshire and Vermont. *Journal of the American Academy of Dermatology*, **24**, 574–9.

Smith, K.C. and Hanawalt D.C. (1969) *Molecular Photobiology*, Academic Press, New York.

Sterenborg, H.J.C.M. and Van Der Leun, J.C. (1992) Tumorigenesis by long wave length UVA, in *Biologic Responses to Ultraviolet A Radiation*, (ed. F. Urbach), Valdenmar Publishing Company, Overland Park.

Stenbeck, K., Bolander, K.P., Williams, M.J. *et al.* (1990) Patterns of treated non-melanoma skin cancer in Queensland – the region with the highest incidence in the world. *Medical Journal of Australia*, **153**, 511–15.

Stern, R.S., Thibodeau, L.A., Kleinerman, R.A. *et al.* (1979) Risk of cutaneous carcinoma in patients treated with oral methoxsalen photochemotherapy for psoriasis. *New England Journal of Medicine*, **300**, 800–13.

Stern, R.S., Weinstein, M.C. and Baker, S.D. (1986) Risk reduction for non-melanoma skin cancer with childhood sunscreen use. *Archives of Dermatology*, **122**, 537–45.

Studniberg, H.M. and Weller, P. (1995) PUVA, UVB, psoriasis and non-melanoma skin cancer. *Journal of the American Academy of Dermatology*, **29**, 1013–22.

Swerdlow, A.J. and Green, A. (1987) Melanocytic naevi and melanoma. An epidemiologic perspective. *British Journal of Dermatology*, **117**, 137–46.

Unna, P. (1894) *Histopathologie der Hautkrankheiten*, Hirschwald, Berlin.

Urbach, F. (1959) Modification of ultraviolet carcinogenesis by photoactive agents. *Journal of Investigative Dermatology*, **32**, 373–8.

Urbach, F. (1969) Geographic pathology of skin cancer, in *The Biologic Effects of Ultraviolet Radiation*, (ed. F. Urbach), Pergamon Press, Oxford, pp. 635–50.

Urbach, F., Rose, D.B. and Bonnem, M. (1972) Genetic and environmental interactions in skin carcinogenesis, in *Environment and Cancer*, M.D. Anderson Hospital Conference Proceedings, Williams and Wilkins, Baltimore, pp. 356–71.

Urbach, F., Forbes, P.D. and Davies, R.E. (1982) Modification of photocarcinogenesis by chemical agents. *Journal of the National Cancer Institute*, **69**, 229–35.

Van Der Leun, J.C., Tang, X and Tevini, M. (1995) Environmental effects of ozone depletion: 1994 assessment. *Ambio*, **24**, 138–96.

Yoshikawa, T., Streilein, J.W., Roe, T.V. *et al.* (1990) Susceptibility to the effects of UVB radiation on induction of contact hypersensitivity as a risk factor for skin cancer in man. *Journal of Investigative Dermatology*, **95**, 530–6.

8

THE IDIOPATHIC PHOTODERMATOSES: POLYMORPHIC LIGHT ERUPTION, ACTINIC PRURIGO AND HYDROA VACCINIFORME

Paul G. Norris and John L.M. Hawk

INTRODUCTION

The delayed-onset acute idiopathic photodermatoses comprise polymorphic light eruption (PLE), actinic prurigo (AP) and hydroa vacciniforme (HV) and are overall more common in females. Polymorphic light eruption is the most common and while precise pathogenic mechanisms are still unclear, increasing evidence points to a delayed-type hypersensitivity immunological reaction. The disorder is characterized by the intermittent, transient occurrence of cutaneous eruptions following ultraviolet (UV) exposure within a half to several hours, consisting of one or more of pruritic erythematous papules, vesicles and plaques of some or all exposed sites, and resolving without scarring over up to a week or two. Actinic prurigo, which may have at least a partly genetic basis to explain its features, is differentiated from polymorphic light eruption by its childhood onset and more persistent and excoriated lesions present on both sun-exposed and, to a lesser extent, covered sites, while the acute intermittent appearance of cutaneous papules following UV exposure is, as in PLE, also not uncommonly described.

Photodermatology. Edited by J.L.M. Hawk. Published in 1998 by Chapman & Hall, London. ISBN 0 412 72460 X.

Finally, hydroa vacciniforme is a very rare disorder generally beginning in childhood and characterized by recurrent crops of sometimes haemorrhagic vesicles on some or all sun-exposed skin with subsequent vacciniform scarring; it thus differs from PLE in its predominance of vesicles and in particular scarring.

POLYMORPHIC LIGHT ERUPTION

Polymorphic light eruption (PLE) is an acquired disorder characterized by the intermittent, transient occurrence of delayed abnormal cutaneous reactions to UV exposure, consisting in particular of one or more of pruritic, erythematous papules, vesicles or plaques on light-exposed skin (Plate 6). In addition, an accompanying densely aggregated perivascular, dermal lymphocytic infiltrate is a consistent histological finding and an immunological basis for the condition seems likely.

PATHOGENESIS

The experimental induction of PLE has been difficult and remains relatively so and the identity of the initiating chromophores for the disorder thus remains uncertain. Attempts to define the inducing action spectrum have also given conflicting results, probably partly attributable to disease heterogeneity and differences in diagnostic criteria, irradiation equipment and testing techniques. Thus although UVA has seemed more effective in the majority of patients (Hölzle *et al.*, 1982; Ortel *et al.*, 1986), several investigators have also successfully produced lesions with UVB irradiation (Cahn *et al.*, 1959; Epstein, 1962; Magnus, 1964; Miyamoto, 1989). In addition, there is a suggestion in some patients that the presence of the shorter UVA wavelengths may perhaps inhibit reactions otherwise evoked by the longer ones (Przybilla *et al.*, 1988). Further, in nearly half of cases, monochromatic irradiation studies may be normal, perhaps because single wavelength exposures are insufficiently energetic, but UVA sensitivity occurs in about two thirds of the abnormal cases, with less commonly UVB sensitivity concurrently or instead (Frain-Bell, 1985). PLE induction by a UVA sunbed at the non-tanning sacral pressure site also suggests that the UV–absorber interaction may be oxygen independent in at least some cases (Tegner and Brudin, 1986).

Epstein (1942) first postulated that PLE might involve cell-mediated immune mechanisms in which a sunlight-induced neoantigen might trigger a delayed-type hypersensitivity response. However, Jansen and Helander (1978) were later unable to detect such antigen in the irradiated epidermal homogenates from any of 16 patients, although PLE, apparently triggered by photo-allergic contact dermatitis to the exogenous allergen, Fentichlor (Norris *et al.*, 1988), then raised the possibility that the Fentichlor exposure had produced an antigenic photoproduct similar to UV-induced endogenous antigen, or else stimulated patient immune responsiveness so as to recognize the latter. The former mechanism is at least theoretically possible, because there is evidence for the photosensitized alteration of carrier protein in an *in vitro* system containing tetrachlorsalicylanilide (Kochevar and Harber, 1977). In addition, more recently

Gonzales-Amaro *et al.* (1991) have demonstrated that high doses of UVB or UVA may induce cultured PLE epidermal cells to stimulate autologous peripheral blood mononuclear cells, thus again suggesting immune sensitization against autologous UV-modified antigen may be possible in PLE.

Characterization of the cells of the PLE infiltrate by the use of monoclonal antibodies in an attempt to provide other evidence for the nature of the PLE reaction has also been attempted, first by Muhlbauer *et al.* (1983), who studied biopsies of naturally occurring lesions of uncertain and varying age but were unable to obtain consistent results. Moncada *et al.* (1984) then carried out a similar study but induced the lesions with 20 times the patients' minimal erythema doses, thus leading to histological interpretation difficulties because of co-existent sunburn changes, which include mononuclear cell infiltration. However, an immunohistochemical study (Norris *et al.*, 1989) of timed biopsies from PLE lesions induced by low doses of solar-simulated radiation finally demonstrated the appearance of a T cell-dominated perivascular infiltrate within five hours of irradiation with a peak at around 72 hours; CD4+ T cells were numerous early on, but CD8+ cells dominated after 72 hours while, significantly increased numbers of dermal and epidermal Langerhans cells were also detected. These cellular changes resembled those seen in allergic contact dermatitis (Scheynius *et al.*, 1984) and the tuberculin reaction (Poulter *et al.*, 1982), already known delayed-type hypersensitivity reactions, while a study of the pattern of adhesion molecule expression in evolving PLE (Norris *et al.*, 1992) also suggested delayed-type hypersensitivity. These observations thus all support a delayed-type hypersensitivity immunological basis for PLE.

Finally, the sometimes striking overlap of the clinical and histopathological features of PLE and the photosensitive condition lupus erythematosus, also considered to be a disorder associated with the induction of UV-induced antigen, perhaps so-called UV-DNA (see Chapter 14), again supports the possibility of a similar pathogenic process for PLE, but very probably with a different putative UV-induced antigen (Murphy and Hawk, 1991; Petzelbauer *et al.*, 1992). Heat shock protein has been speculatively suggested as one candidate for the latter (McFadden *et al.*, 1994).

CLINICAL FEATURES

PLE is the most common photodermatosis. Thus, Morison and Stern (1982) interviewed 271 apparently healthy, consecutive entrants to a medical library in Boston in the Northern United States and found 10% with a history consistent with PLE, while in a survey of 412 employees from a Swedish pharmaceutical company, 21% had such a history (Ros and Wennersten, 1986). Pao *et al.* (1994) then further emphasized that PLE is commoner in temperate climates than nearer the equator, showing an incidence of around 5% in Australia and 15% in the United Kingdom. This is very possibly because of the greater proportion of UVA to UVB in temperate areas, such a higher proportion perhaps reducing inadvertent UVA exposure because of patient susceptibility to earlier sun burning, or else inhibitng of lesion development through the depression of patient immunological reactivity.

PLE affects females more commonly than males and usually has its onset in the first three decades of life (Frain-Bell, 1985); a positive family history is also not uncommon (Ros and Wennersten, 1986). Symptoms typically begin each spring and may moderate as summer progresses, rarely occurring in winter except as a result of UV reflection from lying snow. However, individual patient susceptibility varies considerably, the period of sun exposure necessary to trigger the eruption usually being between 30 minutes and several hours, although up to several days may be required after a period of relative sunlight abstinence. Lesions then appear after a latent interval of minutes to hours and, in the absence of further exposure, subside completely, virtually always without scarring, within 1–14 days or so.

Various attempts have been made to subdivide PLE into several morphological types, papular, papulovesicular, plaque, vesicobullous, eczematous, insect bite-like and erythema multiforme-like variants in particular having been noted. In addition, a mild, often delayed-onset clinical variant, frequently occurring just on vacations, has occasionally been designated as benign summer light eruption (Thomas and Amblard, 1986), while another such variant, sometimes called juvenile spring eruption, is characterized by self-limiting pruritic grouped papules and vesicles of the light exposed helices of usually boys' ears in early spring (Berth-Jones *et al.*, 1989a, b); finally, a pruritic form with no visible eruption at all has also been reported (Dover and Hawk, 1988). However, although it is agreed that papular forms are the commonest and that many of the other variants may also regularly occur, some such as the rare vesicobullous insect bite-like and erythema multiforme-like forms, and in particular all eczematous types, should only be considered as PLE if all other possible diagnoses have first been carefully excluded. In fact, it seems unlikely that such variants represent true pathogenic subgroups since, for example, diffuse facial erythema and swelling not uncommonly accompany the occurrence of typical papular lesions elsewhere.

The PLE eruption in all forms usually occurs symmetrically, but often affects only some exposed, or very rarely relatively unexposed, body sites, particularly those normally covered in winter such as the upper chest and arms. In any one patient, such lesions generally remain morphologically similar from attack to attack and usually occur on the same sites, although they may sometimes spread or recede overall, either gradually with time or with the severity of the individual UV exposure. Associated systemic symptoms are very uncommon but chills, headache, fever and nausea are possible.

INVESTIGATIONS

Negative circulating antinuclear factor and anti-SSA (Ro) and -SSB (La) titres should be confirmed in all patients and negative urinary, stool and red blood cell porphyrins in those where porphyria is a possibility. Irradiation skin testing and biopsy for histology may also assist in uncertain cases.

TREATMENT

Many patients are satisfactorily controlled by the avoidance of excessive UV exposure and the regular application of broad-spectrum high UV-protection sunscreens (Proby *et al.*, 1993). Failing this, however, more severely affected subjects nearly always respond well to prophylactic courses of psoralen photochemotherapy (PUVA) (Ortel *et al.*, 1986), or less reliably broad-band (Murphy *et al.*, 1987b), or more recently narrow-band (312 nm) (Bilsland *et al.*, 1993), phototherapy each spring. In addition, short-course PUVA regimens lasting 2–4 weeks may be as effective as longer ones (Menagé *et al.*, 1992), while one small controlled study has even suggested that UVA alone may be as effective as PUVA (Berg *et al.*, 1994). Such phototherapy may work to some extent by the induction of cutaneous melanogenesis and hyperplasia in responsive patients, but since these do not always occur, alterations in skin immunological reactivity (Strauss *et al.*, 1980), probably partly through UV effects upon Langerhans cells (Friedmann *et al.*, 1983), are likely to be mainly responsible.

Beta-carotene has been advocated from time to time as a prophylactic oral treatment for PLE (Swanbeck and Wennersten, 1972), but has not been shown to be usefully effective in controlled studies (Corbett *et al.*, 1982).

Similarly, chloroquine (Corbett *et al.*, 1982) and hydroxychloroquine (Murphy *et al.*, 1987a) have also been traditionally used, but controlled studies have again demonstrated these to be of mild efficacy at best. Recently, Rhodes *et al.* (1995) have further suggested that dietary fish oil rich in omega-3 polyunsaturated fatty acids may increase the threshold for the UVA provocation of PLE, perhaps by reducing UV-generated prostaglandin levels in irradiated skin, but this preliminary work requires confirmation. On the other hand, although not yet carefully studied, brief courses of systemic corticosteroids for up to several days seem rapidly effective in abating the rash once it begins to develop, but should only be used occasionally for severe disease exacerbations during vacations or photochemotherapy. Finally, low-dose azathioprine therapy has also been effective in two severely affected patients refractory to all other treatments (Norris and Hawk, 1989).

ACTINIC PRURIGO

Actinic prurigo (AP) is a not uncommon, chronic acquired disorder of generally childhood onset and female preponderance, characterized by a persistent, pruritic, excoriated, papular or nodular eruption of the sun-exposed and to a lesser extent non-exposed skin, frequently failing to clear in winter; sometimes an acute erythematous, itchy, papular eruption similar to that of PLE after individual sun exposures is also described. The condition usually arises in childhood and lasts until puberty although later onset and more persistent forms occur; it is also more frequent in native American (Amerindian) populations, where it is often familial (Bernal *et al.*, 1990). AP has been regarded as a variant of PLE by some investigators (Dominguez and Hojyo, 1982) and as a distinct condition by others (Calnan and Meara, 1977), although more recent work suggests that the former is perhaps more likely.

PATHOGENESIS

In about two thirds of patients, the action spectrum for erythema as tested with narrow waveband irradiation has been reported as abnormal, more commonly to UVA than UVB (Frain-Bell, 1985), while other investigations, in particular for circulating antinuclear factor and anti-SSA (Ro) and -SSB (La) antibodies, for lesional direct immunofluorescence and for other usual haematological and biochemical investigations, are uniformly negative. However, Farr and Diffey (1988) have reported the augmentation of cutaneous UVA erythema in AP by the presumed inhibition of cutaneous cyclo-oxygenase activity with topical indomethacin, thus suggesting that the lipoxygenase derivatives of arachidonic acid metabolism might perhaps be involved in the mechanism of AP photosensitivity; however, the repeatability of these findings has not been confirmed nor their relevance clarified. On the other hand, unlike in PLE (Lane *et al.*, 1991), the tissue typing of AP patients has now demonstrated an increased frequency of human leucocyte antigens (HLA) A24 and Cw4 in Colombian Amerindians (Bernal *et al.*, 1990), and of HLA DR4 in around 90%, and in particular its rare subtype, DRB1*0407, in about 60%, of British Caucasoids (Menagé *et al.*, 1996); only about 30% and 6% of normal subjects respectively have these tissue types. As a result, it has been suggested that since the genetic positions 74 and 86 making DRB1*0407 different from other DR4 alleles are intimately involved in peptide binding, this highly characteristic HLA type in AP may determine its skin response to peptide antigen, arguably one induced by UV irradiation, so as to initiate the typical and prolonged AP clinical picture.

CLINICAL FEATURES

AP is more common in females, usually beginning by age ten years and resolving in adolescent or early adult life, although a later onset and longer persistence are possible, particularly in Amerindian types; familial incidence also occurs in just over 50% of patients (Frain-Bell, 1985), and atopy in about 10% (Calnan and Meara, 1977). The condition usually worsens in summer and improves in winter although the opposite is also rarely possible, as well as flares in spring and autumn, while the appearance of lesions only occasionally clearly follows sun exposure, although the apparently unassociated affects of a PLE-like rash are more frequently reported. All exposed sites are usually affected with the AP eruption, along to a lesser extent with the normally covered skin of the limbs and occasionally buttocks, although the part of the forehead under a hair fringe is often spared. The typical rash consists of pruritic, often excoriated papules or nodules, sometimes with associated eczematization, lichenification or crusting (Plate 7); lesions of the face may then heal to leave minute pitted or linear scars. Cheilitis, particularly of the lower lip, is also common, as is conjunctivitis, particularly in Amerindian variants.

INVESTIGATIONS

Negative circulating antinuclear factor and anti-SSA (Ro) and -SSB (La) titres should be confirmed in all patients, as should blood, urinary and stool porphyrins in those few where porphyria might instead be present. Irradiation skin testing, HLA tissue typing and to a much lesser extent biopsy for histology also often contribute to the diagnosis and should be undertaken where possible.

TREATMENT

The restriction of sun exposure and use of high UV-protection sunscreens usually provides inadequate control. In such cases, PUVA or UVB therapy given as for PLE may then sometimes be helpful, the former preferably restricted, except in its bath form to adolescent or adult patients; however, PUVA does not appear to alter the reported abnormal augmentation of UVB erythema by indomethacin in the disorder (Farr and Diffey, 1989), perhaps thus suggesting only moderate efficacy. In otherwise non-responsive patients, however, intermittent courses of low-dose thalidomide, usually given at night since the drug is a hypnotic, in doses of 50–100 mg, are very effective in many patients (Lovell *et al.*, 1983), although careful monitoring is required to avoid teratogenicity and a moderate risk of peripheral neuropathy; otherwise the drug is usually well tolerated, apart from causing occasional drowsiness during the day. Once resolution of the eruption develops over several weeks, the drug may then be reduced in dosage or stopped, particularly in the winter, to be restarted at the first sign of any relapse.

HYDROA VACCINIFORME

Hydroa vacciniforme (HV) is a very rare acquired disorder, usually beginning in childhood and resolving by early adulthood; it is characterized by the intermittent transient occurrence of abnormal cutaneous reactions to UV exposure, consisting in particular of recurrent crops of vesicles on some or all sun-exposed skin, which then settle over days to weeks to leave persistent vacciniform scarring. Distinctive, essentially diagnostic histological changes are initial intraepidermal vesicle formation with later focal epidermal keratinocyte necrosis, along with dermal perivascular neutrophil leucocyte and lymphocyte infiltration.

PATHOGENESIS

Repetitive broad-spectrum UVA (Goldgeier *et al.*, 1982; Halasz *et al.*, 1983) and UVB (Bickers *et al.*, 1978; Schiff and Jillson, 1960) irradiation have been reported to induce lesions indistinguishable from the natural HV eruption, while increased erythemal sensitivity to short wavelength monochromatic UVA has also been noted (Sonnex and Hawk, 1988); blood, urine and stool porphyrin concentrations, however, are always normal, as are lesional viral studies and circulating viral, antinuclear factor, anti-SSA (Ro) and -SSB (La) titres. The cause of the condition is unknown but its acute attacks, symmetrically distributed lesions affecting usually only some exposed sites and its dermal, perivascular lymphocytic infiltrate early on all suggest it may possibly be a scarring variant of PLE and thus conceivably also a delayed type hypersensitivity reaction, the inducing allergen perhaps being at a critical site, or else a toxic photoproduct being produced to cause the scarring.

CLINICAL FEATURES

HV generally begins in childhood, a little more often in males, with resolution usually by early adult life; familial incidence is rare. It is characterized by the intermittent transient occurrence of itching or burning erythematous macules within hours of sun exposure in summer on some or all exposed areas; within 24 hours, these progress to tender papules, also often associated with a severe burning sensation, which later become vesicular, sometimes haemorrhagic, then umbilicated (Plate 8). Crusted lesions next form, and their detachment within 1–6 weeks leaves scattered or confluent, depressed, pock-like scars, sometimes associated with telangiectasia. Occasional associated systemic features include headaches, malaise, fever and generalized aching (Sonnex and Hawk, 1988).

INVESTIGATIONS

Negative circulating antinuclear factor and anti-SSA (Ro) and -SSB (La) titres should be confirmed in all patients, as should normal blood, urinary and stool porphyrin concentrations. Viral studies and histology should also be undertaken on new vesicular lesions, and the latter should strongly suggest the diagnosis if uncertainty persists. In addition, irradiation skin testing may also demonstrate abnormal sensitivity.

TREATMENT

HV symptoms are reported to have been successfully controlled by the regular use of high UV protection broad-spectrum sunscreens (Sonnex and Hawk, 1988), while hydroxychloroquine has also been stated to improve the clinical features and UVA sensitivity of the condition (Goldgeier *et al.*, 1982); however, clinical experience suggests such efficacy is not reliable. In difficult cases, therefore, prophylactic UVB phototherapy and PUVA may instead be tried with some expectation of efficacy, although the latter may precipitate an exacerbation if not given with care (Sonnex and Hawk, 1988). Finally, immunosuppressive therapy, including the intermittent use of oral steroids, might be considered for intractable, particularly adult, cases although its efficacy as yet appears not to have been formally assessed.

REFERENCES

Berg, M., Ros, A-M. and Berne, B. (1994) Ultraviolet A phototherapy and trimethylpsoralen UVA photochemotherapy in polymorphous light eruption – a controlled study. *Photodermatology, Photoimmunology and Photomedicine*, **10**, 139–43.

Bernal, J.E., Duran de Rueda, M.M., Ordonez, C.P. *et al.* (1990). Actinic prurigo among the Chimila Indians in Columbia: HLA studies. *Journal of the American Academy of Dermatology*, **22**, 1049–51.

Berth-Jones, J., Hutchinson, P.E., Burns, D. *et al.* (1989a) Juvenile spring eruption of the ears. A re-examination. *British Journal of Dermatology*, **121** (suppl. 34), 51.

Berth-Jones, J., Norris, P.G., Graham-Brown, R.A.C. *et al.* (1989b) Juvenile spring eruption of the ears. *Clinical and Experimental Dermatology*, **14**, 462–3.

Bickers, D.R., Lemar, L.K. and DeLeo, V. (1978) Hydroa vacciniforme. *Archives of Dermatology*, **114**, 1193–7.

Bilsland, D., George, S., Gibbs, N. *et al.* (1993) A comparison of narrow band phototherapy (TL-01) and photochemotherapy (PUVA) in the management of polymorphic light eruption. *British Journal of Dermatology*, **129**, 708–12.

Cahn, M.M., Levy, E.J., Shafer, B. *et al.* (1959) Experimentally induced reactions to ultraviolet light. Polymorphous light eruption and phototoxicity to drugs. *Journal of Investigative Dermatology*, **32**, 355–61.

Calnan, C.D. and Meara, R.H. (1977) Actinic prurigo. *Clinical and Experimental Dermatology*, **2**, 365–7.

Corbett, M.F., Hawk, J.L.M., Herxheimer, A. *et al.* (1982) Controlled therapeutic trials in polymorphic light eruption. *British Journal of Dermatology*, **107**, 571–81.

Dominguez, L. and Hojyo, M.T. (1982) Actinic prurigo, a variety of polymorphous light eruption. *International Journal of Dermatology*, **21**, 260–1.

Dover, J.S. and Hawk, J.L.M. (1988) Polymorphic light eruption sine eruptione. *British Journal of Dermatology*, **118**, 73–6.

Epstein, J.H. (1962) Polymorphous light eruptions. Phototest technique studies. *Archives of Dermatology*, **85**, 502–4.

Epstein, S. (1942) Studies in abnormal human sensitivity to light. IV. Photoallergic concept of prurigo aestivalis. *Journal of Investigative Dermatology*, **5**, 289–95.

Farr, P.M. and Diffey, B.L. (1988) Augmentation of ultraviolet erythema by indomethacin in actinic prurigo. Evidence of mechanism of photosensitivity. *Photochemistry and Photobiology*, **47**, 413–17.

Farr, P.M. and Diffey, B.L. (1989) Treatment of actinic prurigo with PUVA: mechanism of action. *British Journal of Dermatology*, **120**, 411–18.

Frain-Bell, W. (1985) The idiopathic photodermatoses, in *Cutaneous Photobiology*, Oxford, Oxford University Press, pp. 24–59.

Friedmann, P.S., Ford, G.P., Ross, J. *et al.* (1983) Reappearance of epidermal Langerhans cells after PUVA therapy. *British Journal of Dermatology*, **109**, 301–7.

Goldgeier, M.H., Norlund, J.J., Lucky, A.W. *et al.* (1982) Hydroa vacciniforme. Diagnosis and therapy. *British Journal of Dermatology*, **118**, 588–91.

Gonzales-Amaro, R., Baranda, L., Salazar-Gonzalez, J.F. *et al.* (1991) Immune sensitisation against epidermal antigens in polymorphous light eruption. *Journal of the American Academy of Dermatology*, **24**, 70–3.

Halasz, C.L.G., Leach, E.E., Walthjer, R.R. *et al.* (1983) Hydroa vacciniforme. Induction of lesions with ultraviolet A. *Journal of American Academy of Dermatology*, **8**, 171–6.

Hölzle, E., Plewig, G., Hofmann, C. *et al.* (1982) Polymorphic light eruption. Experimental reproduction of skin lesions. *Journal of the American Academy of Dermatology*, **7**, 111–25.

Jansen, C.T. and Helander, I. (1978) Cell-mediated immunity in chronic polymorphous light eruptions. *Acta Dermatovenereologica (Stockholm)*, **56**, 121–5.

Kochevar, I.E. and Harber, L.C. (1977) Photoreactions of 3,3′,4′,5-tetrachlorsalicylanilide with proteins. *Journal of Investigative Dermatology*, **68**, 151–6.

Lane, P.R., Sheridan, D.P. and Hogan, D.J. (1991) HLAA typing in polymorphous light eruption. *Journal of the American Academy of Dermatology*, **24**, 570–3.

Lovell, C.R., Hawk, J.L.M. and Calnan, C.D. (1983) Thalidomide in actinic prurigo. *British Journal of Dermatology*, **108**, 467–71.

Magnus, I.A. (1964) Studies with a monochromator in the common idiopathic photodermatoses. *British Journal of Dermatology*, **76**, 245–64.

McFadden, J.P., Norris, P.G., Cerio, R. *et al.* (1994) Heat shock protein 65 immunoreactivity in experimentally induced polymorphic light eruption. *Acta Dermatolvenereologica (Stockholm)*, **74**, 253–5.

Menagé, H., Norris, P., Cheong, W. and Hawk, J. (1992). Short course PUVA therapy is effective in polymorphic light eruption. *British Journal of Dermatology*, **127** (suppl 40), 32.

Menagé, H., Vaughan, R.V., Baker, C.S. *et al.* (1996) HLA-DR4 may determine expression of actinic prurigo in British patients. *Journal of Investigative Dermatology*, **106**, 362–4.

Miyamoto, C. (1989) Polymorphous light eruption: successful reproduction of skin lesions, including papulovesicular light eruption, with ultraviolet B. *Photodermatology*, **6**, 69–79.

Moncada, B., Gonzales-Amaro, R., Barcunda, M.L. *et al.* (1984) Immunopathology of polymorphous light eruption. *Journal of the American Academy of Dermatology*, **10**, 970–3.

Morison, W.L. and Stern, R.S. (1982) Polymorphous light eruption: a common reaction uncommonly recognised. *Acta Dermatovenereologica (Stockholm)*, **62**, 237–40.

Muhlbauer, J.E., Bahn, A.K., Harrist, T.J. *et al.* (1983) Papular polymorphic light eruption: an immunoperoxidase study using monoclonal antibodies. *British Journal of Dermatology*, **108**, 153–62.

Murphy, G.M. and Hawk, J.L.M. (1991) The prevalence of antinuclear antibiotics in patients with apparent polymorphic light eruption. *British Journal of Dermatology*, **125**, 448–51.

Murphy, G.M., Hawk, J.L.M. and Magnus, I.A. (1987a) Hydroxychloroquine in polymorphic light eruption: a controlled trial with drug and visual sensitivity monitoring. *British Journal of Dermatology*, **116**, 379–86.

Murphy, G.M., Logan, R.A., Lovell, C.R. *et al.* (1987b) Prophylactic PUVA and UVB therapy in polymorphic light eruption – A controlled trial. *British Journal of Dermatology*, **116**, 531–538.

Norris, P.G. and Hawk, J.L.M. (1989) Successful treatment of severe polymorphous light eruption with azathioprine. *Archives of Dermatology*, **124**, 80–3.

Norris, P.G., Hawk, J.L.M. and White, I.R. (1988) Photoallergic contact dermatitis from Fentichlor. *Contact Dermatitis*, **18**, 318–20.

Norris, P.G., Morris, J., McGibbon, D.M. *et al.* (1989) Polymorphic light eruption: an immunopathological study of evolving lesions. *British Journal of Dermatology*, **120**, 173–83.

Norris, P.G., Barker, J.N.W.N., Allen, M.H. *et al.* (1992) Adhesion molecule expression in polymorphic light eruption. *Journal of Investigative Dermatology*, **99**, 504–8.

Ortel, B., Tanew, H. and Hönigsmann, H. (1986) Polymorphous light eruption. Action spectrum and photoprotection. *Journal of the American Academy of Dermatology*, **14**, 748–53.

Pao, C., Norris, P.G., Corbett, M. *et al.* (1994) Polymorphic light eruption: prevalence in Australia and England. *British Journal of Dermatology*, **130**, 62–4.

Petzelbauer, P., Binder, M., Nikolakis, P. *et al.* (1992) Severe sun sensitivity and the presence of antinuclear antibodies in patients with polymorphous light eruption-like lesions. *Journal of the American Academy of Dermatology*, **26**, 68–74.

Poulter, L.W., Seymour, G.J., Duke, O. *et al.* (1982) Immunohistological analysis of delayed-type hypersensitivity in man. *Cell Immunology*, **74**, 358–69.

Proby, C., Baker, C., Morton, O. and Hawk, J. (1993) New broad-spectrum sunscreen for polymorphic light eruption. *Lancet*, **341**, 1347–8.

Przybilla, B., Galosi, A., Heppeler, M. *et al.* (1988) Polymorphous light eruption: eliciting and inhibiting wavelengths. *Acta Dermatovenereologica (Stockholm)*, **68**, 173–6.

Rhodes, L., Durham, B., Fraser, W. *et al.* (1995) Dietary fish oil reduces basal and ultraviolet B-generated PGE_2 levels in skin. *Journal of Investigative Dermatology*, **105**, 532–5.

Ros, A. and Wennersten, G. (1986) Current aspects of polymorphous light eruptions in Sweden. *Photodermatology*, **3,** 298–302.

Scheynius, A., Fischer, T., Forsum, U. *et al.* (1984) Phenotypic characterisation *in situ* of inflammatory cells in allergic and irritant contact dermatitis in man. *Clinical and Experimental Immunology*, **55,** 81–90.

Schiff, M. and Jillson, O.F. (1960) Photoskin tests in hydroa vacciniforme. *Archives of Dermatology*, **82,** 812–15.

Sonnex, T.S. and Hawk, J.L.M. (1988) Hydroa vacciniforme. A review of ten cases. *British Journal of Dermatology*, **118,** 101–8.

Strauss, G.H., Greaves, M.W., Price, N. *et al.* (1980) Inhibition of delayed hypersensitivity reaction in skin (DNCB test) by methoxypsoralen photochemotherapy. Possible basis for pseudopromoting action in skin carcinogenesis. *Lancet*, **2,** 556–9.

Swanbeck, G. and Wennersten, G. (1972) Treatment of polymorphous light eruptions with beta-carotene. *Acta Dermatovenereologica* (*Stockholm*), **54,** 491–4.

Tegner, E. and Brudin, A.M. (1986) Polymorphous light eruption in hypopigmented pressure areas with a UVA sunbed. *Acta Dermatovenereologica* (*Stockholm*), **66,** 446–8.

9

THE IDIOPATHIC PHOTODERMATOSES: SOLAR URTICARIA

Erhard Hölzle

Solar urticaria is a rare but often incapacitating photodermatosis, probably an immediate-type hypersensitivity reaction against photoactivated endogenous allergen. Itching, erythema and usually wealing occur after exposure to generally small amounts of sunlight or artificial ultraviolet or visible radiation within a few minutes, persisting for an hour or two; rarely, such wealing is confined to circumscribed skin sites, a variety termed fixed solar urticaria. The action spectrum encompasses diverse, usually broad portions of the electromagnetic spectrum, mostly in the UVA and visible regions, a variability probably reflecting a similar diversity in possible chromophores responsible for initiating the reaction, presumably by leading to photoallergen production. Rarely, certain portions of the ultraviolet and visible spectrum instead inhibit wealing, probably by photoinactivation of the putative photoallergen, which may be demonstrated in some patients. The development of hours to a day or so of tolerance to wealing by repeated skin exposure to the eliciting wavelengths is not uncommon in solar urticaria, perhaps because IgE-binding sites on mast cells remain blocked by photoallergen already present. The classification of solar urticaria into two types has been proposed, patients with type I having a specific photoallergen present only in them and those with type II a non-specific allergen also present in normal subjects. Histamine probably represents the major mediator of the reaction, but antihistamines are of therapeutic value in only about half of patients. Broad- or narrow-band UVB phototherapy or psoralen photochemotherapy (PUVA) may help others, while plasmapheresis may be helpful in those resistant to conventional therapy in whom a circulating photoallergen is present.

INTRODUCTION

Solar urticaria (SU) is a rare, often extremely disabling photosensitivity disorder of unknown aetiology first described in 1904 by Merklen *et al.* Reproduction of the wealing by sun exposure under controlled conditions was first carried out by Ward in 1905 and the designation 'solar urticaria' was proposed by Duke in 1923, before finally Wucherpfennig (1928) quantitatively investigated the response with increasing irradiation doses at different wavelengths. SU belongs to the group of urticarias elicited by physical agents, in this case ultraviolet or visible radiation, and is generally accepted as having an immunological basis. Thus, it appears likely that a putative photoallergen formed by irradiation in skin, or in many patients' serum or plasma (Horio, 1978; Horio *et al.*, 1984; Kojima *et al.*, 1986), leads to a type I immunoreaction. However, many questions still exist regarding the exact pathogenesis of SU (Horio, 1987),

Photodermatology. Edited by J.L.M. Hawk. Published in 1998 by Chapman & Hall, London. ISBN 0 412 72460 X.

particularly because action spectra in the condition, which should theoretically provide clues concerning the initiating chromophores, are usually broad and lacking in specific absorption maxima, while for safety reasons it is no longer feasible to perform passive and reverse passive serum transfer tests between subjects. In addition, there is no animal model for the disease.

PATHOGENESIS AND WORKING CLASSIFICATION OF SOLAR URTICARIA

In 1942, Rajka passively transferred SU to normal subjects in a patient's serum, this passive transfer test (the Prausnitz–Küstner test) providing clear evidence for an immediate-type hypersensitivity reaction as the basis of SU pathogenesis; later, in 1949, Epstein also showed that reverse passive transfer was possible. In such experiments, the skin of normal subjects was first irradiated and patient serum then intradermally injected into the exposed sites. Different investigators obtained different results, thus suggesting that the mechanisms involved were variable. In addition, an awareness of variations in SU action spectra led to a careful classification by Harber *et al.* (1963), which has since needed complete revision as a result of steadily accumulating experimental evidence (Table 9.1). Thus, type 6 SU in the Harber classification is in fact erythropoietic protoporphyria and a broadening of the SU action spectrum during the course of the disease in

another instance indicated a transition from one SU type to another (Murphy and Hawk, 1987). Therefore in 1989, Leenutaphong and co-workers reviewed all the available evidence from patient reports and developed from these a working classification distinguishing just two SU types.

In spite of this new classification, the nature of the pathogenic mechanism in SU remains largely hypothetical. Thus, it is assumed that a precursor in patient skin absorbs the activating ultraviolet or visible radiation to form a putative photoallergen. Thereafter, IgE specifically directed against this allergen may be generated and bound to mast cells in the skin, following which, in the presence of further radiation-induced allergen, immediate-type hypersensitivity reaction with weals and flare formation occurs in association with mast cell histamine release (Fig. 9.1).

A search for putative SU chromophores then ensued, Horio being the first to demonstrate that such a molecule present in the serum or plasma of patients may be activated by irradiation *in vitro* to form photoallergen (Horio, 1987; Horio and Minami, 1977); thereafter, such serum factors were identified in many (Duschet *et al.*, 1987; Horio, 1978; Kojima *et al.*, 1986; Leenutaphong *et al.*, 1990; Sams, 1970; Sams *et al.*, 1969) but not all (Leenutaphong *et al.*, 1988a) patients. Kojima *et al.* (1986) as well as our group (Leenutaphong *et al.*, 1990) also observed patients whose precursor was present only in plasma but not serum. We also investigated a patient without precursor in either serum or plasma who reacted to eluates of irradiated isolated epidermis from his own skin although unirradiated samples failed to induce wealing. This therefore suggested that precursor was probably present only in the epidermis (Leenutaphong *et al.*, 1988a). Torinuki and Tagami (1986) then demonstrated both photoallergen and reaginic antibodies in the serum, while heating of the serum was shown to destroy its capacity for passive transfer (Van Hecke, 1979).

Table 9.1 Classification of solar urticaria according to Harber *et al.* (1963)

Type	Action spectrum	Passive transfer	Reverse passive transfer
I	285–320 nm	Positive	Positive
II	320–400 nm	Negative	Negative
III	400–500 nm	Negative	Negative
IV	400–500 nm	Positive	Negative
V	280–500 nm	Negative	Negative
VI	400 nm	Not done	Not done

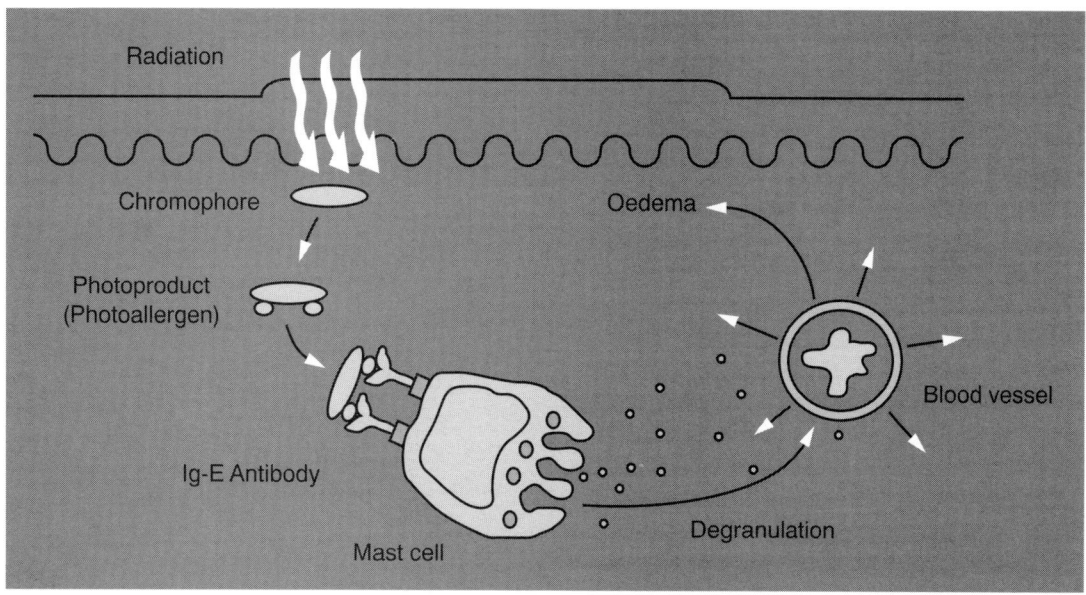

Figure 9.1 Pathogenesis of solar urticaria. A precursor (chromophore) is activated by ultraviolet or visible irradiation, thus forming photoproduct (photoallergen). Specific IgE directed against photoallergen is bound to the surface of the mast cell. Bridging of IgE molecules by photoallergen leads to release of histamine and probably also other mediators.

Kojima *et al.* (1986) then proceeded to investigate the nature of the photoallergen, separating the *in vitro*-activated serum or plasma by gel filtration and assessing the molecular weight of the photoallergen as between 25 and 45 kD in three patients with action spectra in the short visible range (400–500 nm). However, in other patients with wider action spectra, the values ranged instead between 300 and 1000 kD and it was therefore felt that the diversity of action spectrum between patients derived from differences in chromophores.

In response to this further information, Leenutaphong *et al.* (1989) then proposed that their two SU types appeared to differ only in the nature of their precursors. Thus, in type I SU, the precursor is apparently an abnormal endogenous substance present only in the patient, while in type II it is a normal factor present in both patients and unaffected subjects.

IN VITRO PRECURSOR ACTIVATION STUDIES TO DETERMINE SU TYPE

SU type may be determined by the injection of *in vitro*-irradiated patient and normal serum or plasma into patient or normal subject skin (Table 9.2). Such studies, however, are no longer considered ethical.

TYPE I

If wealing develops in patient or normal skin after injection of patient but not normal irradiated serum or plasma, the SU is of type I, the precursor occurring only in the patient.

TYPE II

If wealing develops in patient or normal skin after injection of both patient and normal irradiated serum or plasma, the SU is of type II, the precursor occurring in both patients and normal subjects.

Table 9.2 Results of *in vitro* activation studies and passive and reverse passive transfer tests, according to type of solar urticaria

Experimental procedure	Type I	Type II
In vitro activation studies		
Reaction of patient to irradiated serum or plasma of patient	Wealing	Wealing
Reaction of normal subject to irradiated serum or plasma of patient	No effect	No effect
Reaction of patient to irradiated serum or plasma of normal subject	No effect	Wealing
Reaction of normal subject to irradiated serum or plasma of normal subject	No effect	No effect
Passive transfer test	Variable	Wealing
Reverse passive transfer test	No effect	Variable

EARLY PASSIVE AND REVERSE PASSIVE TRANSFER TESTS TO ELUCIDATE NATURE OF SU

Passive and reverse passive transfer both refer to the injection of only patient serum into only normal subject skin; in each instance, however, this skin is also irradiated, after injection for the former and before the latter. Such studies, however, are no longer considered ethical.

In 1970, Sams demonstrated that the presumed passively transferred factor in two SU patients was neither IgG nor IgM and was therefore probably IgE, while disease unable to be so transferred was considered probably phototoxic instead. However, Kojima *et al.* (1986) then found that the irradiated serum from such patients induced wealing after intradermal injection into their own skin, thus suggesting an allergic mechanism after all.

Epstein (1949) went further by introducing the reverse passive transfer test, the results of which are negative in patients with type I SU (Horio, 1978; Horio and Minami, 1977; Torinuki and Tagami, 1986), its precursor being absent from normal human skin. In contrast, however, the type II allergen is produced by normal skin irradiation and if transferred patient serum IgE adheres to mast cells before it disappears, the reverse transfer test is positive (Kojima *et al.*, 1986) (see Table 9.2).

For correct interpretation of the passive and reverse transfer tests, several factors must be taken into account. First, samples of patient serum or plasma contain photoallergen precursor as well as specific IgE against that allergen. Second, a lag period between serum injection and skin irradiation is required, during which transferred serum IgE adheres to skin mast cells; thus, Kojima *et al.* (1986) reported negative results for irradiations undertaken 30 minutes after serum injection, but positive for those postponed for 2–6 hours. Third, in type I SU allergen precursor concomitantly transferred with IgE antibody must remain in the receptor skin until IgE binding to mast cells; thus, passive transfer may be successful in some (Epstein *et al.*, 1963; Murphy and Hawk, 1987) but not other (Kojima *et al.*, 1986) type I SU patients. Fourth, passive transfer is always successful in type II SU, IgE being transferred, binding to mast cells and enabling histamine release following irradiation-induced formation of the ubiquitous non-specific photoallergen. However, an adequate lag period between serum injection and skin irradiation is still essential.

CLINICAL FEATURES

SU is a relatively rare disease (although exact incidence figures are not available) but is often incapacitating because of the associated exquisite photosensitivity; in such instances, even small amounts of sunlight, often of only a few minutes' duration, or of artificial lighting in patients sensitive to visible irradiation may suffice to elicit the unpleasant symptoms. The disorder occurs worldwide, affecting all races and ethnic groups, including black-skinned subjects (Ravits *et al.,* 1982), with a slight female preponderance (Stevanovic, 1960); age of onset also varies, ranging from one year to the eighth decade (Ferguson, 1988), but mostly being between the ages of 20 and 40 years. There are no known predisposing genetic factors, only one familial case having been reported (Polano, 1948), and the disease occurs almost exclusively in otherwise healthy individuals. Thus, there is no clear relationship with other disorders except other physical urticarias such as cold urticaria (Rantanen and Suhonen, 1980), dermographism (Rantanen and Suhonen, 1980), heat urticaria (Willis and Epstein, 1974) and pressure urticaria (personal observation).

Within minutes of sunlight or appropriate artificial radiation exposure, intense itching followed by erythema and wealing occurs on exposed sites, fading spontaneously back to normal within an hour or so, although residual erythema may last a little longer. Very rarely, onset delayed by a few hours has also been reported (Monfrecola *et al.,* 1988), while if lesions not only develop slowly but persist for days, a form of solar urticarial vasculitis should be considered (Armstrong *et al.,* 1985). Other differential diagnoses include relatively transient plaque forms of polymorphic light eruption and erythropoietic protoporphyria, in which immediate urticaria is a very rare feature (Beljaards and Bruynzeel, 1991); in addition, the experimental induction of immediate wealing has also been reported once in porphyria cutanea

tarda (Ichihashi *et al.,* 1985b). All body areas including the mucous membranes (Illig and Born, 1964) are sensitive to light, but chronically sun-exposed skin such as the face and backs of hands are sometimes less so because of tolerance occurring as a result of repeated exposure.

One patient has been reported with solar urticaria caused by intake of the drug repirinast, an antiallergic medication introduced in Japan in 1987 (Kurimaji, and Shono, 1994); this was confirmed by provocation tests demonstrating immediate wealing following irradiation with wavelengths between 320 and 350 nm. Passive and reverse passive transfer was negative, however, although the intradermal injection of patient serum irradiated *in vitro* led to wealing in both the patient and a healthy individual and a non-allergic mechanism was considered possible. Drug-related urticarial responses have also been reported in patients exposed to tar and pitch (Crow *et al.,* 1961), benoxaprofen (Frain-Bell, 1985; Keahey *et al.,* 1982) and chlorpromazine (Horio, 1975; Lovell *et al.,* 1986), all agents already known to induce other immediate phototoxic reactions in sunlight.

The exposure of large skin areas in SU may lead to systemic collapse as a result of presumed massive mediator release, probably mainly histamine (Hawk *et al.,* 1980; Hölzle *et al.,* 1980; Keahey *et al.,* 1984; Soter *et al.,* 1979); other symptoms such as dizziness, sleepiness and muscle aching are also possible, particularly in patients with extreme light sensitivity. The natural course of SU is not well documented but in most patients, onset is sudden, after which the condition generally persists for years (Ferguson, 1988), spontaneous remission being relatively rare. In a few patients, however, gradual improvement seems to occur. A variant of classic SU, so-called fixed SU as described above, has also been reported, in which wealing occurs in a strictly localized but patchy pattern (Reinauer *et al.,* 1993). In three such patients, circumscribed wealing was reliably reproducible by irradiation with the wavebands 320–700, 320–585 and 400–560 nm, respectively, while intradermal injections of irradiated patient plasma induced wealing only at the affected sites. Differences in the mast cell population between the afflicted and non-afflicted sites may account for the irregular distribution of the lesions. Fixed SU appears to be associated with only moderate photosensitivity, patients being able to manage their disease by themselves, often with graduated exposures to natural sunlight to induce tolerance. In addition, systemic symptoms are absent, probably because of the relatively small skin areas and mediator release involved. Thus, this form of SU may be largely underreported.

HISTOPATHOLOGY AND ULTRASTRUCTURAL FINDINGS

The histopathology of SU wealing largely reveals the features of other urticarias, with some dermal oedema and a scanty mononuclear inflammatory infiltrate with admixed neutrophils and eosinophils. Time course studies demonstrate that the neutrophils and eosinophils appear in a dose-dependent way, predominantly perivascularly, at around five minutes and increase for up to two hours after the eliciting irradiation, while at 24 hours, mononuclear cell numbers (Norris *et al.*, 1988) are also increased. There is also tissue deposition of eosinophil major basic protein as a result of eosinophil degranulation (Leiferman *et al.*, 1989). Some case reports also suggest that vasculitis may be a feature of solar urticaria (Armstrong *et al.*, 1985) in some patients documented by immunoelectron microscopy (Plewig *et al.*, 1980); however, this contention remains controversial.

Sequential ultrastructural analysis in SU demonstrates the margination and activation of platelets, the formation of interendothelial clefts and the alteration of nerve fibres as primary events preceding mast cell degranulation (Behrendt *et al.*, 1989); in addition, mediators other than histamine may also be involved in these early stages. However, once a weal is formed, the presence of degranulated mast cells is clearly evident from the dissolution of their granular matrices, fusion of their perigranular membranes with labyrinth formation and their connections with the extracellular space. This degranulation is then followed by the extravasation of eosinophils, their connections with neutrophils mentioned above, while the nerve fibres go on to demonstrate partial swelling, then oedema of the endoneurium (Behrendt *et al.*, 1989). In fixed SU, the mast cells at affected sites may also contain numerous cytoplasm lipid bodies (Reinauer *et al.*, 1993).

HISTAMINE AND OTHER MEDIATORS

A number of investigators have found increased serum histamine levels in the venous blood draining wealed skin in SU (Hawk *et al.*, 1980; Keahey *et al.*, 1984; Soter *et al.*, 1979), while mast cell degranulation has also been confirmed electron microscopically (Behrendt *et al.*, 1989; Hawk *et al.*, 1980; Keahey *et al.*, 1984). Nevertheless, classic H1 receptor-blocking antihistamines have been of little therapeutic value in SU in the past, at best reducing light sensitivity by a factor of two to three (Michell *et al.*, 1980); however, modern agents of this sort with little sedative effect, such as terfenadine and astemizole, are now relatively effective in high doses (Bilsland and Ferguson, 1991; Diffey *et al.*, 1984; Ferguson, 1988; Monfrecola *et al.*, 1990; Rajatanavin and Bernhard, 1987), although erythema may not be diminished. Thus mediators other than histamine may be involved in the erythemal response, a hypothesis supported by the electron microscopic finding that the interendothelial clefting of dermal blood vessels precedes mast cell degranulation. Candidates as mediators for this immediate erythema are neurotransmitters such as substance P and vasoactive intestinal protein, while leukotrienes may also conceivably be involved (Armstrong, 1986), the mast cell lipid bodies in fixed SU perhaps containing such lipid mediators.

ACTION SPECTRA, INHIBITION SPECTRA AND AUGMENTATION SPECTRA

The confirmation of a diagnosis of SU and patient screening for action, inhibition and augmentation spectra in the disease may be undertaken by the phototesting of susceptible skin (Hölzle *et al.*, 1987) with broad-band irradiation sources emitting in the UVB 280–315 nm (Philips TL-12), UVA 315–400 nm (Philips TL-09) and visible 400–800 nm) spectra (e.g. a conventional slide projector with a Schott WG 420 filter), in combination if necessary with appropriate cut-off filters. For more precise action spectrum determina-

tion, however, the use of an irradiation monochromator is necessary.

The action spectrum for SU induction varies greatly between patients (Table 9.3), but usually includes a broad band of wavelengths. Thus, it may stretch across the UVC, UVB, UVA and visible light wavelengths in some (Harber *et al.*, 1963), although in most, it is confined to UVA or visible light regions or both (Hasei and Ichihashi, 1982; Horio, 1978; Kojima *et al.*, 1986; Ramsay, 1977). The minimal urticaria doses elicited are usually small, generally equating to sun exposure over only a few minutes.

An unusual feature of some SU is the presence of a band of inhibiting radiation, the usual activating wavelengths in such patients being in the UVA or short visible region and the inhibiting ones in the longer visible

Table 9.3   Synopsis of phototest results in solar urticaria

Sex, age	Action spectrum (nm)	MUD (J/cm²)	Inhibition spectrum (nm)	Plasma/ serum factor	Distribution of weals
F, 30	Vis 400–800	5.0	n.d.	n.d.	Generalized
F, 69	Vis 400–520	40.0	–	Positive	Generalized
M, 22	Vis 400–500	0.8	–	Positive	Generalized
M, 17	Vis 400–500	3.0	320–400	Positive	Generalized
M, 47	Vis 400–430	20.0	–	Negative	Generalized
	UVA 330–400	6.0			
F, 21	Vis 400–560	n.d.	–	n.d.	Fixed
	UVA 330–400	2.0			
M, 55	Vis 400–700	7.0	280–320	Positive	Fixed
	UVA 330–400	5.0			
F, 51	Vis 400–585	10.0	n.d.	Positive	Fixed
	UVA 330–400	3.0			
M, 36	Vis 580 ± 10	0.4	–	Negative	Generalized
	UVA 360 ± 10	0.1			
	UVB 300 ± 5	0.01			
	UVC 250 ± 5	0.01			
F, 40	UVA 330–400	0.5	–	Positive	Generalized
	UVB 280–320	0.0025			
F, 41	UVA 360 ± 5	1.0	n.d.	n.d.	Generalized
	UVB 300 ± 5	0.0015			
	UVC 250 ± 5	0.01			
M, 25	UVA 360 ± 5	0.025	n.d.	n.d.	Generalized
	UVB 300 ± 5	0.001			
	UVC 250 ± 5	0.01			

n.d., not investigated; MUD, minimal urticaria dose; vis, visible light range (Hasei and Ichihashi, 1982; Horio *et al.*, 1984; Ichihashi *et al.*, 1985a); however, two patients have had inhibition spectra shorter than the eliciting one (Leenutaphong, 1993; Leenutaphong *et al.*, 1988b, 1991) (Table 9.4). In most patients such inhibition occurs only if the skin is activated and inhibited simultaneously or consecutively in that order (Hasei and Ichihashi, 1982; Horio *et al.*, 1984; Ichihashi *et al.*, 1985a; Leenutaphong *et al.*, 1988b), but exceptionally inhibition by pre-irradiation has been reported (Ichihashi *et al.*, 1985a; Torinuki and Tagani, 1986); inhibitory effects can also be produced by the *in vitro* irradiation of patient serum or plasma and its subsequent injection into patient skin (Leenutaphong *et al.*, 1988b). A likely mechanism is that photoallergen is first generated by the SU-inducing wavelengths and then broken down by the inhibiting ones, rather than there being any interaction with allergen precursor (Horio *et al.*, 1984; Leenutaphong *et al.*, 1988b); however, the mechanism of inhibition by preirradiation remains unknown. An enhancement or augmentation of SU by wavelengths other than the inducing spectrum has also been described, wealing

Table 9.4 Action, inhibition and augmentation spectra (nm)

Author, year	Action spectrum	Inhibition spectrum	Augmentation spectrum
Hasei *et al.* 1982	400–500	> 503	
Torinuki *et al.* 1983	400–500	> 660	
Horio *et al.* 1984	400–500	> 530	
Leenutaphong *et al.* 1988b	400–500	320–400	
Leenutaphong 1993	320–400	400–460	
Reinauer *et al.* 1993	320–700	280–320	
Horio and Fujigaki 1988	320–420		450–500

elicited by the visible wavelengths being increased by UVA irradiation (Horio and Fujigaki, 1988); such an augmentation spectrum presumably increases photoallergenic activity.

MECHANISMS OF TOLERANCE DEVELOPMENT

In most physical urticarias, including SU, tolerance, namely a temporary decrease in the wealing response, may be induced by repeated cutaneous exposure to the inducing stimulus (Ramsay, 1977). The mechanism by which such tolerance develops is not fully understood, but simple explanations would be the occurrence of end-organ fatigue against histamine or complete degranulation of mast cells with exhaustion of their mediator reserves; however, these seem not to be responsible. Thus, if histamine or histamine-releasing agents (e.g. substance 48/80, codeine) are injected into tolerant skin, the weal and flare responses are as for non-tolerant skin (Keahey *et al.*, 1984; Leenutaphong *et al.*, 1990), while ultrastructural studies (Behrendt *et al.*, 1989; Keaney *et al.*, 1984) have also demonstrated that mast cells in tolerant skin still contain histamine. Further, *in vitro*-irradiated activated plasma or serum containing photoallergen produces wealing in unexposed patient skin but not at tolerant sites, thus also proving tolerance is not due to cutaneous photoallergen exhaustion (Leenutaphong *et al.*, 1990). In addition, repeated injections of *in vitro*-irradiated activated serum or plasma also induce tolerance to irradiation, but again not to intradermal codeine or substance 48/80. Thus, the likely mechanism of tolerance development in SU is not elevation of the mast cell degranulation threshold by their direct irradiation, as proposed by Keahey *et al.* (1984), but rather mast cell IgE-binding site blocking by photoallergen until new IgE is generated. Table 9.5 outlines a set of experiments confirming this notion.

TREATMENT

As soon as irradiation ceases, wealing in SU spontaneously fades. More useful, however, is the prevention of such wealing and the choice of treatment and response to it depend on two main factors, namely the patient SU action spectrum and the severity of patient wealing as expressed by the minimal urticarial dose.

PHOTOPROTECTION BY CLOTHING AND SUNSCREENS

Photoprotection by the use of appropriate clothing or highly protective sunscreening preparations is theoretically possible but rarely helpful in practice. Thus, absorbent chemical sunscreens are of little value in view of their relative narrow spectrum of efficacy compared with the usually broad SU action spectrum, reaching frequently into the visible light region, and the often exquisite photosensitivity of the disease, while the broader spectrum reflectant preparations are little better and usually cosmetically unsatisfactory as well. Hence the effective use of sunscreens is generally limited to patients with a relatively narrow SU action spectrum in the UVB or short UVA ranges combined with only mild photosensitivity.

SYSTEMIC MEDICATION

Reports on the effectiveness of systemic medications in SU are equivocal. Thus, there are sporadic observations of benefit from antimalarial drug therapy (Hasei and Ichihashi, 1982), perhaps not borne out by experience, while indomethacin and β-carotene have been disappointing (Horio, 1978; Kobza et al., 1973). On the other hand, H1 receptor antagonist antihistamines clearly provide protection to some degree, only modest (Michell et al., 1980) with the earlier sedating preparations but much greater, helping the majority of patients, with modern high-potency, non-sedative products such as terfenadine (Diffey et al., 1984; Ferguson, 1988; Reinauer et al., 1993). However, only the weal and flare, not the immediate erythema, were suppressed by this drug, although astemizole, another highly potent H1 receptor antagonist, appears to have suppressed the erythema as well (Monfrecola et al., 1990; Reinauer et al., 1993). Further studies are now needed to determine the efficacy of even newer antihistamines of this type. In our experience, however, all antihistamines fail in highly photosensitive patients, although they may be helpful in combination with other therapies; patients with low or moderate photosensitivity may, on the other hand, respond. Recent reports

Table 9.5 Experimental investigations on mechanism of tolerance

Mode of inducing tolerance	Type of challenge	Result
Eliciting radiation	Eliciting radiation	No response
Eliciting radiation	Histamine	Wealing
Eliciting radiation	Codeine	Wealing
Eliciting radiation	*In vitro*-irradiated patients' plasma*	No response
In vitro-irradiated patients' plasma*	*In vitro*-irradiated patients' plasma*	No response
In vitro-irradiated patients' plasma*	Eliciting radiation	No response
In vitro-irradiated patients' plasma*	Codeine	Wealing

*In most patients serum can also be used

of occasional life-threatening cardiac arrhythmias with high-dose terfenadine and astemizole necessitate great care in their use (Bernhard, 1993), although the new drug, fexofenadine, as yet untried in SU, may be safe in this respect.

PHOTOTHERAPY AND PHOTOCHEMOTHERAPY

The induction of tolerance by recurrent sunlight exposure is a well-known feature of some SU (Duke, 1923) and a similar outcome from phototherapy offers some patients a means of treatment. This may be repeated by patient exposure to narrow-band UVB (Collins and Ferguson, 1995), broad-band UVB (Kalimo and Jansen, 1986), broad-band UVA (Bernhard *et al.*, 1984) or a combination of UVB and UVA; in rare cases visible light has also been used (Diffey and Farr, 1988). As a prerequisite for successful treatment of this sort, the wavelengths used must include the patient's action spectrum, but therapeutic efficacy is usually short-lived, often for less than 72 hours, thus necessitating further treatment before the end of this period (Bernhard *et al.*, 1984; Ramsay, 1977). However, in selected patients this therapy, sometimes combined with antihistamine medication, may be very helpful, as demonstrated by Rubin *et al.* as early as 1947.

Psoralen photochemotherapy (PUVA) is superior to the tolerance induction described above, often providing protection lasting for several weeks (Hölzle *et al.*, 1980; Plewig *et al.*, 1986). It is probably the treatment of choice and was first introduced by Ramsay *et al.* in 1970, who used 8-methoxypsoralen in combination with natural sunlight. From 1980 (Hölzle *et al.*, 1980; Parrish *et al.*, 1982), however, artificial sources in combination with the psoralen medication have been employed, sometimes in a modified regimen proposed by Roelandts (1985) incorporating a tolerance induction procedure before the PUVA. In this, multiple partial-body or subthreshold whole-body exposures induce complete tolerance, before PUVA is carried out following standard techniques, a procedure generally eliminating the cumbersome initial treatment phase and shortening the PUVA course. The mechanism by which PUVA exerts its effects is unknown, but since patients reacting to visible light alone fail to respond to UVA phototherapy (Bernhard *et al.*, 1984) and do respond to PUVA (Plewig *et al.*, 1986) and since the PUVA protective effect lasts markedly longer than that of UVA alone, other mechanisms than tolerance induction appear involved. Thus, photoprotection by pigment formation and thickening of the stratum corneum, immunosuppression and perhaps the downregulation of IgE production may play a role; certainly in atopic patients, UVB irradiation decreases plasma IgE levels (Barlag *et al.*, 1991). On the other hand, UVA and UVB irradiation decrease normal mast cell histamine release *in vivo* after codeine challenge (Gollhausen *et al.*, 1985) and direct mast cell effects may thus also be important.

PLASMAPHERESIS

The rationale for the use of plasmapheresis (Table 9.6) in SU is the elimination of putative photoallergen from patient plasma. However, experimental evidence is sparse, few treated patients having been reported (Duschet *et al.*, 1987, 1989; Leenutaphong *et al.*, 1991), but the procedure appears effective only in patients demonstrating a serum factor. Even then, most experience only a partial and transient remission, while just two have remained completely free of symptoms. Nevertheless, a protocol employing plasmapheresis followed by PUVA has also been proposed (Hudson-Peacock *et al.*, 1993), its hypothetical mechanism of action perhaps being the elimination of photoallergen, followed by the induction of photoprotection and downregulation of cutaneous and systemic immunological reactivity.

Table 9.6   Plasmapheresis for treatment of solar urticaria

Author	Patient age, sex	Serum factor	Therapeutic effect Immediate	2 months
Leenutaphong *et al.* (1991)	17, M	Present	+++	+++
Duschet *et al.* (1987)	41, F	Present	+++	+++
Leenutaphong *et al.* (1991)	49, F	Present	++	—
Unpublished	40, F	Present	++	n.d.
Leenutaphong *et al.* (1991)	36, M	Absent	—	—
Duschet *et al.* (1989)	39, F	Absent	—	—

REFERENCES

Armstrong, R.B. (1986) Solar urticaria. *Dermatologic Clinics*, **4**, 253–9.

Armstrong, R.B., Horan, D.B. and Silver, D.N. (1985) Leukocytoclastic vasculitis in urticaria induced by ultraviolet irradiation. *Archives of Dermatology*, **121**, 1145–8.

Barlag, K., Hölzle, E., Schürer, N. and Goerz, G. (1991) UVB-phototherapy reduces total serum IgE levels in patients with atopic dermatitis. *Archives of Dermatology Research*, **283**, 23–4.

Behrendt, H., Lehmann, P., Leenutaphong, V., Hölzle, E. and Plewig, G. (1989) Sequential ultrastructural analysis of solar urticaria: inflammatory cells, blood vessels, and nerve fibers. *Journal of Investigative Dermatology*, **92**, 400 (A).

Beljaards, R.C. and Bruynzeel, D.P. (1991) Solar urticaria and disturbed metabolism of porphyrins. *Dermatologica*, **182**, 231–2.

Bernhard, J.D. (1993) Treatment of solar urticaria with terfenadine. *Journal of the American Academy of Dermatology*, **28**(10), 668.

Bernhard, J.D., Jaenicke, K., Momtaz, T.K. and Parrish, J.A. (1984) Ultraviolet A phototherapy in the prophylaxis of solar urticaria. *Journal of the American Academy of Dermatology*, **10**, 29–33.

Bilsland, D. and Ferguson, J. (1991) A comparison of cetirizine and terfenadine in the management of solar urticaria. *Photodermatology, Photoimmunology and Photomedicine*, **8**, 62–4.

Collins, P. and Ferguson, J. (1995) Narrow-band UVB (TL-01) phototherapy: an effective preventative treatment for the photodermatoses. *British Journal of Dermatology*, **132**, 956–63.

Crow, K.D., Alexander, E., Buck, W.H.L. *et al.* (1961) Photosensitivity due to pitch. *British Journal of Dermatology*, **73**, 220–32.

Diffey, B.L. and Farr, P.M. (1988) Treatment of solar urticaria with terfenadine. *Photodermatology*, **5**, 25–9.

Diffey, B.L., Farr, P.M. and Ive, F.A. (1984) Home phototherapy of solar urticaria. *Photodermatology*, **1**, 145–6.

Duke, W.W. (1923) Urticaria caused by light. *Journal of the American Medical Association*, **80**, 1835–8.

Duschet, P., Leyen, P., Schwarz, T. *et al.* (1987) Solar urticaria: effective treatment by plasmapheresis. *Clinical and Experimental Dermatology*, **12**, 185–8.

Duschet, P., Schwarz, T. and Gschnait, F. (1989) Plasmapherese bei Lichturtikaria. Ein rationales Therapiekonzept in Fällen mit nachgewiesenem Serumfaktor. *Hautarzt*, **40**, 553–5.

Epstein, J.H., Vandenberg, J.J. and Wright, W.L. (1963) Solar urticaria. *Archives of Dermatology*, **88**, 135–41.

Epstein, S. (1949) Urticaria photogenica: report of two cases, one of them associated with purpura photogenica. *Annals of Allergy*, **7**, 443–57.

Ferguson, J. (1988) Idiopathic solar urticaria: natural history and response to non-sedative antihistamine therapy. A study of 26 cases. *British Journal of Dermatology*, **119** (suppl 33), 16.

Frain-Bell, W. (1985) Drug induced photosensitivity: benoxaprofen, in *Cutaneous Photobiology*, (ed. W. Frain-Bell), Oxford University Press, Oxford, pp. 136–9.

Gollhausen, R., Kaidbey, K. and Schechter, N. (1985) UV suppression of mast cell-mediated wealing in human skin. *Photodermatology*, **2**, 58–67.

Harber, L.C., Holloway, R.M., Wheatley, V.R. and Baer, R.L. (1963) Immunologic and biophysical studies in solar urticaria. *Journal of Investigative Dermatology*, **41**, 439–43.

Hasei, K. and Ichihashi, M. (1982) Solar urticaria: determinations of action and inhibition spectra. *Archives of Dermatology*, **118**, 346–50.

Hawk, J.L.M., Eady, R.A.J., Challoner, A.V.J. *et al.* (1980) Elevated blood histamine levels and mast cell degranulation in solar urticaria. *British Journal of Clinical Pharmacology*, **9**, 183–6.

Hölzle, E., Hofmann, C. and Plewig, G. (1980) PUVA-treatment for solar urticaria and persistent light reaction. *Archives of Dermatology Research*, **269**, 87–91.

Hölzle, E., Plewig, G. and Lehmann, P. (1987) Photodermatoses – diagnostic procedures and their interpretation. *Photodermatology*, **4**, 109–14.

Horio, T. (1975) Chlorpromazine photoallergy: coexistence of immediate and delayed type. *Archives of Dermatology*, **111**, 1469–71.

Horio, T. (1978) Photoallergic urticaria induced by visible light: additional cases and further studies. *Archives of Dermatology*, **114**, 1761–4.

Horio, T. (1987) Solar urticaria – sun, skin and serum. *Photodermatology*, **4**, 115–17.

Horio, T. and Fujigaki, K. (1988) Augmentation spectrum in solar urticaria. *Journal of the American Academy of Dermatology*, **18**, 1189–93.

Horio, T. and Minami, K. (1977) Solar urticaria: photoallergen in a patient's serum. *Archives of Dermatology*, **113**, 157–60.

Horio, T., Yoshioka, A. and Okamoto, H. (1984) Production and inhibition of solar urticaria by light exposure. *Journal of the American Academy of Dermatology*, **11**, 1094–9.

Hudson-Peacock, M.J., Farr, P.M., Diffey, B.L. and Goodship, T.H. (1993) Combined treatment of solar urticaria with plasmapheresis and PUVA. *British Journal of Dermatology*, **128**(4), 440–2.

Ichihashi, M., Hasei, K. and Hayashibe, K. (1985a) Solar urticaria: further studies on the role of inhibition spectra. *Archives of Dermatology*, **112**, 503–7.

Ichihashi, M., Hasei, K. and Horikawa, T.A. (1985b) A case of porphyria cutanea tarda with experimental light urticaria. *British Journal of Dermatology*, **113**, 745–50.

Illig, I. and Born, W. (1964) Untersuchungen zur Pathogenese der Lichturticaria. *Archives of Dermatological Research*, **220**, 19–37.

Kalimo, K. and Jansen, C. (1986) Severe solar urticaria: active and passive action spectra and hyposensitizing effect of different UV modalities. *Photodermatology*, **3**, 194–5.

Keahey, T.M., Webster, G.F., Kaidbey, K.H. *et al.* (1982) Photourticaria from Benoxaprofen. *Journal of Investigative Dermatology*, **78**, 355.

Keahey, T.M., Lavker, R.M., Kaidbey, K.H., Atkins, P.C. and Zweiman, B. (1984) Studies on the mechanism of clinical tolerance in solar urticaria. *British Journal of Dermatology*, **110**, 327–38.

Kobza, A., Ramsay, C.A. and Magnus, I.A. (1973) Oral beta-carotene therapy in actinic reticuloid and solar urticaria. Failure to demonstrate a photoprotective effect against long wave ultraviolet and visible radiation. *British Journal of Dermatology*, **88**, 157–66.

Kojima, M., Horiko, T., Nakamura, Y. and Aoki, T. (1986) Solar urticaria: relationship of photoallergen and action spectrum. *Archives of Dermatology*, **122**, 550–5.

Kurumaji, Y. and Shono, M. (1994) Drug-induced solar urticaria due to repirinast. *Dermatology*, **188**, 117–21.

Leenutaphong, V. (1993) Solar urticaria induced by UVA and inhibited by visible light. *Journal of the American Academy of Dermatology*, **29**, 337–40.

Leenutaphong, V., Hölzle, E. and Plewig, G. (1988a) Evidence for an epidermal photoallergen in solar urticaria. *Journal of Investigative Dermatology*, **91**, 408.

Leenutaphong, V., Hölzle, E. and Plewig, G. (1988b) Solar urticaria induced by visible light and inhibition by UVA. *Photodermatology*, **5**, 170–4.

Leenutaphong, V., Hölzle, E. and Plewig, G. (1989) Pathomechanism and classification of solar urticaria: a new concept. *Journal of the American Academy of Dermatology*, **21**, 237–40.

Leenutaphong, V., Hölzle, E. and Plewig, G. (1990) Solar urticaria: study on mechanisms of tolerance. *British Journal of Dermatology*, **122**, 601–6.

Leenutaphong, V., Hölzle, E., Plewig, G., Kutkuhn, B. and Grabensee, B. (1991) Plasmapheresis in solar urticaria. *Dermatologica*, **182**, 35–8.

Leiferman, K.M., Norris, P.G., Murphy, G.M., Hawk, J.L. and Winkelmann, R.K. (1989) Evidence for eosinophil degranulation with deposition of granule major basic protein in solar urticaria. *Journal of the American Academy of Dermatology*, **21**, 75–80.

Lovell, C.R., Cronin, E. and Rhodes, E.L. (1986) Photocontact urticaria from chlorpromazine. *Contact Dermatitis*, **14**, 290–1.

Merklen, P. (1904) Urticae, in *La Pratique Dermatologique*, (eds E. Besnièr, L. Brocq and L. Jacquet), Masson, Paris, pp. 728 71.

Michell, P., Hawk, J.L.M., Shafir, A., Corbett, M.F. and Magnus, I.A. (1980) Assessing the treatment of solar urticaria. The dose-response as a quantifying approach. *Dermatologica*, **160**, 198–207.

Monfrecola, G., Nappa, P. and Pini, D. (1988) Solar urticaria with delayed onset: a case report. *Photodermatology*, **5**, 103–4.

Monfrecola, G., Nappa, P. and Pini, D. (1990) Solar urticaria in the visible spectrum successfully treated with astemizole. *Dermatologica*, **180**, 154–6.

Murphy, G.M. and Hawk, J.L.M. (1987) Broadening of action spectrum in a patient with solar urticaria. *Clinical and Experimental Dermatology*, **12**, 455–6.

Norris, P.G., Murphy, G.M., Hawk, J.L.M. and Winkelmann, R.K. (1988) A histological study of the evolution of solar urticaria. *Archives of Dermatology*, **124**, 80–3.

Parrish, J.A., Jaenicke, K.F., Morison, W.L., Momtaz, K. and Shea, C. (1982) Solar urticaria: treatment with PUVA and mediator inhibitors. *British Journal of Dermatology*, **106**, 575–80.

Plewig, G., Wolff, H.H. and Hölzle, E. (1980) Solar urticaria: immunoelectron microscopic study of leukocytoclastic vasculitis. *Archives of Dermatology Research*, **267**, 209.

Plewig, G., Hölzle, E. and Lehmann, P. (1986) Phototherapy for photodermatoses, in *Therapeutic Photomedicine*, (eds H. Hönigsmann and G. Stingl), Karger, Basel, pp. 254–64.

Polano, G. (1948) Urticaria solaris. *Dermatologica*, **97**, 327–8.

Rajatanavin, N. and Bernhard, J.D. (1987) Solar urticaria: treatment with terfenadine. *Journal of the American Academy of Dermatology*, **18**, 574.

Rajka, E. (1942) Passive transfer in light urticaria. *Journal of Allergy and Clinical Immunology*, **13**, 327–45.

Ramsay, C.A. (1977) Solar urticaria treatment by inducing tolerance to artificial radiation and natural light. *Archives of Dermatology*, **113**, 1222–5.

Ramsay, C.A., Scrimenti, R.J. and Cripps, D.J. (1970) Ultraviolet and visible action spectrum in a case of solar urticaria. *Archives of Dermatology*, **101**, 520–3.

Rantanen, T. and Suhonen, R. (1980) Solar urticaria: a case with increased skin mast cells and good therapeutic response to an antihistamine. *Acta Dermato-venereologica (Stockholm)*, **60**, 363–5.

Ravits, M., Armstrong, R.B. and Harber, L.C. (1982) Solar urticaria: clinical features and wavelength dependence. *Archives of Dermatology*, **118**, 228–31.

Reinauer, S., Leenutaphong, V. and Hölzle, E. (1993) Fixed solar urticaria. *Journal of the American Academy of Dermatology*, **29**, 161–5.

Roelandts, R. (1985) Pre-PUVA UVA desensitization for solar urticaria. *Photodermatology*, **2**, 174–6.

Rubin, L., Beal, P.L. and Rothman, S. (1947) A method for protection of patients with solar urticaria. *Journal of Investigative Dermatology*, **8**, 189.

Sams, W.M. (1970) Solar urticaria: studies of the active serum factor. *Journal of Allergy*, **45**, 295–301.

Sams, W.M., Epstein, J.H. and Winkelmann, R.K. (1969) Solar urticaria. Investigation of pathogenetic mechanisms. *Archives of Dermatology*, **99**, 390–7.

Soter, N.A., Wassermann, S.L., Pathak, M.A. *et al.* (1979) Solar urticaria: release of mast cell mediators into the circulation after experimental challenge. *Journal of Investigative Dermatology*, **72**, 282.

Stevanovic, D.V. (1960) Urticaria solaris. A clinical and experimental study. *Acta Medica Yugoslavia*, **14**, 144–53.

Torinuki, W. and Tagami, H. (1986) Solar urticaria without inhibitory spectrum: demonstration of both circulating photoallergen and reaginic antibodies. *Dermatologica*, **173**, 116–19.

Torinuki, W., Kumai, N. and Miura, T. (1983) Solar urticaria inhibited by visible light. *Dermatologica*, **166**, 151–5.

Van Hecke, E. (1979) Solar urticaria. *Archives of Dermatology*, **115**, 759.

Ward, S.B. (1905) Erythema and urticaria with a condition resembling angioneurotic edema caused by exposure to sun's rays. *New York Medical Journal*, **81**, 742–3.

Willis, I. and Epstein, J.H. (1974) Solar- vs heat-induced urticaria. *Archives of Dermatology*, **110**, 389–92.

Wucherpfennig, V. (1928) Pathologische Lichtüberempfindlichkeit in qualitativer und quantitativer Hinsicht, nebst Untersuchungen zur Pathogenese der Lichtquaddel. *Archiv für Dermatologie u. Syphilis*, **156**, 520–44.

Hélène du P. Menagé and John L.M. Hawk

EVOLUTION OF THE TERM CHRONIC ACTINIC DERMATITIS

The term chronic actinic dermatitis (CAD), originally coined by Hawk and Magnus (1979), is now precisely synonymous with the term photosensitivity dermatitis/actinic reticuloid syndrome (PD/AR), as proposed by Frain-Bell and colleagues (1974), and in fact encompasses four diagnoses, namely persistent light reactivity (reaction) (Wilkinson, 1962), actinic reticuloid (Ive *et al.*, 1969), photosensitive eczema (Ramsay and Kobza-Black, 1973) and photosensitivity dermatitis (Frain-Bell *et al.*, 1974), all originally described as distinct conditions but now accepted as variants of CAD. As a result the four latter terms, although explained for clarity below, are no longer in general use.

Persistent light reactivity (PLR) was first described by Wilkinson in 1962 and referred to a continuing eczema of the light-exposed sites following an apparently completed episode of topical photoallergic contact dermatitis. This disorder then remained despite avoidance of the original photocontact allergen and irrespective of whether the affected sites

had previously been exposed to allergen. The wavelengths responsible for the induction of such lesions lay not only in the UVA (315–400 nm) waveband, generally responsible for photoallergenic responses, but extended into the UVB (280–315 nm) wavelengths as well, thereby fulfilling the requirements later defined for CAD. PLR has been reported to develop following photoallergic contact sensitization to halogenated phenols (tetrachlorsalicylanilide and tribromosalicylanilide) (Wilkinson, 1962), to certain antibacterial agents used in soaps, antiseptics and toiletries in the 1960s and early 1970s (Fentichlor and bithionol) (Jillson and Baughman, 1963), and to the fragrance musk ambrette, a synthetic musk formerly used widely in aftershave preparations. As a result, these products have now been withdrawn, after which only a few isolated cases of PLR have been reported following patient contact sensitization to quinoxaline-N-dioxide in animal foodstuffs (Zaynoun *et al.*, 1976), to zinc pyrithione (Yates and Finn, 1980) and to certain bleaching agents (Burckhardt, 1957). Generally speaking, however, the disorder now appears to be vanishingly rare.

Actinic reticuloid was first referred to by Ive *et al.* in 1969, its clinical hallmark being

Photodermatology. Edited by J.L.M. Hawk. Published in 1998 by Chapman & Hall, London. ISBN 0 412 72460 X.

infiltrated erythematous, hence reticuloid, plaques arising on a base of eczematous, erythematous or normal skin in elderly males; in addition, the histopathological features were similar to those of cutaneous T-cell lymphoma (CTCL). A clinical likeness to the appearance of severe photoallergic contact dermatitis was noted, but photopatch tests were generally negative and the eruption was found to be inducible by UVB, UVA and sometimes visible irradiation as may also occur in CAD. Such infiltrated disease is still observed from time to time as part of the CAD spectrum, but its frequency appears to have diminished; a heightened clinical awareness of the condition has probably led to its much earlier diagnosis and treatment before its severe forms can develop.

Photosensitive eczema, first noted by Ramsay and Kobza-Black in 1973, referred to an eczematous eruption of the exposed areas, also with no preceding photoallergy. Some features of actinic reticuloid were also observed in a few patients but the action spectrum differed and was largely in the UVB region alone.

Photosensitivity dermatitis, originally reported by Frain-Bell and colleagues (1974), also described an eczematous eruption of the exposed areas but with photosensitivity often also extending to include the UVA wavelengths.

In 1979, however, Hawk and Magnus showed that there was significant overlap between the features of photosensitive eczema and actinic reticuloid, describing patients with the clinical and histological changes of eczema and the photobiological abnormalities of actinic reticuloid. They also noted that transitions could be observed between these disease states (Frain-Bell *et al.*, 1974; Hawk and Magnus, 1978) and therefore unified all the variants of what appeared to be the same condition within the term CAD. More recently, it has also been observed that a transition occurs from PLR to actinic reticuloid (Horio, 1982) and that there may be overlap between PLR and the CAD spectrum. In 1990, it was therefore proposed that PLR should also be encompassed within the term CAD (Lim *et al.*, 1990; Norris and Hawk, 1990), thus making the terms PLR, actinic reticuloid, photosensitive eczema and photosensitivity dermatitis of predominantly historical interest. In addition, the introduction of unifying diagnostic criteria has led to a better understanding of the condition and facilitated its recognition (Lim *et al.*, 1990; Mude *et al.*, 1991; Roelandts, 1993). Thus CAD is an eczema of the exposed areas induced by UVB, sometimes also UVA and occasionally by visible light as well.

CLINICAL ASPECTS

PREDISPOSING OR ASSOCIATED FEATURES (TABLE 10.1)

CAD is an uncommon but possibly underdiagnosed condition, unpublished observations in the Tayside region of Scotland estimating its incidence at 1:6000 (Ferguson, 1990); males are more often affected, women making up only 10% (Ferguson, 1990) to 22% (Menagé *et al.*, 1995b) of all sufferers. In addition, patients are generally middle aged to elderly with an average age of 65 years (Menagé *et al.*, 1995b),

Table 10.1   Factors predisposing to or associated with CAD

Male sex

Increasing age

Outdoor activities

Human immunodeficiency virus infection (probable)

Atopic eczema (early-onset disease)

Allergic contact dermatitis

Topical photoallergic contact dermatitis (previously known as persistent light reactivity; now rarely observed, if at all)

Systemic drug photosensitivity (controversial)

sufferers under 50 years of age being exceptional apart from a few with co-existent atopic eczema (Kurumaji *et al.*, 1994), and of white Caucasian race, although Japanese (Horio, 1982), Afro-Caribbeans (Kingston *et al.*, 1987; Menagé *et al.*, 1995b) and Asians (Menagé *et al.*, 1995b) may also be affected. However, there is also a suggestion of geographical variation in the incidence of CAD, the peak incidence perhaps occurring in more temperate climates. Familial incidence is not reported. Outdoor workers, particularly gardeners, appear most likely to be affected, very likely because they are simultaneously exposed at length to both sunlight and apparently predisposing allergens. CAD has also occasionally been observed in patients previously treated with potentially photosensitizing systemic drugs such as thiazide diuretics (Robinson *et al.*, 1985), but since the intake of potentially photosensitizing medication is common in the affected age group, it remains unclear whether such systemic agents predispose to the disorder. CAD has further been reported in association with human immunodeficiency (HIV) virus infection and predating the onset of acquired immune deficiency syndrome (AIDS)-defining disorders; however, the mechanisms for this are not understood (Pappert *et al.*, 1994).

Allergic contact dermatitis to ubiquitous allergens frequently co-exists with CAD (Ferguson, 1990) and may precede the development of photosensitivity (Murphy *et al.*, 1990) or complicate its management. Thus, positive responses to one or more allergens are found consistently in about 75% of patients (Menagé *et al.*, 1995b; Frain-Bell, 1986; Hannuksela *et al.*, 1981) and to two or more in 65% (Menagé *et al.*, 1995b), the main culprits being Compositae plant extracts and to a lesser extent fragrance compounds, colophony, metals and rubber and occasionally epoxy resins, phosphorus sesquisulphide, medicaments, preservatives and vehicle bases (Addo *et al.*, 1982, 1985; Menagé *et al.*, 1995b; Frain-Bell *et al.*, 1979; Green *et al.*, 1991; Hannuksela *et al.*, 1981; Thune, 1977); rarely, contact

dermatitis to sunscreen constituents also develops during the course of the disease (Green *et al.*, 1991). These reactions have been shown to be persistent and reproducible, not simply representing an increased cutaneous reactivity in association with the disease (Addo and Frain-Bell, 1987). Photoallergic contact dermatitis is also historically associated with CAD, the condition known as PLR having been reported to evolve from this. Finally, a proportion of patients with CAD, including those with associated contact and photocontact allergies, have a history of endogenous eczema such as, for example, the atopic, palmar and plantar forms (Ramsay and Kobza-Black, 1973). Thus, in our experience, only 12% of patients have neither associated contact or photocontact allergies, nor endogenous eczema (Menagé *et al.*, 1995b).

CLINICAL FEATURES

Although CAD is generally worse in the spring and summer months, its relationship to ultraviolet exposure is not always evident to the patient or physician. Thus worsening of the eruption may not be apparent for hours to days following exposure, while the condition may also persist into the winter months, become generalized or be complicated by the associated features of contact dermatitis. Classic cases show chronic or subacute eczema, predominantly of the light-exposed sites, most notably the face, back and sides of the neck, upper chest, scalp and backs of the hands, characteristically with a clear cut-off where clothing begins (Plates 9, 10, 11). In addition, the upper eyelids, submental area, skin protected by the earlobes, skin creases and finger webs (Plate 12) are often but not always spared. In patients with severe disease, the eruption frequently spreads to affect the covered areas as well and erythroderma may sometimes develop (Plate 13). Lichenification is often observed in chronic cases while in more severely affected patients, infiltrated papules and plaques mimicking those of cutaneous lymphoma may develop (Ive *et al.*, 1969) (Plate 14); palmar and occasionally plantar eczema may also be a feature. Further, areas of hyper- or hypopigmentation may sometimes occur during the course of the disease, the latter occasionally closely resembling widespread vitiligo and having been attributed to the cytotoxic destruction of melanocytes (von den Driesch *et al.*, 1992), while the loss of eyebrow and scalp hair may occur through rubbing or scratching and scalp hair may perhaps become grey prematurely.

CRITERIA FOR DIAGNOSIS (TABLE 10.2)

The diagnosis of chronic actinic dermatitis is suggested by the clinical findings, supported where necessary by the histological features of eczema, sometimes pseudolymphomatous in severe cases (Plate 15), while the irradiation phototesting of unaffected skin with broad-band or monochromatic irradiation is virtually always abnormal. Very rarely, such phototest abnormalities appear not to become manifest for some months after onset of the disorder, such that retesting may be advisable in patients with clinically suggestive disease.

Thus, there is a reduction in the minimum ultraviolet dose required to induce an erythemal response at 24 hours and the response is often of abnormal morphology, demonstrating papular or eczematous lesions characteristic of the disease itself (Frain-Bell *et al.*, 1974) (Plate 16). Further, virtually all patients react abnormally to the UVB wavelengths and the majority also the UVA; a minority respond to the visible wavelengths as well (Menagé *et al.*, 1995b; Frain-Bell *et al.*, 1974). Occasionally, however, abnormalities have been reported to the UVA wavelengths alone and such cases, although not fulfilling the original diagnostic criteria (Hawk and Magnus, 1979; Norris and Hawk, 1990), are now increasingly but still rarely being suggested to occur in otherwise typical CAD (Healy and Rogers, 1995; Lim *et al.*, 1994).

DIFFERENTIAL DIAGNOSIS (TABLE 10.3)

Contact dermatitis, particularly to airborne allergens, and photocontact dermatitis may closely mimic CAD, but are distinguished by their normal monochromatic irradiation tests; however, both may also occur in association with CAD.

Table 10.2   Diagnosis of CAD

Clinical features	Mainly eczematous eruption of exposed areas, with or without cutaneous T-cell lymphoma-like features
Histology of lesional skin (not a prerequisite for diagnosis)	Chronic eczema, with or without cutaneous T-cell lymphoma-like changes
Phototest responses (essential for diagnosis)	*Irradiation monochromator*: reduction in 24-hour MED and exaggerated papular responses to UVB, usually UVA and rarely visible wavelengths; occasionally UVA alone seems possible instead *Broad-band source*: reduction in the 24-hour MED; induction of eczema is also possible
Patch and photopatch testing (essential ancillary investigation)	Abnormalities frequently detected, often to ubiquitous airborne allergens or topical medications
Blood, urine and faecal porphyrin concentrations	Normal
Antibodies to DNA, Ro (anti-SSA) and La (anti-SSB)	Not detected

Table 10.3 Differential diagnosis of CAD (modified from Arndt *et al. Cutaneous Medicine and Surgery: An Integrated Programme in Dermatology, Volume 1*, Table 87.3, W.B. Saunders)

Disease	Distinguishing features
Allergic or photoallergic contact dermatitis	Normal cutaneous irradiation tests in absence of antigen and abnormalities generally to UVA alone; eruption localized only to sites of photoallergen contact
Systemic drug-induced photosensitivity	Normal cutaneous irradiation tests or abnormalities usually to UVA alone. Resolution of clinical and photo-test abnormalities within six months of withdrawal of drug; eruption not usually eczematous
Light-exacerbated atopic eczema	Normal cutaneous irradiation tests; other features of atopic eczema
Light-exacerbated seborrhoeic eczema	Normal cutaneous irradiation tests; other features of seborrhoeic eczema
Erythroderma of non-CAD aetiology	Normal cutaneous irradiation tests, undertaken after erythroderma is settled
Cutaneous T-cell lymphoma	Normal cutaneous irradiation tests or only minor abnormalities, predominantly in UVA Predominance of CD4+ circulating lymphocytes, as against CD8+ in severe CAD Predominance of CD4+ lymphocytes in epidermis, as against CD8+ in CAD Discordance between CD3+ and BF1+ expression may be present T-cell receptor and immunoglobin gene rearrangement studies positive

Light-exacerbated atopic or seborrhoeic eczema (see Chapter 14) can also generally be distinguished clinically, but in more difficult cases, cutaneous irradiation tests are necessary, generally being normal or at most minimally abnormal in the light-exacerbated conditions. Again, both may occur in association with CAD. Erythrodermic CAD may be distinguished from other erythrodermas by the abnormal irradiation tests; in the former, however, clearance of the eruption in darkened conditions is necessary prior to testing to avoid false-negative responses.

Systemic drug-induced (see Chapter 12) photosensitivity may resemble CAD in demonstrating an erythema but generally not usually eczema of the light-exposed areas, but is associated with either normal cutaneous irradiation tests or abnormalities in the UVA range only. In addition, withdrawal of the drug generally results in steady resolution of the clinical and phototest abnormalities, generally within six months (Bilsland and Ferguson, 1991).

CTCL may also occasionally be clinically and histologically indistinguishable from severe CAD, whether erythrodermic or not, while some patients with the erythrodermic form may even have circulating Sézary cells (Neild *et al.*, 1982). However, lymphocyte morphometry by electron microscopy and image analysis generally distinguishes the reactive cells of CAD from the malignant ones in the Sézary syndrome (Preesman *et al.*, 1995). Further, the cutaneous irradiation tests are generally at most mildly positive in CTCL, principally to the UVA wavelengths (Volden and Thune, 1977), thus being out of keeping with the severity of the clinical disease. In difficult cases, however, the CD4+:CD8+ circulating lymphocyte ratio may be helpful in distinguishing the conditions, CD8+ cells being predominant in CAD, particularly the severe variants (Menagé *et al.*, 1992b), and CD4+ in CTCL (Chu *et al.*, 1986), while T-cell receptor gene studies may also be helpful, abnormalities having only been reported in CTCL. Finally, quantitative phenotypic analysis of the cutaneous T-cell infiltrate may also be of value, epidermal CD8+ predominance having again been reported in CAD and CD4+ in CTCL, while a discordance between CD3+ and BF-1 expression occurs in CTCL but not CAD (Heuer *et al.*, 1994). In spite of these differences between the conditions, however, there remain isolated reports of the development of cutaneous lymphoma in patients with CAD (Ashinoff *et al.*, 1989; Jensen and Sneddon, 1970; Meynardier *et al.*, 1984; Thestrup-Pedersen *et al.*, 1988; Thomsen, 1977) and it is as yet unclear whether these rarities are coincidental occurrences, confusions in diagnosis or causal associations. It has been suggested that an unrelenting cellular response to antigen, such as is postulated to occur in CAD, may predispose to CTCL (Tan *et al.*, 1974) but neither clinical (Ferguson, 1990) nor experimental evidence supports such a transformation as a regular phenomenon. Thus, a comparison of the incidence of CTCL in CAD patients with that obtained from sex-matched national morbidity data has not confirmed such an increased risk (Bilsland *et al.*, 1993), while a flow cytometric study showed no evidence of DNA aneuploidy in the cutaneous infiltrate of patients with CAD (Norris *et al.*, 1989), and T-cell receptor and immunoglobulin gene rearrangement studies likewise demonstrated no evidence of a clonal lymphoid population in the disorder (Menagé *et al.*, 1992b). Thus, if present at all, the risk of lymphomatous transformation in CAD must be extremely small.

MANAGEMENT (TABLE 10.4)

CAD is a severely disabling condition which before the introduction of immunosuppressive therapy was associated with significant psychological morbidity, leading on occasion even to suicide. Ultraviolet avoidance remains the cornerstone of management, although the longer, UVA wavelengths are still particularly difficult to protect against. Thus, outdoor exposure should be minimized, particularly during the middle of the day in summer when solar irradiance is high, and appropriately protective clothing should be worn in conjunction with the regular use of high sun protection factor sunscreens; non-irritant reflectant sunscreen preparations are generally preferable in view of the risk of irritation

Table 10.4   Management of CAD (modified from Arndt *et al. Cutaneous Medicine and Surgery: An Integrated Programme in Dermatology, Volume 1*, Table 87.3, W.B. Saunders)

1. All patients	Avoidance of exposure to inducing ultraviolet wavelengths through restriction of solar exposure when ultraviolet irradiance is high, use of suitably protective clothing, regular application of non-irritant, reflectant sunscreen preparations. Avoidance of associated contact or photocontact allergens. Regular use of emollients and topical corticosteroid preparations as adjunctive therapy.
2. Acute flares	Nursing in light-protected cubicles or inside with drawn blinds. Short-term oral corticosteroid therapy.
3. Resistant cases	Oral azathioprine 1–2.5 mg/kg/d. Oral cyclosporin 3.5–5 mg/kg/d. Therapy should be discontinued if possible in winter months. Oral psoralen photochemotherapy (PUVA) (with initial oral corticosteroid cover if necessary early on), gradually reducing in frequency as resolution supervenes.

and contact allergy to chemical preparations. Ultraviolet screening blinds in the home and car may also be helpful to limit solar UVA exposure further, while the avoidance of prolonged exposure to fluorescent lamps for room lighting is also necessary in sensitive subjects, although computer and television screens are safe (Moseley *et al.*, 1989). It is also essential to avoid potentially exacerbating contact allergens and any apparent worsening of CAD may be due to the development of new or additional contact or photocontact sensitivities, sunscreen allergy being particularly notorious in this regard (Green *et al.*, 1991).

Acute flares of CAD may require patient nursing in light-protected cubicles, an effective but time-consuming and costly measure thus generally available only in specialist units, while emollients and topical or short-term oral corticosteroids are generally helpful adjunctive therapy. However, care should be taken to stop oral and local topical corticosteroid therapy several days before patient phototesting to avoid any inhibition of the response (Lowe and Ferguson, 1989).

For severe, persistent or frequently relapsing disease, psoralen photochemotherapy (PUVA) or oral immunosuppressive therapy may also be required. PUVA may eventually be very effective but is often poorly tolerated in the early phases of treatment, even under systemic steroid cover, while maintenance therapy, possibly just to the light-exposed sites, is generally also required (Hindson *et al.*, 1984, 1990). The mode of action of such treatment is uncertain, but may well involve a modification of the cutaneous immune response, with some slight additional assistance perhaps from the induction of protective skin thickening and melanogenesis. Oral azathioprine, on the other hand, is often moderately effective, if tolerated, in doses of 1.0–2.5 mg/kg (Murphy *et al.*, 1989), as is cyclosporin A at 3.5–5.0 mg/kg (Norris *et al.*, 1989a), perhaps by preventing the clonal expansion of activated T cells through the inhibition of interleukins 1 and 2. Danazol

has also been reported to be effective on one occasion in a patient with associated α1-antitrypsin deficiency, but this awaits confirmation (Humbert *et al.*, 1991), while there are two isolated reports of the possible efficacy of α-interferon, which downregulates suppressor T cells (Parodi *et al.*, 1995). Although immunosuppressive therapy indeed appears to control the CAD inflammatory response, it seems unlikely that such treatments significantly modify the underlying photosensitivity; however, the therapy certainly improves the lot of many otherwise disabled sufferers.

OUTCOME

CAD is a persistent disorder, although occasional clinical improvement occurs, sometimes with continuing phototest abnormalities in spite of this (Ferguson, 1990). Nevertheless, careful management can generally allow the patient to maintain a satisfactory lifestyle, while long-term life expectancy is probably unaffected, except perhaps for the few with erythroderma (Sigurdsson *et al.*, 1996).

PATHOGENESIS

DISEASE SUSCEPTIBILITY

There is no evidence to date for a genetic susceptibility to the development of CAD. Thus, a positive family history is not reported in patients with the disease, while preliminary observations have also failed to reveal any significant HLA association (authors' unpublished observations). However, anecdotal evidence suggests that continuing solar and ambient allergen exposure may predispose to cutaneous sensitization to later ultraviolet irradiation in many patients, as suggested by a tendency for the condition to develop more readily in those with outdoor occupations or hobbies, while a report of onset after accidental UVC exposure suggests that any form of excessive ultraviolet exposure may be contributory (Roelandts and Huys, 1993).

Thus, environmental rather than significant genetic factors might largely explain why patients develop CAD, as well perhaps as the male and elderly predominance of the disorder.

NATURE OF THE RESPONSE

The clinical response of CAD to T-cell immunodulatory drugs supports an immunological basis for the disease, although it is unclear if this is a primary or secondary phenomenon. However, a number of immunohistochemical studies of lesional skin have shown cellular responses and time courses for such responses, compatible with delayed-type hypersensitivity, thus suggesting a primary immunological disorder. On the other hand, a cellular hypersensitivity to ultraviolet irradiation has also been briefly suggested as a possible pathogenic basis for the disease; however, such a claim appears largely to have been refuted.

EVIDENCE FOR A DELAYED-TYPE HYPERSENSITIVITY REACTION

Humoral immunity appears to be normal in CAD (Mentor *et al.*, 1974), occasionally reported raised peripheral IgA, IgE and IgG concentrations and eosinophilia being unlikely to be primary phenomena (Ehlers and Scharr, 1979; Johnson *et al.*, 1979). On the other hand, CAD is clinically, histologically and experimentally compatible with a process of cell mediated hypersensitivity. Thus, while the lesions clinically resemble those of allergic contact dermatitis, so do the histological changes, demonstrating epidermal spongiosis and variable acanthosis, along with a predominantly upper dermal perivascular mononuclear cell infiltrate containing occasional plasma cells and eosinophils and extending into the epidermis. In the pseudolymphoma or actinic reticuloid stage, however, the infiltrate is much heavier, often containing atypical lymphocytes with convoluted Sézary cell-like

nuclei, while Pautrier-like microabscesses may be present in the epidermis. Such changes have also been reported in certain forms of chronic contact dermatitis, the so-called lymphomatoid type (Orbeneja *et al.*, 1976), thus suggesting that the pseudolymphomatous lesions of CAD represent a severe stage in the disease spectrum, arguably the result of persistent putative antigenic stimulation.

Finally, a number of experimental studies have also produced evidence in favour of a delayed-type hypersensitivity immunological reaction for CAD. Thus, various immunohistochemical studies have characterized the dermal infiltrate in the condition, showing it to contain predominantly T cells, both in fully evolved (Braathen *et al.*, 1979; Norris *et al.*, 1989b; Ralfkiaer *et al.*, 1986; Takigawa *et al.*, 1987; Toonstra *et al.*, 1989) and induced lesions (Menagé *et al.*, 1993; Fujita *et al.*, 1990), together with Langerhans cells, interdigitating reticulum cells and monocyte-macrophages, including in particular CD36+ (OKM5+), factor XIIIa+, CD11b+, CD11c+ and CD14+ cells (Menagé *et al.*, 1993; Fujita *et al.*, 1990); leucocyte epidermotropism is also observed, while keratinocytes express MHC class II antigens in induced lesions (Menagé *et al.*, 1993; Fujita *et al.*, 1990). The dermal T-cell proportions have varied between studies, a predominance of CD4+ (helper/inducer) cells having been reported in some (Menagé *et al.*, 1993; Ralfkiaer *et al.*, 1986), but in others equal ratios (Ralfkiaer *et al.*, 1986; Takigawa *et al.*, 1987) or a predominance of CD8+ (suppressor/cytotoxic) cells (Fujita *et al.*, 1990; Toonstra *et al.*, 1989), the last particularly in lesions with more florid histological changes (Norris *et al.*, 1989b). Most studies agree that CD4+ cells predominate over CD8+ in the early stages of the allergic contact dermatitis and tuberculin responses (Gawkrodger *et al.*, 1986; Poulter *et al.*, 1982), with an increase in CD8+ cells occurring in the later stage (Fujita *et al.*, 1990). The kinetics of the inflammatory cell infiltrate in the induced lesions of CAD are thus also consistent with such delayed-type hypersensitivity responses (Poulter *et al.*, 1982), particularly in view of the peak in infiltrating cell numbers, particularly dermal and epidermal activated T-cells, epidermal Langerhans cells and monocyte-macrophages at 24–48 hours (Menagé *et al.*, 1993), and the fact that the pattern of the infiltrate is distinct from that following the UVB irradiation of normal skin, in which T- and Langerhans-cell epidermotropism is not observed (Vandervleuten *et al.*, 1996).

Analysis of the circulating lymphocyte subsets in CAD has also given variable results, being normal in some patients (Kofoed *et al.*, 1986; Norris *et al.*, 1989b), whilst in others demonstrating a reduction in the CD4+:CD8+ ratio (Fujita *et al.*, 1990; Norris *et al.*, 1989b; Takigawa *et al.*, 1987), generally because of a predominance of CD8+ cells, particularly in the actinic reticuloid CAD variant (Menagé *et al.*, 1992b). This latter finding thus correlates with the reported increase in CD8+ cells in the cutaneous infiltrate of florid CAD (Norris *et al.*, 1989b).

Specific changes in the kinetics and pattern of cell surface adhesion molecule expression have also been reported in delayed-type hypersensitivity and similar changes have been documented in CAD. Thus, following cutaneous purified protein derivative (PPD) injection, prolonged endothelial cell E-selectin expression has been noted, as well as the expression of vascular cell adhesion molecule (VCAM)-1 by perivascular and dermal interstitial cells and early intercellular adhesion molecule (ICAM)-1 expression by keratinocytes (Norris *et al.*, 1990). Similar changes also occur in allergic contact dermatitis, keratinocyte ICAM-1 expression appearing in early lesions, along with upregulated ICAM-1, VCAM-1 and E-selectin on dermal perivascular cells (Griffiths *et al.*, 1991). In addition, timed biopsies following 8–10 minimal lesion-inducing doses of solar-simulated irradiation (less than 1 MED in normals) in five patients with CAD have revealed upregulated perivascular ICAM-1, VCAM-1 and E-selectin, along with dermal interstitial VCAM-1 and ICAM-1, from one to five hours up to 5–7 days; there is also increased basal and focal epidermal keratinocyte ICAM-1 expression from one hour up to 5–7 days (Menagé *et al.*, 1996). Again, these changes are not simply a normal function of ultraviolet irradiation; thus, following UVB, the expression of E-selectin is less prolonged, while VCAM-1 and keratinocyte ICAM-1 are not expressed, and following combined UVB and UVA, keratinocyte ICAM-1 expression *in vitro* is delayed by 48 hours (Norris *et al.*, 1990, 1991). Thus, the pattern of adhesion molecule expression in CAD is likely to be of pathogenic significance and by its resemblance to the pattern in similar, already classified responses, suggests delayed-type hypersensitivity.

CYTOKINE EXPRESSION

Cytokine production by keratinocytes plays an important role in the initiation and maintenance of the allergic contact dermatitis reaction. However, studies on the role of cytokines in the pathogenesis of CAD lesions are limited, although an immunohistochemical time course study of induced lesions supports a proinflammatory role for interleukin-1α, regulated by its receptor and receptor antagonist (Menagé *et al.*, 1992a).

FUNCTIONAL STUDIES

Preliminary studies of dermal and epidermal extracts of lesional skin from CAD patients have shown no suggestion of proliferation in response to antigen in the autologous mixed epidermal cell leucocyte culture reaction (Sepulveda-Merill *et al.*, 1994). However, these negative findings may reflect the handling of specimens, leading to the possible destruction or alteration of any hypothetical antigen therein. Confirmatory evidence of an antigen-driven process is thus still awaited.

INDUCTION OF THE CAD RESPONSE

A number of different possible triggers have been proposed historically for the observed cellular responses in CAD patients, including in particular:

- the persistence of previous photocontact allergens in the skin;
- an autosensitization to skin proteins following an episode of photoallergic contact dermatitis;
- a reaction to kynurenic acid acting as an endogenous photosensitizer;
- an alteration in normal cutaneous immune regulation.

The persistence of previous photocontact allergens in the skin

Willis and Kligman in 1968 induced local cutaneous photosensitivity to halogenated salicylanilides and related compounds and by subsequent study of the ultraviolet absorption spectra of skin extracts from these patients, showed persistence of the original photosensitizer in the skin for many months, occasionally up to a year or more. They therefore proposed that persistent small amounts of exogenous photoallergen in the skin were the trigger for the photosensitivity in CAD, particularly since *in vitro* studies with tetrachlorsalicylanilide showed it to bind to human serum albumin (Kochevar and Harber, 1977), and since binding to the epidermal proteins of guinea pigs has also been demonstrated (Nakayama and Pathak, 1976). However, this theory does not explain the development of generalized cutaneous photosensitivity in CAD nor extension of the original UVA elicitation spectrum of the preceding photoallergic contact dermatitis to include UVB sensitivity, nor the fact that CAD arises in all but the occasional patient in the absence of any documented exogenous photoallergy.

Autosensitization to skin proteins following an episode of photoallergic contact dermatitis

In 1964, Baer and Kopf proposed that a carrier protein, namely albumin or another skin protein, binding to exogenous photoallergen during the process of induction of photocontact dermatitis, might alter to become a neoantigen itself capable of stimulating the immune system. Support for this theory was again lent by Kochevar and Harber in 1977, who showed that tetrachlorsalicylanilide may bind strongly *in vitro* to human albumin and promote oxidation of the histidine moiety of albumin, thus rendering it weakly antigenic; the subsequent absorption of ultraviolet radiation by the altered albumin alone then produced the oxidized protein. The same phenomenon could therefore presumably occur *in vivo*, and since albumin is universally distributed throughout the skin, could explain the potential for development of a delayed-type hypersensitivity response at all skin sites in the absence of an initial photosensitizer. However, this does not explain the development of CAD in the absence of documented exogenous photoallergy, although unrecognized photoallergens could perhaps be involved.

Reaction to kynurenic acid acting as an endogenous photosensitizer

Kynurenic acid is a byproduct of endogenous tryptophan metabolism and has been shown to induce the phototoxic oxidation of histidine *in vitro* (Swanbeck and Wennersten, 1973). In addition, elevated kynurenic acid concentrations were reported in the skin of two patients with CAD, one with apparently abnormal tryptophan metabolism (Binazzi and Calandra, 1971; Swanbeck and Wennersten, 1973). However, these findings have not been reproducible (Vonderheid *et al.*, 1987).

Alteration in normal cutaneous immune regulation

Ultraviolet irradiation in general diminishes cutaneous immune responsivity and in particular, the induction phase of delayed-type hypersensitivity (Baadsgaard, 1991). It is therefore conceivable that CAD may result from a fundamental dysregulation of such suppressor mechanisms, which might thus enable the easy development of cutaneous hypersensitivity to ultraviolet radiation-induced antigens generally not recognized by the immune system, as well as of ordinary contact allergy.

It now seems unlikely that any of these theories is precisely able to account for the pathogenesis of CAD, although a combination of certain aspects of them in addition to other factors appears very possible. Thus, it currently seems most likely that a photo-induced endogenous antigen, perhaps produced more readily or recognized more easily as a result of the concomitant presence of contact allergy, leads to a delayed-type hypersensitivity eczematous response in CAD indistinguishable from that of contact allergy. The contribution of any associated contact allergy and the possible nature of the endogenous photoallergen are now discussed below.

THE ROLE OF ASSOCIATED CONTACT ALLERGY IN CAD

Contact, and much more rarely photocontact, allergy appear to play a significant role in the development of CAD but are not absolute prerequisites for it. Thus, photocontact allergy was predominant in early reports of the condition but is now rarely observed, while contact allergy in contrast is now frequent. There are a number of possible explanations for this association. First, contact allergens may conceivably have a direct role in CAD pathogenesis, the more prevalent of these associated with the disease, namely the

Compositae oleoresins, fragrance materials and colophony, all apparently having a photo-toxic potential (Addo *et al.*, 1982; Frain-Bell *et al.*, 1979), which might enable them to convert endogenous protein into allergen. Alternatively, both the CAD and contact dermatitis states might reflect an altered immune reactivity and heightened tendency to the development of delayed type hypersensitivity responses. On the other hand, CAD has been reported to develop in other conditions associated with persistent T-cell stimulation, notably long-standing endogenous eczema and rarely long-standing PLE and it is therefore possible that any contact allergy may play a facilitative rather than causal role in pathogenesis of the condition by enhancing cutaneous immune function and facilitating endogenous, perhaps otherwise weak, photoantigen recognition. Finally, a combination of these hypotheses is also possible and all are indeed supported to some extent by the fact that many CAD patients are outdoor enthusiasts constantly exposed to both airborne allergens and sunlight, thereby continually being at risk simultaneously for the development of contact allergy and of endogenous photoallergen production.

THE POSSIBLE NATURE OF THE PUTATIVE ENDOGENOUS PHOTOALLERGEN IN CAD

The action spectrum for induction of the CAD response resembles that for the induction of ultraviolet-induced sunburn inflammation in normal subjects (Menagé *et al.*, 1995a), for which the chromophore is considered to be DNA; this thus suggests that DNA or a similar or related molecule may be the absorber and therefore the presumed photoallergen leading to the delayed type hypersensitivity response, in at least some CAD patients. In addition, sesquiterpene lactones, allergens known to be associated with the Compositae contact sensitivity often present in CAD, have been proposed in one study to be photoreactive with DNA under UVA irradiation (Berl *et al.*, unpublished observations, presented at the Jadassohn Centenary Congress on Contact Dermatitis, London, October 1996) and this may conceivably explain how photoallergen might be produced in sufficient quantities for cutaneous immunological recognition in CAD patients; other such allergens now need similar study.

POSSIBLE HYPERSENSITIVITY OF CAD CELLS TO UVA-INDUCED KILLING

In 1983, Gianelli and co-workers reported an enhanced sensitivity to the UVA killing of fibroblast cell lines in CAD, findings which have since been unconfirmed (Johnson *et al.*, 1988), apparently confirmed in certain strains only (Gibbs *et al.*, 1988) or considered to be at most slight (Applegate *et al.*, 1994). Other studies have also pursued this matter (Francis and Gianelli, 1991; Kondo and Nishioka, 1991; Kralli and Moss, 1987; Luy *et al.*, 1994) but in the end no clear differences between CAD and normal cells have been established and it seems most unlikely that any inherent abnormality in CAD cells themselves contributes to pathogenesis of the condition.

CONCLUSION

CAD is a disorder characterized by an extreme cutaneous sensitivity to ultraviolet irradiation, which thereby initiates an eczematous inflammatory process apparently indistinguishable from that of delayed-type hypersensitivity. It is an uncommon, often disabling and persistent disorder predominantly affecting middle-aged to elderly males and responds satisfactorily to immuno-modulatory therapy. An endogenously produced photoallergen, conceivably photoaltered DNA or associated molecule, in at least some patients, may be responsible for the process, but there is as yet no direct demonstration of this. A state of heightened reactivity of cutaneous immune function as a result of concomitant or preceding contact allergic or endogenous eczema in subjects who are persistently sun exposed may predispose to disease development, but the precise mechanisms as yet remain uncertain.

REFERENCES

Addo, H.A. and Frain-Bell, W. (1987) Persistence of allergic contact sensitivities in subjects with the photosensitive dermatitis and actinic reticuloid syndrome. *British Journal of Dermatology*, **117**, 555.

Addo, H.A., Ferguson, J., Johnson, B.E. *et al.* (1982) The relationship between exposure to fragrance materials and persistent light reaction in the photosensitivity dermatitis with actinic reticuloid syndrome. *British Journal of Dermatology*, **107**, 261.

Addo, H.A., Sharma, S.C., Ferguson, J. *et al.* (1985) A study of Compositae plant extract reactions in photosensitivity dermatitis. *Photodermatology*, **2**, 68.

Applegate, I.A., Frenk, E., Gibbs, N. *et al.* (1994) Cellular sensitivity to oxidative stress in the photosensitivity dermatitis/actinic reticuloid syndrome. *Journal of Investigative Dermatology*, **102**, 762–7.

Ashinoff, R., Buchness, M.R. and Lim, H.W. (1989) Lymphoma in a black patient with actinic reticuloid treated with PUVA: possible aetiologic considerations. *Journal of the American Academy of Dermatology*, **21**, 1134.

Baadsgaard, O. (1991) *In vivo* ultraviolet irradiation causes profound perturbation of the immune system. *Archives of Dermatology*, **127**, 99.

Baer, R.L. and Kopf, A.W. (1964) Editor's comment, in *Yearbook of Dermatology, 1963–64*, (eds R.L. Baer and A.W. Kopf), Yearbook Medical Publishers, Chicago, p. 133.

Bilsland, D. and Ferguson, J. (1991) Management of chronic photosensitive eczema. *Archives of Dermatology*, **127**, 1065.

Bilsland, D., Crombie, I.K. and Ferguson, J. (1993) Is the photosensitivity dermatitis/actinic reticuloid syndrome associated with cutaneous lymphoma? *British Journal of Dermatology*, **129** (suppl 42), 42.

Binazzi, M. and Calandra, P. (1971) Actinic reticuloid: pathogenic aspects. *Archiv für Dermatologische Forschung*, **241**, 391.

Braathen, L.R., Førre, Ø. and Natvig, J.B. (1979) An anti-human T-lymphocyte antiserum: *in situ* identification of T-cells in the skin of delayed type hypersensitivity reactions, chronic photosensitivity dermatitis, and mycosis fungoides. *Clinical Immunology and Immunopathology*, **13**, 211.

Burckhardt, W. (1957) Photoallergic eczema due to blankophores (optic brightening agents). *Hautarzt*, **8,** 486.

Chu, A.C., Robinson, D., Hawk, J.L.M. *et al.* (1986) Immunologic differentiation for the Sézary syndrome due to cutaneous T-cell lymphoma and chronic actinic dermatitis. *Journal of Investigative Dermatology*, **98**(4), 134.

Ehlers, G. and Scharr, K. (1979) Aktinisches Reticuloid. *Z. Hautkr.*, **55,** 1443.

Ferguson, J. (1990) Photosensitivity dermatitis and actinic reticuloid syndrome (chronic actinic dermatitis). *Seminars in Dermatology*, **9,** 47.

Frain-Bell, W. (1986) Photosensitivity and Compositae dermatitis. *Clinics in Dermatology*, **4**(2), 122.

Frain-Bell, W., Lakshmipathi, T., Rogers, J. *et al.* (1974) The syndrome of chronic photosensitivity dermatitis and actinic reticuloid. *British Journal of Dermatology*, **91,** 617.

Frain-Bell, W., Hetherington, A. and Johnson, B.E. (1979) Contact allergic sensitivity to chrysanthemum and the photosensitivity dermatitis and actinic reticuloid syndrome. *British Journal of Dermatology*, **101,** 491.

Francis, A.J. and Gianelli, F. (1991) Cooperation between human cells sensitive to UVA radiations: a clue to the mechanism of cellular hypersensitivity associated with different clinical conditions. *Experimental Cell Research*, **195,** 47–52.

Fujita, M., Miyachi, Y., Horio, T. *et al.* (1990) Immunohistochemical comparison of actinic reticuloid with contact dermatitis. *Journal of Dermatological Science*, **1,** 289.

Gawkrodger, D.J., McVittie, E., Carr, M.M. *et al.* (1986) Phenotypic characterisation of the early cellular responses in allergic and irritant contact dermatitis. *Clinical and Experimental Immunology*, **66,** 590.

Gianelli, F., Botcherby, P.K., Marimo, B. *et al.* (1983) Cellular hypersensitivity to UVA: a clue to the aetiology of actinic reticuloid? *Lancet* **1,** 88–91.

Gibbs, N.K., Botcherby, P.K., Morris, R.W. *et al.* (1988) UVA dose response of normal and actinic reticuloid cell fibroblasts: a statistical analysis. *British Journal of Dermatology*, **118,** 289.

Green, C., Catterall, M. and Hawk, J.L.M. (1991) Chronic actinic dermatitis and sunscreen allergy. *Clinical and Experimental Dermatology*, **16,** 70.

Griffiths, C.E.M., Barker, J.N.W.N., Kunkel, S. *et al.* (1991) Modulation of leucocyte adhesion molecules, a T-cell chemotactin (IL-8), and a regulatory cytokine (TNF-a) in allergic contact dermatitis (rhus dermatitis). *British Journal of Dermatology*, **124,** 519.

Hannuksela, M., Suhonen, R. and Forstrom, L. (1981) Delayed contact allergies in patients with photosensitivity dermatitis. *Archives of Dermatovenereology (Stockholm)*, **61,** 303.

Hawk, J.L.M. and Magnus, I.A. (1978) Resolution of actinic reticuloid with transition to photosensitive eczema. *Journal of the Royal Society of Medicine*, **71,** 608.

Hawk, J.L.M. and Magnus, I.A. (1979) Chronic actinic dermatitis – an idiopathic photosensitivity syndrome including actinic reticuloid and photosensitive eczema. *British Journal of Dermatology*, **101** (suppl 17), 24.

Healy, F. and Rogers, S. (1995) Photosensitivity dermatitis/actinic reticuloid syndrome in an Irish population: a review and some unusual features. *Acta Dermatovenereologica (Stockholm)*, **75**(1), 72–4.

Heller, P., Wieczorek, R., Waldo, L. *et al.* (1994) Chronic actinic dermatitis: an immunohistochemical study of its T-cell antigenic profile, with comparison to T-cell lymphoma. *American Journal of Dermatopathology*, **165**(5), 510–16.

Hindson, C., Spiro, J. and Downey, A. (1984) PUVA therapy of chronic actinic dermatitis. *British Journal of Dermatology*, **113,** 156.

Hindson, C., Downey, A., Sinclair, S. *et al.* (1990) PUVA therapy of chronic actinic dermatitis: a 5 year follow-up. *British Journal of Dermatology*, **123,** 264.

Horio, J. (1982) Actinic reticuloid via persistent light reactivity from photoallergic contact dermatitis. *Archives of Dermatology*, **118,** 339.

Humbert, P., Drobacheff, C., Vigan, M. *et al.* (1991) Chronic actinic dermatitis responding to danazol. *British Journal of Dermatology*, **124,** 195.

Ive, F.A., Magnus, I.A., Warin, R.P. *et al.* (1969) 'Actinic reticuloid': a chronic dermatosis associated with severe photosensitivity and the histological resemblance to lymphoma. *British Journal of Dermatology*, **81,** 469.

Jensen, N.E. and Sneddon, I.B. (1970) Actinic reticuloid with lymphoma. *British Journal of Dermatology*, **82,** 287.

Jillson, O.F. and Baughman, R.D. (1963) Contact photodermatitis from bithionol. *Archives of Dermatology*, **88,** 409.

Johnson, B.E., Walker, E.M., Ferguson, J. *et al.* (1988) Cellular sensitivity to UVA in photosensitivity dermatitis/actinic reticuloid (PD/AR). *British Journal of Dermatology*, **118,** 286.

Johnson, S.C., Cripps, D.J. and Norbach, D.H. (1979) Actinic reticuloid, a clinical, pathological and action spectrum study. *Archives of Dermatology*, **115**, 1078.

Kingston, T.P., Lowe, N.J., Sofen, H.L. *et al.* (1987) Actinic reticuloid in a black man: successful treatment with azathioprine. *Journal of the American Academy of Dermatology*, **16**, 1079.

Kochevar, I.E. and Harber, L.C. (1977) Photo-reactions of 3',3',4',5'-tetrachlorsalicylanilide with proteins. *Journal of Investigative Dermatology*, **68**, 151.

Kofoed, M.L., Munch-Petersen, B., Larsen, J.K. *et al.* (1986) Non-replicative DNA synthesis detected in peripheral lymphocytes from a patient with actinic reticuloid. *Photodermatology*, **3**, 158.

Kondo, S. and Nishioka, K. (1991) Hypersensitivity of skin fibroblasts from patients with chronic actinic dermatitis to ultraviolet B (UVB), UVA and superoxide radical. *Photodermatology, Photoimmunology and Photomedicine*, **8**, 212–17.

Kralli, A. and Moss, S.H. (1987) The sensitivity of an actinic reticuloid cell strain to near ultraviolet radiation and its modification by Trolox-C, a vitamin E analogue. *British Journal of Dermatology*, **116**, 761–72.

Kurumaji, Y., Kondo, S., Fukuro, S. *et al.* (1994) Chronic actinic dermatitis in a young patient with atopic dermatitis. *Journal of American Academy of Dermatology*, **31**(4), 667–9.

Lim, H.W., Buchness, M.R., Ashinoff, R. *et al.* (1990) Chronic actinic dermatitis: study of the spectrum of chronic photosensitivity in 12 patients. *Archives of Dermatology*, **126**, 317.

Lim, H.W., Morison, W.L., Kamide, R. *et al.* (1994) Chronic actinic dermatitis: an analysis of 51 patients evaluated in the United States and Japan. *Archives of Dermatological Research*, **130**, 1284–9.

Lowe, J.G. and Ferguson, J. (1989) A double blind control study to assess the effect of pre-treatment with a potent topical steroid on the phototest response of photosensitivity dermatitis and actinic reticuloid syndrome (PD/AR). *Scottish Medical Journal*, **34**, 509.

Luy, H., Frenk, E. and Applegate, L.A. (1994) Ultraviolet A-induced cellular membrane damage in the photosensitivity dermatitis/actinic reticuloid syndrome. *Photodermatology, Photoimmunology and Photomedicine*, **10**, 126–33.

Menagé, H. du P., Kristensen, M., Chu, C.Q. *et al.* (1992a) Upregulation of interleukin 1, its receptor and interleukin 1 receptor antagonist levels in induced lesions of chronic actinic dermatitis. *British Journal of Dermatology*, **127** (suppl), 429.

Menagé, H. du P., Whittaker, S.J., Ng, Y.I. *et al.* (1992b) Analysis of T-cell receptor genes in chronic actinic dermatitis: no evidence of clonality. *Journal of Investigative Dermatology*, **98**(4), 456.

Menagé, H. du P., Sattar, N., Hawk, J.L.M. *et al.* (1993) Immunophenotyping of the inflammatory cell infiltrate during the evolution of induced lesions of chronic actinic dermatitis. *Journal of Investigative Dermatology*, **100**(4), 482.

Menagé, H. du P., Harrison, G.I., Potten, C.S. *et al.* (1995a) The action spectrum for induction of chronic actinic dermatitis is similar to that for sunburn inflammation. *Photochemistry and Photobiology*, **62**(6), 976–9.

Menagé, H. du P., Ross, J., Hawk, J.L.M. *et al.* (1995b) Contact and photocontact sensitisation in chronic actinic dermatitis: sesquiterpene lactone mix is an important allergen. *British Journal of Dermatology*, **132**, 543–7.

Menagé, H. du P., Sattar, N., Haskard, D.O. *et al.* (1996) A study of the kinetics and pattern of adhesion molecule expression in induced lesions of chronic actinic dermatitis. *British Journal of Dermatology*, **134**, 262–8.

Mentor, M.A., McKerron, R.A. and Amos, H.E. (1974) Actinic reticuloid: an immunological investigation providing evidence of basement membrane damage. *British Journal of Dermatology*, **90**, 507.

Meynadier, J., Peyron, J.I., Barneon, G. *et al.* (1984) Hodgkin's disease complicating actinic reticulosis. *Annals of Dermatology and Venereology*, **111**(11), 999.

Milde, P., Hölzle, E., Neumann, N. *et al.* (1991) Chronic actinic dermatitis. Concept and case examples. *Hautarzt*, **42**, 617–22.

Moseley, H., Johnston, S. and Susskind, W. (1989) Is viewing television harmful to actinic reticuloid patients? *Photodermatology*, **6**, 191–3.

Murphy, G.M., Maurice, P.M., Norris, P.G. *et al.* (1989) Azathioprine in the treatment of chronic actinic dermatitis: a double-blind controlled trial with monitoring of exposure to ultraviolet radiation. *British Journal of Dermatology*, **121**, 639.

Murphy, G.M., White, I.R. and Hawk, J.L.M. (1990) Allergic airborne dermatitis to Compositae with photosensitivity – CAD in evolution. *Photodermatology, Photoimmunology and Photomedicine*, **7**, 38.

Nakayama, Y. and Pathak, M.A. (1976) Photoconjugation of 3',4',5'-tetrachlorsalicylanilide to proteins of guinea-pig skin. *Journal of Investigative Dermatology*, **66**, 273.

Neild, V.S., Hawk, J.L.M., Eady, R.A.J. *et al.* (1982) Actinic reticuloid with Sézary cells. *Clinical and Experimental Dermatology*, **7**, 143.

Norris, D.A., Bradley-Lyons, M., Middleton, M. *et al.* (1990) Ultraviolet radiation can either suppress or induce expression of intercellular adhesion molecule 1 on the surface of cultured human keratinocytes. *Journal of Investigative Dermatology*, **95**, 132.

Norris, P.G. and Hawk, J.L. (1990) Chronic actinic dermatitis: a unifying concept. *Archives of Dermatology*, **126**, 376.

Norris, P.G., Camp, R.D.R. and Hawk, J.L.M. (1989a) Actinic reticuloid: response to cyclosporin. *Journal of the American Academy of Dermatology*, **307**, 21.

Norris, P.G., Morris, J., Smith, N.P. *et al.* (1989b) Chronic actinic dermatitis: an immunohistologic and photobiologic study. *Journal of the American Academy of Dermatology*, **21**, 966.

Norris, P.G., Newton, J.A., Camplejohn, R.S. *et al.* (1989c) A flow cytometric study of actinic reticuloid. *Clinical and Experimental Dermatology*, **14**, 128.

Norris, P.G., Poston, R.N., Thomas, D.S. *et al.* (1991) The expression of endothelial leukocyte adhesion molecule-1 (ELAM-1), intercellular adhesion molecule-1 (VCAM-1) in experimental cutaneous inflammation: a comparison of ultraviolet B erythema and delayed type hypersensitivity. *Journal of Investigative Dermatology*, **96**, 763.

Orbaneja, J.G., Diez, L.I., Lozano, J.I.S. *et al.* (1976) Lymphomatoid contact dermatitis: a syndrome produced by epicutaneous hypersensitivity with clinical features and a histopathologic picture similar to that of mycosis fungoides. *Contact Dermatitis*, **2**, 139.

Pappert, A., Grossman, M. and DeLeo, V. (1994) Photosensitivity as the presenting illness in four patients with human immunodeficiency viral infection. *Archives of Dermatological Research*, **130**, 618–23.

Parodi, A., Gallo, R., Guarrera, M. *et al.* (1995) Natural alpha interferon in chronic actinic dermatitis. *Acta Dermatovenereologica (Stockholm)*, **75**(1), 80.

Poulter, L.W., Seymour, G.J., Duke, O. *et al.* (1982) Immunohistological analysis of delayed type hypersensitivity in man. *Cellular Immunology*, **74**, 358.

Preesman, A.H., Schrooyen, S.J., Toonstra, J. *et al.* (1995) The diagnostic value of morphometry in blood lymphocytes in erythrodermic actinic reticuloid. *Archives of Dermatology*, **131**(11), 1298–303.

Ralfkiaer, E., Lange Wantzin, G., Stein, H. *et al.* (1986) Photosensitive dermatitis with actinic reticuloid syndrome: an immunohistological study of the cutaneous infiltrate. *British Journal of Dermatology*, **114**, 47.

Ramsay, C.A. and Kobza-Black, A. (1973) Photosensitive eczema. *Transactions of the St John's Hospital Dermatological Society*, **59**, 152.

Robinson, H.N., Morison, W.I. and Hood, A.F. (1985) Thiazide diuretic therapy and chronic photosensitivity. *Archives of Dermatology*, **121**, 522.

Roelandts, R. (1993) Chronic actinic dermatitis. *Journal of the American Academy of Dermatology*, **28**, 240–9.

Roelandts, R. and Huys, I. (1993) Broad-band and persistent photosensitivity following accidental ultraviolet C overexposure. *Photodermatology, Photoimmunology and Photomedicine*, **9**, 144–6.

Sepulveda-Merill, C., Menagé, H.P., Hawk, J.L.M. *et al.* (1994) Functional studies of antigen presentation in induced lesions of chronic actinic dermatitis. *Journal of Investigative Dermatology*, **102**, 603.

Sigurdsson, V., Toonstra, J., Hezemans-Boer, M. *et al.* (1996) Erythroderma. A clinical and follow-up study of 102 patients, with a special emphasis on survival. *Journal of the American Academy of Dermatology*, **35**(1), 53–7.

Swanbeck, G. and Wennersten, G. (1973) Evidence for kynurenic acid as a potential photosensitiser in actinic reticuloid. *Acta Dermatovenereologica (Stockholm)*, **53**, 109.

Takigawa, M., Tokura, Y., Shirahama, S. *et al.* (1987) Actinic reticuloid: an immunohistochemical study. *Archives of Dermatology*, **123**, 296.

Tan, R.S.H., Butterworth, C.M., McLaughlin, H. *et al.* (1974) Mycosis fungoides – a disease of antigen persistence. *British Journal of Dermatology*, **91**, 607.

Thestrup-Pedersen, K., Zachariae, C., Kaltoft, K. *et al.* (1988) Development of cutaneous pseudolymphoma following cyclosporin therapy of actinic reticuloid. *Dermatologica*, **177**, 376.

Thomsen, K. (1977) The development of Hodgkin's disease in a patient with actinic reticuloid. *Clinical and Experimental Dermatology*, **2**, 209.

Thune, P. (1977) Allergy to lichens with photosensitivity. *Contact Dermatitis*, **3**, 213.

Toonstra, H., Van Der Putte, S.C.J., Van Wichen, D.F. *et al.* (1989) Actinic reticuloid: immunohistochemical analysis of the cutaneous infiltrate in 13 patients. *British Journal of Dermatology*, **120**, 779.

Vandervleuten, C.J.M., Kroot, E.J.A., Dejong, E.M.J. *et al.* (1996) The immunohistochemical effects of a single challenge with an intermediate dose of ultraviolet B on normal human skin. *Archives of Dermatological Research*, **288**(9), 510–16.

Volden, G. and Thune, P.O. (1977) Light sensitivity in mycosis fungoides. *British Journal of Dermatology*, **97**, 279.

Von den Driesch, P., Fartasch, M. and Hornstein, O.P. (1992) Chronic actinic dermatitis with vitiligo-like depigmentation. *Clinical and Experimental Dermatology*, **17**, 38.

Vonderheid, F.C., Sobel, F.L., Hoeldtke, R.D. *et al.* (1987) Kynurenic acid and xanthurenic acid excretion after tryptophan loading in actinic reticuloid. *International Journal of Dermatology*, **26**, 33.

Wilkinson, D.S. (1962) Patch test reactions to certain halogenated salicylanilides. *British Journal of Dermatology*, **74**, 295.

Willis, I. and Kligman, A.M. (1968) The mechanism of the persistent light reactor. *Journal of Investigative Dermatology*, **51**, 385.

Yates, V.M. and Finn, O.A. (1980) Contact allergic sensitivity to zinc pyrithione followed by the photosensitivity dermatitis and actinic reticuloid syndrome. *Contact Dermatitis*, **6**, 349.

Zaynoun, S., Johnson, B.E. and Frain-Bell, W. (1976) The investigation of quindoxin photosensitivity. *Contact Dermatitis*, **2**(6), 343.

THE DNA REPAIR-DEFICIENT PHOTODERMATOSES

11

Paul G. Norris and Alan R. Lehmann

INTRODUCTION

The maintenance of genetic stability is essential to the viability of all multicellular organisms. However, structural alterations are continually appearing in their cellular DNA, either spontaneously or as a result of environmental insult. Such organisms have therefore evolved a range of DNA repair mechanisms to protect the cell from the accumulation of deleterious mutations. The proteins involved in such repair are inevitably encoded by the very DNA they protect and consequently, mutations at those DNA sites can impair the repair processes themselves. In such circumstances, the unchecked accumulation of mutations becomes possible, often with consequent accelerated tumorigenesis.

The understanding of cellular DNA repair mechanisms has been advanced by study of the inherited disorders in which these repair processes are defective. Such disorders are all rare autosomal recessive multisystem complaints and, in particular, currently comprise xeroderma pigmentosum (XP), Cockayne's syndrome (CS), trichothiodystrophy (TTD) and Bloom's syndrome (BS). While XP is characterized by a greatly increased incidence of skin cancer and BS by an increased susceptibility to internal neoplasms, such an association with malignancy has not been

Photodermatology. Edited by J.L.M. Hawk. Published in 1998 by Chapman & Hall, London. ISBN 0 412 72460 X.

reported in CS or TTD. Study of these disorders has therefore provided useful insights into the complex association between defective DNA repair and the presence or absence of cancer susceptibility. The conditions will now be discussed in detail.

XERODERMA PIGMENTOSUM

XP is a rare autosomal recessive disorder of all races worldwide, affecting around four per million live births. Approximately 75% of patients have so-called classic XP, associated with a defect in DNA nucleotide excision repair (NER); genetic variants detected by complementation tests have now identified seven excision-defective so-called complementation groups, designated by the letters A–G (Hoeijmakers, 1993), while the remaining 25% have excision-proficient XP variants with a deficient but ill-characterized, post-replicative repair process.

CLINICAL FEATURES

XP patients usually first present with dermatological manifestations between one and two years of age (Kraemer and Slor, 1984). The commonest initial symptom is markedly exaggerated sunburning for the degree of exposure, even minimal irradiation often leading to blistering which may take several days or weeks to resolve. Later clinical abnormalities include pigmented macules of variable intensity from light brown to black, predominantly of the sun-exposed areas but sometimes also the palms, soles and mucous membranes. In addition, patients also frequently exhibit 1–5 mm diameter vitiligo-like hypopigmented spots, both interspersed with the pigmented lesions and also affecting the non-sunexposed sites, particularly the buttocks (Césarini *et al.*, 1975). Other common abnormalities, particularly of the exposed skin, include progressive dryness, telangiectasia, atrophy and scarring (Plate 17).

A comprehensive survey by Kraemer *et al.* (1987) of 830 published cases showed that:

- individuals with XP generally die about 30 years earlier than the US population as a whole;
- the median age for a first skin malignancy in XP is approximately 50 years earlier than that of the normal population;
- 50% of XP patients in the 10–14 age group had skin cancers.

The predominant skin malignancies in XP are squamous and basal cell carcinomas, although the incidence of malignant melanoma is also significantly elevated, while other reported skin tumours are actinic keratoses, fibromas, angiomas, keratoacanthomas and fibrosarcomas. The cancers occur predominantly on exposed sites, including the tip of the tongue, while there is also some evidence for an elevated incidence of internal malignancies (Kraemer *et al.*, 1984). Clinical features are variable, however, and may be mild, for example in complementation groups E and F.

Ocular abnormalities in XP are also common and generally confined to the areas exposed to ultraviolet (UV) radiation, namely eyelids, conjunctiva and cornea. Initial photophobia may proceed to later conjunctival inflammatory lesions such as pinguecula, keratitis and ectropion, followed by various benign and malignant neoplasms. In addition, approximately 20% of patients develop neurological disorders, generally beginning in infancy but occasionally in the second decade, as a result of progressive neuronal loss from the cerebral cortex and sometimes also cerebellum, medulla and spinal cord (Hakamada *et al.*, 1982; Roytta and Anttinan, 1986). Such neurological abnormalities may be mild or severe and include, for example, hypo- and areflexia, abnormal speech, seizures, sensorineural deafness, abnormal motor activity and mental retardation. In the most extreme cases, however, severe and progressive neurological features are combined with microcephaly, dwarfism and immature sexual development (Reed *et al.*, 1965) a combination sometimes called the De Sanctis–Cacchione syndrome.

There is an uneven overall distribution of the XP complementation groups, both on the basis of their frequency and their worldwide occurrence. Thus groups A, C, D and variant are the most common in Europe and the USA, while in Japan, groups A and variant are the most common, groups C and D being only rarely observed. On the other hand, there are only two known group B XP families, both having the features of both XP and CS, while five other individuals with XP and CS are also known, two in group D and three in group G (Hoeijmakers, 1993; Moriwaki *et al.*, 1996). Considerable variability in clinical severity also exists both between and within complementation groups, correlating only roughly with the magnitude of the DNA repair defect. Thus, group A patients frequently develop neurological disease, often severe, during the first decade, while group D generally do so during the second; group C patients are usually neurologically normal. Further, XP variants are free of neurological disease and present clinically either in a form indistinguishable from classic XP or with late-onset pigmentation, neoplasms and occasionally photosensitivity. Skin cancer susceptibility also varies between groups; thus, squamous cell carcinoma predominates in group C, lentigo maligna melanoma in group D and basal cell carcinoma in groups E and variant (Jung, 1986).

IMMUNE FUNCTION

Impaired adaptive T cell-mediated immune responses have been reported in XP, including in particular reduced responses to recall antigens and dinitrochlorobenzene (DNCB), a reduction in the ratio of T helper to suppressor cells and a reduced response to the phytohaemagglutinin stimulation of lymphocytes (Berkel and Kiran, 1974; Dupuy and Lafforet, 1974; Morison *et al.*, 1985; Salaman *et al.*, 1975; Wysenbeek *et al.*, 1986); there is again considerable variation amongst patients with regard to these effects. Natural killer (NK) cell number and function have also been found to be reduced in some but not all XP patients (Gaspari *et al.*, 1993; Norris *et al.*, 1990) while in one interesting case, an individual aged 65 years with self-healing melanomas had reduced NK cellular function but a greater number of such cells (Anstey *et al.*, 1991). Turner *et al.* (1993) have recently reported a case where intralesional α-interferon injections were effective in the treatment of melanomas in an XP patient, while it is also of interest that following UVB irradiation, XP cells have a reduced capacity to mount γ-interferon stimulation of ICAM-1 expression, as compared with normal individuals (Krutmann *et al.*, 1994). Finally, XP group A knockout mice have recently been shown to undergo the normal induction of contact hypersensitivity but then to demonstrate greatly enhanced UVB-induced local and systemic immunosuppression (Miyauchi-Hashimoto *et al.*, 1996).

MOLECULAR ABNORMALITIES

Cells cultured from XP patients of all genetic complementation groups except the variant show a 2–15-fold increase in hypersensitivity to both the lethal and mutagenic effects of UVC irradiation. Such hypersensitivity results from a partial or total deficiency in the excision repair of UV- and otherwise induced bulky adducts within cellular DNA, the cells

in each complementation group having a characteristic level of residual excision repair, although variations occur. Thus, interestingly, XPC cells are able to carry out so-called transcription-coupled repair, a particular subpathway of NER defective in CS cells and discussed in more detail on p. 148.

In recent years, there has been dramatic progress in our understanding of the functions of the different gene products represented by the seven XP complementation groups. Thus, all the XP genes have now been cloned, the encoded proteins characterized biochemically and the many associated mutations identified in affected patients. Further, the roles of most of the proteins in NER have now been characterized (Lehmann, 1995) (Plate 18). In the first step, DNA damage, such as for example a UV-induced photoproduct, is recognized by the XPA protein in association with the single-stranded binding protein, RPA (Plate 18). The next step is then recruitment of the transcription factor TFIIH complex (see below), composed of several subunits, two of which are the XPB and XPD proteins. Both of these have DNA helicase activity and it is thought that they unwind the DNA on either side of the damaged site (Plate 18), such that two nucleases can then cut out the damaged material (Plate 18); one of these is the XPG protein, which cuts on the 3′ side of the damage, the other a protein with two subunits, one of which is the XPF protein, which cuts on the 5′ side. The roles of XPC and XPE are not yet understood. Following the action of the nucleases, a piece of DNA of about 29 nucleotides, including the damaged bases, is removed, thus completing the incision steps. Subsequently, repair synthesis is brought about by a DNA polymerase with its accessory proteins (Plate 18) and ligation by a DNA ligase (Plate 18) (Aboussekhra *et al.*, 1995).

Mutations in XP genes have now been identified in a number of patients by molecular genetic analysis, in many cases enabling clinical features to be explained by the mutation positions. Thus, in Japan, over 80% of XPA patients have the same mutation, the result of a founder effect, in which the mutation arose many generations ago and has since spread through the population; this causes the production of a truncated protein, as a result of which all patients are severely affected, while another causes only a single amino acid change, leading to relatively mild clinical features (Nishigori *et al.*, 1994).

Approximately 25% of the XP patients studied are XP variants, who show only slight hypersensitivity to the lethal effects of UVC irradiation and no defects in excision repair. Instead, they have a deficiency in an ill-characterized daughter-strand repair process (Lehmann *et al.*, 1975) which, however, also results in hypermutability of the cells following UV irradiation.

Thus, all XP cells studied to date have both defective DNA repair and also a secondary enhanced mutability following UV irradiation. This hypermutability, probably in combination with the immune abnormalities described above, presumably accounts for most of the cutaneous abnormalities found in XP. Thus, the p53 tumour suppressor gene is mutated in 50% of human cancers and, in non-melanoma skin cancers, has a spectrum of mutations characteristic of that produced by UV irradiation (Ziegler *et al.*, 1993); that spectrum is the same as that seen in skin tumours from most XP patients (Dumaz *et al.*, 1993). These observations thus strongly support the hypothesis that sunlight-induced p53 mutations are an important step in skin carcinogenesis in both normal and XP individuals.

DIAGNOSIS

Phototesting

Following monochromatic UVB (280–315 nm) irradiation, frequently observed findings include low minimal erythemal doses, abnormal papular and vesicular reactions and the delayed development of the minimal erythemal reactions beyond the normal time of 24 hours to as long as 72 hours (Cripps *et al.*, 1971; Ichihashi and Fujiwara, 1981; Ramsay and Gianelli, 1975).

Cellular diagnosis

The characteristic defect in excision repair can be assessed in a number of ways, measurement of the repair synthesis step (Plate 18) being easiest, differing from replicative DNA synthesis in that it occurs throughout the cell cycle and is relatively resistant to inhibitors of the latter, such as hydroxyurea. Thus, by the radioactive labelling of cells with irrited thymidine after UV irradiation followed by autoradiography, such synthesis can be measured by the counting of grains over the nuclei of non-S phase cells, all of which are thus undergoing unscheduled DNA synthesis (UDS); a large reduction in UDS confirms the XP defect. Alternatively, non-dividing cells may be treated with hydroxyurea, irradiated and labelled with tritiated thymidine, under which conditions replicative DNA synthesis is abolished and the incorporated radioactivity, mostly from repair synthesis, may be measured by scintillation counting. Both techniques give similar results and can be applied to fibroblasts, keratinocytes, lymphocytes, amniocytes and villus cells, so that both pre- and postnatal diagnosis is possible (Halley *et al.*, 1979; Ramsay *et al.*, 1974). On the other hand, XP variant can be diagnosed only by measurement of the defect in daughter-strand repair which, although possible both pre- and postnatally, is relatively sophisticated, requiring centrifugation of the cellular DNA through alkaline sucrose gradients to enable measurement of the molecular weights of the daughter DNA strands (Halley *et al.*, 1979; Lehmann *et al.*, 1975). However, Itoh *et al.* (1996) have recently described an alternative method for the diagnosis of XP variant, involving the autoradiographic measurement of three cellular markers for DNA repair after UV irradiation, namely, unscheduled DNA synthesis, the recovery of RNA synthesis and the recovery of replicative DNA synthesis.

TREATMENT

Protection from UV exposure should be life-long by the adoption of a lifestyle to minimize UV exposure, the wearing of protective clothing and sunglasses and the use of highly protective, broad-spectrum sunscreens. In addition, oral isotretinoin has been shown to reduce the incidence of skin cancer in XP patients significantly, although side effects are common and high rates of tumour development occur following any cessation of treatment, suggesting drug action at a relatively late stage in carcinogenesis (Kraemer *et al.*, 1988). Finally, a topically applied, bacterio-phage-derived, liposome-encapsulated DNA repair enzyme preparation has recently shown promise as an XP treatment, improving DNA repair rates at artificially irradiated skin sites by perhaps 30%; patient user studies are now in progress (Yarosh *et al.*, 1996).

COCKAYNE'S SYNDROME

CLINICAL FEATURES

This rare disorder (Nance and Berry, 1992) shows a pattern of inheritance consistent with a recessive status and after apparently normal initial development, CS patients develop clinical abnormalities usually between six and 24 months of age. Photosensitivity is a common presenting feature and may be char-acterized by a scaly erythematous dermatitis of the exposed sites, particularly cheeks and nose, aggravated by sun exposure (Cockayne, 1936; Paddison *et al.*, 1963), a susceptibility to severe sunburning similar to that in XP, sometimes with pigmentation and atrophic scarring of the exposed skin (MacDonald *et al.*, 1960) or an erythematous papular eruption, particularly of facial skin, with onset within hours of sun exposure. In addition, a combination of prognathism, sunken eyes, thin prominent nose and lack of subcutaneous fat may often result in a characteristic, bird-headed facies or prema-turely senile, wizened, appearance (Plate 19). Growth retardation, too, is generally early and severe, while disproportionately large hands and feet, long limbs and a compara-tively small trunk also commonly occur. Neurological abnormalities are also charac-teristic and include microcephaly, progressive mental retardation, sensorineural hearing loss, choreoathetosis, normal pressure hydro-cephalus, ataxia and myoclonus spasticity (MacDonald *et al.*, 1960; Paddison *et al.*, 1963), while ocular lesions such as optic atrophy, pigmentary retinal degeneration and cataracts are also common, frequently resulting in blindness. Considerable variation in CS clinical features is possible; for example, a 25-year-old woman patient was reported to have acute photosensitivity but otherwise mild features, such that she was able to grad-uate from high school and have a successful pregnancy (Kennedy *et al.*, 1980), while at the other end of the spectrum, extremely severe disease has been described with symptoms already evident at birth (see Nance and Berry, 1992).

IMMUNE FUNCTION

There have been only very limited investiga-tions concerning the immunological status of CS patients, with two patients demonstrating adaptive cell-mediated immunity and NK cell function within normal limits (Norris *et al.*, 1990).

MOLECULAR ABNORMALITIES

As in XP, the photosensitivity of CS patients is reflected at the cellular level by hypersen-sitivity to the lethal and mutagenic effects of UVC irradiation (Wade and Chu, 1979), but in CS this cannot be attributed to any defi-ciency in UV-induced DNA excision repair which in fact appears normal by several criteria. Nevertheless, a biochemical abnormality following the UV irradiation of CS cells can be detected in DNA replicative synthesis and RNA synthesis rates (Lehmann *et al.*, 1979; Mayne and Lehmann, 1982), the UV-induced DNA damage causing a rapid depression in both. Thus, in normal but not CS cells, RNA synthesis recovers within 1–2 (Mayne and Lehmann, 1982) and DNA synthesis within 5–7 (Lehmann *et al.*, 1979) hours of a UVC exposure dose of 4 J/m^2.

It is now known that although the bulk of UV-induced DNA pyrimidine dimers are repaired relatively slowly in normal subjects (about half within eight hours), damage to active DNA regions, namely those being transcribed into RNA, is removed much more rapidly and completely (Bohr *et al.*, 1985) and it is this preferential repair that has been shown to be defective in CS (Venema *et al.*, 1990). Furthermore, it is the transcribed strand of active genes that is repaired rapidly in normal cells (transcription-coupled repair), but this is not the case in CS cells (Van Hoffen *et al.*, 1993). Clearly, it is imperative for a cell to undergo the rapid removal of damage to genes actually being used, the specific defect in this process in CS thus being associated with its failure of RNA synthesis recovery and its pronounced hypersensitivity to UV light, even though the bulk of the DNA is normal. Cell fusion studies have shown two complementation groups for CS, namely CSA and CSB, the majority (about 80%) of patients falling into the CSB group (Stefanini *et al.*, 1996). Both the CSA (Henning *et al.*, 1995) and CSB (Troelstra *et al.*, 1992) genes have been cloned, but the precise functions of the proteins are not yet understood. However, the genes do not appear to be essential for life, many of the mutations found in patients completely abolishing the protein function. In addition, as mentioned above, there are seven patients reported with the features of both CS and XP, the defects in these patients

falling instead into the XPB, D and G complementation groups.

DIAGNOSIS

Both the pre- and postnatal diagnosis of CS can be carried out by demonstration of the lack of recovery of RNA synthesis in CS cells following UV irradiation (Lehmann *et al.*, 1985, 1993; Mayne and Lehmann, 1982). Typically, non-dividing cells are irradiated, their RNA synthesis being measured by uridine incorporation the following day. It should be noted that a similar defect is found in XP, although in this case accompanied by the excision-repair defect.

TREATMENT

No specific treatments are available.

TRICHOTHIODYSTROPHY

CLINICAL FEATURES

This rare autosomal recessive condition is characterized by brittle, unruly and sparse scalp hair, eyelashes and eyebrows (Baden *et al.*, 1976; Coulter *et al.*, 1982; Jackson *et al.*, 1974; Jorizzo *et al.*, 1982; Lucky *et al.*, 1984; Pollit *et al.*, 1968; Price *et al.*, 1980), while pili torti and trichoschisis (clean transverse fractures of the scalp hair shafts) are revealed by light microscopy, a banded appearance being seen under polarized light. In addition, patients are generally of short stature (Jackson *et al.*, 1974; Jorizzo *et al.*, 1982), many with an unusual facial appearance characterized by a receding chin and protruding ears, while a variable degree of mental retardation is also common (Jackson *et al.*, 1974; Jorizzo *et al.*, 1982; Price *et al.*, 1980). Other possible features are cataracts, dental caries, decreased fertility, hypoplastic nails and, in about 50% of cases, an XP-like photosensitivity (Coulter *et al.*, 1982; Jackson *et al.*, 1974; Jorizzo *et al.*, 1982; Lucky *et al.*, 1984), but there are no reports of skin cancer.

IMMUNE FUNCTION

Mariani *et al.* (1992) have recently demonstrated impaired NK cell lytic activity in some patients and their families, similar to that in XP, thus suggesting that the relationship between immune surveillance and elevated cancer risk in the DNA repair-defective disorders is very complex.

MOLECULAR ABNORMALITIES

Stefanini *et al.* (1986) first demonstrated a DNA repair defect in TTD fibroblasts, after which a detailed analysis of cells from several patients showed a varied response to UV irradiation (Broughton *et al.*, 1990; Lehmann *et al.*, 1988). Thus, cells from some patients have a totally normal response by several criteria, while those from many others show the hypersensitivity to irradiation and excision-repair defect characteristic of XP. This defect is of variable severity but cell fusion studies have remarkably shown that it is usually the same complementation group as XPD (Stefanini *et al.*, 1993a); in one case, however, it is in the XPB group (Vermeulen *et al.*, 1994), while in another it appears to be a new group altogether, named TTDA (Stefanini *et al.*, 1993b). From the foregoing, it would thus appear that defects in the XPD gene may be associated with three different clinical entities, namely XP, TTD and XP with CS, and a clue to the understanding of this paradox has now come with the discovery that the transcription factor TFIIH has two roles in the cell, namely in RNA transcription and in NER (Hoeijmakers *et al.*, 1996) (see Plate 18). Thus, as mentioned above on p. 145, the XPD, XPB and TTDA proteins are subunits of TFIIH, such that mutations in these genes may in turn variably affect TFIIH repair and transcription. A currently widely held view, therefore, is that mutations that severely diminish repair activity but have little effect on transcription result clinically in XP but if transcription is also affected, TTD occurs instead (Bootsma and Hoeijmakers, 1993). TTD is thus proposed as a 'transcription syndrome' (Vermeulen *et al.*, 1994) and in support of these ideas, the XPD gene mutations in XP and TTD are at different sites (Broughton *et al.*, 1994; Takayama *et al.*, 1995, 1996); however, why TTD patients do not get skin cancer, as in XP, despite the similar DNA repair defects remains a mystery.

DIAGNOSIS

Amino acid hair analysis, as determined by oxygen combustion, for example, demonstrates a diagnostic reduction in the cysteine/cystine concentration ratio to 15–50% of normal; the diagnosis can then be confirmed in the majority of cases by the measurement of unscheduled DNA or RNA synthesis following UV irradiation. Cutaneous irradiation testing is usually normal.

TREATMENT

No specific treatments are available.

BLOOM'S SYNDROME

CLINICAL FEATURES

A rare autosomal recessive disorder most common in males (Bloom, 1966; German and Passarge, 1989), BS is most prevalent amongst Ashkenazi Jews (carrier rate 1:20). It is characterized by the appearance of a variably severe, telangiectatic erythema, generally between the ages of two weeks and three years, on the cheeks, nose, eyelids, lips, forehead, ears and in some cases dorsa of the hands and forearms, but typically not the trunk, buttocks and lower extremities (Bloom, 1966; German and Passarge, 1989); this then tends to fade after puberty. However, sun exposure frequently exacerbates the facial redness, often leading to bullae, crusting and bleeding, while *café au lait* or larger pigmented macules are frequently present, at times accompanied by adjacent depigmented areas (German and Passarge, 1989).

BS is associated with an up to 300-fold increase in malignant neoplasm incidence, approximately 20% of patients being affected, usually at an early age. Carcinomas, for example of the gastrointestinal tract, breast and skin, occur most frequently, lymphatic and non-lymphatic leukaemias and lymphosarcomas being next most common. A susceptibility to multiple and severe gastrointestinal and respiratory infections is also often evident in childhood, frequently improving with age, however, although chronic lung disease is possible later. Children with BS are usually of low birth weight and remain small thereafter; however, they are generally well proportioned, although a characteristic facial appearance with receding chin, narrow prominent nose and hypoplastic malar areas is common. Learning difficulties are also common but overt mental deficiency is unusual, while diabetes mellitus is a recognized association and males are generally infertile because of defective spermatogenesis.

IMMUNE FUNCTION

Immunological abnormalities are variable, but deficiencies in both B- and T-cell function are possible. Thus, diminished immunoglobulin levels are common, while T-cell proliferative responses in the mixed leucocyte reaction and to mitogens or antigens may also be impaired (Weemaes *et al.*, 1979).

MOLECULAR AND CELLULAR ABNORMALITIES

In contrast to the disorders discussed above, cultured cells in BS are not hypersensitive to UV irradiation, their most marked feature instead being a high frequency of chromosome aberrations (German, 1974) and sister chromatid exchanges (SCE) (Chaganti *et al.*, 1974), a particular feature of the former being quadriradials, structures rarely found in other cells. In spite of this, BS cells are not especially sensitive to other DNA damaging agents either, except mildly to certain alkylating agents (Kurihara *et al.*, 1987), but there is evidence instead for a high spontaneous mutation frequency, both in lymphocytes *in vivo* (Langlois *et al.*, 1989) and in cultured fibroblasts (Warren *et al.*, 1981). Along with this, fibre autoradiographic and biochemical studies have shown the rate of progression of the DNA replication fork in BS to be slower than normal (Gianelli *et al.*, 1977; Hand and German, 1975).

Several studies have reported a deficiency in DNA ligase efficacy in BS cells (Chan *et al.*, 1987; Willis *et al.*, 1987), but it is now clear that this is not after all the primary defect. Thus, the BLM gene defective in BS was cloned in 1995 (Ellis *et al.*, 1995) and the sequence of its encoded protein shown to be similar to that of several DNA helicases in the so-called RecQ family. It is likely, therefore, that the basic protein defective in BS is a helicase, but precise biochemical studies on its function have not yet been carried out.

DIAGNOSIS

BS may be confused with the Rothmund–Thomson syndrome in young children, but useful distinguishing features in the latter include skin atrophy, frequent cataract development, sparse scalp and body hair and an extension of the characteristic telangiectasia and reticulate pigmentation to the skin of the buttocks and legs. In addition, an increased frequency of SCEs in BS is unique and a valuable confirmation of the diagnosis, both post- and prenatally (German *et al.*, 1979). Finally, some workers have demonstrated an increased sensitivity to monochromatic UVB irradiation in BS patients (Fitzpatrick *et al.*, 1963), although others have not (Bloom, 1966); Rothmund-Thomson patients however, are generally normal in this respect.

TREATMENT

No specific treatments are available.

REFERENCES

Aboussekhra, A., Biggerstaff, M., Shivji, M.K.K., *et al.* (1995) Mammalian DNA nucleotide excision repair reconstituted with purified components. *Cell*, **80**, 859–68.

Anstey, A., Arlett, C.F., Cole, J. *et al.* (1991) Long term survival and preservation of natural killer cell activity in a xeroderma pigmentosum patient with spontaneous regression and multiple deposits of malignant melanoma. *British Journal of Dermatology*, **125**, 272–8.

Baden, H.P., Jackson, C.E., Weiss, L. *et al.* (1976) The physicochemical properties of hair in the IBIDS syndrome. *American Journal of Human Genetics*, **27**, 514–21.

Berkel, A.I. and Kiran, O. (1974) Immunological studies in children with xeroderma pigmentosum. *Turkish Journal of Paediatrics*, **16**, 43–52.

Bloom, D. (1966) The syndrome of congenital telangiectatic erythema and stunted growth. *Journal of Paediatrics*, **68**, 102–13.

Bohr, V.A., Smith, C.A., Okumoto, D.S. *et al.* (1985) DNA repair in an active gene. Removal of pyrimidine dimers from the DHFR gene of CHO cells is much more efficient than in the genome overall. *Cell*, **40**, 359–69.

Bootsma, D. and Hoeijmakers, J.H.J. (1993) Engagement with transcription. *Nature*, **363**, 114–15.

Broughton, B.C., Lehmann, A.R., Harcourt, S.A. *et al.* (1990) Relationship between pyrimidine dimers, 6-4 photoproducts, repair synthesis and cell survival. Studies using cells from patients with trichothiodystrophy. *Mutation Research*, **235**, 33–40.

Broughton, B.C., Steingrimsdottir, H., Weber, C. and Lehmann, A.R. (1994) Mutations in the xeroderma pigmentosum group D DNA repair gene in patients with trichothiodystrophy. *Nature Genetics*, **7**, 189–94.

Césarini, J.P., Biovka, P., Moreno, G. *et al.* (1975) Hypopigmented macules of unexposed skin in xeroderma pigmentosum. *Journal of Cutaneous Pathology*, **2**, 28–139.

Chaganti, R.S.K., Schonberg, S. and German, J. (1974) A many fold increase in sister chromatid exchanges in Bloom's syndrome lymphocytes. *Proceedings of the National Academy of Sciences of the USA*, **71**, 4508–12.

Chan, J.Y.H., Becker, F.F., German, J. *et al.* (1987) Altered DNA ligase 1 activity in Bloom's syndrome cells. *Nature*, **325**, 357–9.

Cockayne, E.A. (1936) Dwarfism with retinal atrophy and deafness. *Archives of Diseases of Childhood*, **11**, 1–8.

Coulter, D.L., Beals, T.F. and Allen, R.J. (1982) Neurotrichosis. Hairshaft abnormalities associated with neurological diseases. *Developmental Medicine and Child Neurology*, **24**, 634–44.

Cripps, D.J., Ramsey, C.A. and Ruch, D.M. (1971) Xeroderma pigmentosum, abnormal monochromatic action spectrum and autoradiographic studies. *Journal of Investigative Dermatology*, **56**, 281–6.

Dumaz, N., Drougar, C., Sarasin, A. and Daya-Grosjean, L. (1993) Specific UV-induced mutation spectrum in the p53 gene of skin tumors from DNA repair deficient xeroderma pigmentosum patients. *Proceedings of the National Academy of Sciences of the USA*, **90**, 10529–33.

Dupuy, J.M. and Lafforet, D. (1974) A defect of cellular immunity in xeroderma pigmentosum. *Clinical Immunology and Immunopathology*, **3**, 52–8.

Ellis, N.A., Groden, J., Ye, T.-Z. *et al.* (1995) The Bloom's syndrome gene product is homologous to RecQ helicases. *Cell*, **83**, 655–66.

Fitzpatrick, T.B., Pathak, M.A., Magnus, I.A. *et al.* (1963) Abnormal reactions of man to light. *Annual Reviews in Medicine*, **14**, 195–9.

Gaspari, A.A., Fleisher, T.A. and Kraemer, K.H. (1993) Impaired interferon production and natural killer cell activation in patients with the skin cancer prone disorder, xeroderma pigmentosum. *Journal of Clinical Investigation*, **92**, 1135–42.

German, J. (1974) Bloom's syndrome. II. The prototype of human genetic disorders predisposing to chromosome instability and cancer, in *Chromosomes and Cancer* (ed. J. German), Wiley, New York, pp. 601–17.

German, J. and Passarge, E. (1989) Bloom's syndrome XI. Report from the Registry for 1987. *Clinical Genetics*, **35**, 57–69.

German, J., Bloom, D. and Passarge, E. (1979) Bloom's syndrome. VII. Progress report for 1978. *Clinical Genetics*, **15**, 361–7.

Gianelli, F., Benson, P.F., Pawsey, S.A. *et al.* (1977) Ultraviolet light sensitivity and delayed DNA-chain maturation in Bloom's syndrome fibroblasts. *Nature*, **265**, 466–9.

Hakamada, S., Watanabe, K., Soboe, G. *et al.* (1982) Xeroderma pigmentosum. Neurological, neurophysiological and morphological studies. *European Neurology*, **21**, 69–76.

Halley, D.J.J., Keijzer, W., Jaspers, N.G.J. *et al.* (1979) Prenatal diagnosis of xeroderma pigmentosum (group C) using assays of unscheduled DNA synthesis and postreplication repair. *Clinical Genetics*, **16**, 137–46.

Hand, R. and German, J. (1975) A retarded rate of DNA chain growth in Bloom's syndrome. *Proceedings of the National Academy of Sciences of the USA*, **72**, 758–62.

Henning, K.A., Li, L., Iyer, N. *et al.* (1995) The Cockayne-syndrome group-A gene encodes a WD repeat protein that interacts with CSB protein and a subunit of RNA-polymerase-II TFIIH. *Cell*, **82**, 555–64.

Hoeijmakers, J.H.J. (1993) Nucleotide excision repair II, from yeast to mammals. *Trends in Genetics*, **9**, 21–27.

Hoeijmakers, J.H.J., Egly, J.-M. and Vermeulen, W. (1996) TFIIH: a key component in multiple DNA transactions. *Current Opinion in Genetics and Development*, **6**, 26–33.

Ichihashi, M. and Fujiwara, Y. (1981) Clinical and photobiological characteristics of Japanese xeroderma pigmentosum variant. *British Journal of Dermatology*, **105**, 1–12.

Itoh, T., Tomomichi, O. and Yamaizumi, M. (1996) A simple method for diagnosing xeroderma pigmentosum variant. *Journal of Investigative Dermatology*, **107**, 349–53.

Jackson, C.E., Weiss, C. and Watson, J.H.L. (1974) 'Brittle' hair with short stature, intellectual impairment and decreased fertility. An autosomal recessive syndrome in an Amish kindred. *Pediatrics*, **54**, 201–8.

Jorizzo, J.L., Atherton, D.J., Crounse, R.G. *et al.* (1982) Ichthyosis, brittle hair, impaired intelligence, decreased fertility and short stature (IBIDS syndrome). *British Journal of Dermatology*, **106**, 705–10.

Jung, E. (1986) Xeroderma pigmentosum. *International Journal of Dermatology*, **25**, 629–33.

Kennedy, R.M., Rowe, V.D. and Kepes, J.J. (1980) Cockayne's syndrome. An atypical case. *Neurology*, **30**, 1268–72.

Kraemer, K.H. and Slor, H. (1984) Xeroderma pigmentosum. *Clinics in Dermatology*, **2**, 33–69.

Kraemer, K.H., Lee, M.M. and Scotto, J. (1984) DNA repair protects against cutaneous and internal neoplasia. Evidence from xeroderma pigmentosum. *Carcinogenesis*, **5**, 511–14.

Kraemer, K.H., Lee, M.M. and Scotto, J. (1987) Xeroderma pigmentosum. Cutaneous, ocular and neurologic abnormalities in 830 published cases. *Archives of Dermatology*, **123**, 241–50.

Kraemer, K.H., Digiorama, J.J., Moshell, A.N. *et al.* (1988) Prevention of skin cancer in xeroderma pigmentosum with the use of oral isotretinoin. *New England Journal of Medicine*, **318**, 1633–7.

Krutmann, J., Bohnert, J.E. and Jung, E.G. (1994) Evidence that DNA damage is a mediate in ultraviolet B radiation-induced inhibition of human gene expression: ultraviolet B radiation effects in intercellular adhesion molecule-1 (ICAM-1) expression. *Journal of Investigative Dermatology*, **102**, 428–32.

Kurihara, T., Inoue, M. and Tatsumi, K. (1987) Hypersensitivity of Bloom's syndrome fibroblasts to N-ethyl-N-nitrosourea. *Mutation Research*, **184**, 147–51.

Langlois, R.G., Bigbee, W.L., Jensen, R.H. *et al.* (1989) Evidence for increased *in vivo* mutation and somatic recombination in Bloom's syndrome. *Proceedings of the National Academy of Sciences of the USA*, **86**, 670–4.

Lehmann, A.R. (1995) Nucleotide excision repair and the link with transcription. *Trends in Biochemistry*, **20**, 402–5.

Lehmann, A.R., Kirk-Bell, S., Arlett, C.F. *et al.* (1975) Xeroderma pigmentosum cells with normal levels of excision repair have a defect in DNA synthesis after UV-irradiation. *Proceedings of the National Academy of Sciences of the USA*, **72**, 219–23.

Lehmann, A.R., Kirk-Bell, S. and Mayne, L. (1979) Abnormal kinetics of DNA synthesis in ultraviolet light-irradiated cells from patients with Cockayne's syndrome and xeroderma pigmentosum. *Cancer Research*, **39**, 4237–41.

Lehmann, A.R., Francis, A.J. and Giannelli, F. (1985) Prenatal diagnosis of Cockayne's syndrome. *Lancet*, **1**, 486–8.

Lehmann, A.R., Arlett, C.F., Broughton, B.C. *et al.* (1988) Trichothiodystrophy, a human DNA repair disorder with heterogeneity in the cellular response to ultraviolet light. *Cancer Research*, **48**, 6090–6.

Lehmann, A.R., Thompson, A.F., Harcourt, S.A. *et al.* (1993) Cockayne's syndrome: correlation of clinical features with cellular sensitivity of RNA synthesis to UV-irradiation. *Journal of Medical Genetics*, **30**, 679–82.

Lucky, P.A., Kirsch, N., Lucky, A.W. *et al.* (1984) Low-sulfur hair syndrome associated with UVB photosensitivity and testicular failure. *Journal of the American Academy of Dermatology*, **11**, 340–6.

MacDonald, W.B., Fitch, K.L. and Lewis, K. (1960) Cockayne's syndrome. A heredofamilial disorder of growth development. *Paediatrics*, **25**, 997–1007.

Mariani, E., Facchini, A., Honorati, M.C. *et al.* (1992) Defects in families and patients with xeroderma pigmentosum and trichothiodystrophy. *Clinical and Experimental Immunology*, **88**, 376–82.

Mayne, L.V. and Lehmann, A.R. (1982) Failure of RNA synthesis to recover after UV-irradiation. An early defect in cells from individuals with Cockayne's syndrome and xeroderma pigmentosum. *Cancer Research*, **42**, 1473–8.

Miyauchi-Hashimoto, H., Tanaka, K. and Horio, T. (1996) Enhanced inflammation and immunosuppression by ultraviolet radiation in xeroderma pigmentosum group A (XPA) model mice. *Journal of Investigative Dermatology*, **107**, 343–8.

Morison, W.L., Bucana, C., Hasem, N. *et al.* (1985) Impaired immune function in patients with xeroderma pigmentosum. *Cancer Research*, **45**, 3929–31.

Moriwaki, S.-I., Stefanini, M., Lehmann, A.R. *et al.* (1996) DNA repair and ultraviolet mutagenesis in cells from a new patient with xeroderma pigmentosum group G and Cockayne syndrome. *Journal of Investigative Dermatology*, **107**, 647–53.

Nance, M.A. and Berry, S.A. (1992) Cockayne syndrome: review of 140 cases. *American Journal of Medical Genetics*, **42**, 68–84.

Nishigori, C., Moriwaki, S.-I., Takebe, H., Tanaka, T. and Imamura, S. (1994) Gene alterations and clinical characteristics of xeroderma pigmentosum group A patients in Japan. *Archives of Dermatology*, **130**, 191–7.

Norris, P.G., Limb, G.A., Hamblin, A.S. *et al.* (1990) Immune function, mutant frequency and cancer risk in the DNA repair defective genodermatoses xeroderma pigmentosum, Cockayne's syndrome and trichothiodystrophy. *Journal of Investigative Dermatology*, **94**, 94–100.

Paddison, R.M., Moosy, J., Derbes, V.J. *et al.* (1963) Cockayne's syndrome. A report of five new cases with biochemical, chromosomal, genetic and neuropathologic observations. *Dermatologia Tropica*, **2**, 195–203.

Pollitt, R.J., Fenner, F.A. and Davies, M. (1968) Sibs with mental and physical retardation and trichorrhexis nodosa with abnormal amino acid composition of the hair. *Archives of Diseases of Childhood*, **43**, 21–216.

Price, V.H., Odom, R.B., Ward, W.H. *et al.* (1980) Trichothiodystrophy. Sulfur deficient brittle hair as a marker for a neuroectodermal symptom complex. *Archives of Dermatology*, **16**, 1375–84.

Ramsay, C.A. and Gianelli, F. (1975) The erythemal action spectrum and deoxyribunucleic acid repair synthesis in xeroderma pigmentosum. *British Journal of Dermatology*, **92**, 49–56.

Ramsay, C.A., Coltart, T.M., Blunt, S. *et al.* (1974) Prenatal diagnosis of xeroderma pigmentosum. *Lancet*, **1**, 1109–12.

Reed, W.B., May, S.B. and Nickel, W.B. (1965) Xeroderma pigmentosum with neurological complications. The de Sanctis–Cacchione syndrome. *Archives of Dermatology*, **91**, 224–6.

Roytta, M. and Anttinan, A. (1986) Xeroderma pigmentosum with neurological abnormalities. A clinical and neuropathological study. *Acta Neurologica Scandinavica*, **73**, 191–9.

Salaman, T., Stojakov, M. and Bogdanovic, B. (1975) Delayed hypersensitivity in xeroderma pigmentosum. *Archives of Dermatological Research (Berlin)*, **251**, 277–80.

Stefanini, M., Lagomarsini, P., Arlett, C.F. *et al.* (1986) Xeroderma pigmentosum (complementation group D) mutation is present in patients affected by trichothiodystrophy with photosensitivity. *Human Genetics*, **74**, 107–12.

Stefanini, M., Lagomarsini, P., Gilianai, S. *et al.* (1993a) Genetic heterogeneity of the excision repair defect associated with trichothiodystrophy. *Carcinogenesis*, **14**, 1101–5.

Stefanini, M., Vermeulen, W., Weeda, G. *et al.* (1993b) A new nucleotide excision repair gene associated with the genetic disorder trichothiodystrophy. *American Journal of Human Genetics*, **53**, 817–21.

Stefanini, M., Fawcett, H., Botta, E. *et al.* (1996) Genetic analysis of twenty-two patients with Cockayne syndrome. *Human Genetics*, **97**, 418–23.

Takayama, K., Salazar, E.P., Lehmann, A.R. *et al.* (1995) Defects in the repair and transcription gene *ERCC2* in the cancer-prone disorder xeroderma pigmentosum. *Cancer Research*, **55**, 5656–63.

Takayama, K., Salazar, E.P., Broughton, B.C. *et al.* (1996) Defects in the DNA repair and transcription gene *ERCC2(XPD)* in trichothiodystrophy. *American Journal of Human Genetics*, **58**, 263–70.

Troelstra, C., Van Gool, A., De Wit, J. *et al.* (1992) ERCC6, a member of a subfamily of putative helicases, is involved in Cockayne's syndrome and preferential repair of active genes. *Cell*, **71**, 939–53.

Turner, M.L., Moshell, A. and Corbett, D.W. (1993) Clearing of melanoma-*in-situ* with intralesional-interferon in a patient with xeroderma pigmentosum. *Journal of Investigative Dermatology*, **100**, 538.

Van Hoffen, A., Natarajan, A.T., Mayne, L.V. *et al.* (1993) Deficient repair of the transcribed strand of active genes in Cockayne's syndrome cells. *Nucleic Acids Research*, **21**, 5890–5.

Venema, J., Mullenders, L.H.F., Natarajan, A.T. *et al.* (1990) The genetic defect in Cockayne's syndrome is associated with a defect in repair of uv-induced DNA damage in transcriptionally active DNA. *Proceedings of the National Academy of Sciences of the USA*, **87**, 4707–11.

Vermeulen, W., Van Vuuren, A.J., Chipoulet, M. *et al.* (1994) Three unusual repair deficiencies associated with transcription factor BTF2(TFIIH): evidence for the existence of a transcription syndrome. *Cold Spring Harbor Symposium on Quantitative Biology*, **59**, 317–29.

Wade, M.H. and Chu, E.H.Y. (1979) Effects of DNA damaging agents on cultured fibroblasts derived from patients with Cockayne's syndrome. *Mutation Research*, **59**, 49–60.

Warren, S.T., Schultz, R.A., Chang, C.C. *et al.* (1981) Elevated spontaneous mutation rate in Bloom syndrome fibroblasts. *Proceedings of the National Academy of Sciences of the USA*, **78**, 3133–7.

Weemaes, C.M.R., Bakkeren, J., Ter Haar, B. *et al.* (1979) Immune responses in four patients with Bloom syndrome. *Clinical Immunology and Immunopathology*, **12**, 12–19.

Willis, A.E., Welsberg, R., Tomlinson, S. *et al.* (1987) Structural alterations of DNA ligase 1 in Bloom's syndrome. *Proceedings of the National Academy of Sciences of the USA*, **84**, 8016–20.

Wysenbeek, A.J., Weiss, H., Duczyminer-Kahana, M. *et al.* (1986) Immunologic alterations in xeroderma pigmentosum patients. *Cancer*, **58**, 219–21.

Yarosh, D., Klein, J., Kibitel, J. *et al.* (1996) Enzyme therapy of xeroderma pigmentosum: safety and efficacy of T4N5 liposome lotion containing a prokaryotic DNA repair enzyme. *Photodermatology, Photoimmunology and Photomedicine*, **12**, 122–30.

Ziegler, A., Leffell, D.J., Kunala, S. *et al.* (1993) Mutation hotspots due to sunlight in the p53 gene of nonmelanoma skin cancers. *Proceedings of the National Academy of Sciences of the USA*, **90**, 4216–20.

DRUG AND CHEMICAL PHOTOSENSITIVITY

12

James Ferguson

As new chemicals and drugs emerge, photosensitization becomes an ever-increasing problem. However, we have steadily increased our understanding of the range of mechanisms involved, drug sites of action and possible methods of disease prevention. Phototoxicity from drugs presents in a variety of defined forms that require recognition in the clinic, while photoallergy, an immune-mediated eczema, is now being seen with increasing frequency as a result of the use of chemical sunscreen agents and cosmetics. A greater knowledge, as the result of a better quality of information, is now required by all involved parties at drug preregistration and postmarketing surveillance levels. Interested physicians and scientists thus need to combine with greater effort to improve the current incomplete level of understanding.

INTRODUCTION

Abnormal skin responses resulting from the combination of natural or artificial ultraviolet radiation (UVR) or visible wavelength exposure, with the presence in the skin of an ever-enlarging list of topically or systemically administered chemicals, are being increasingly recognized.

This chapter comments on information in this regard which has emerged in recent

Photodermatology. Edited by J.L.M. Hawk. Published in 1998 by Chapman & Hall, London. ISBN 0 412 72460 X.

years, particularly in the expanding areas of photosensitization by fluoroquinolone antibiotics and sunscreens.

Regulatory and pharmaceutical interest has developed as new, more effective study techniques have become available to answer key questions concerning suspected photosensitizers, ideally before their release as approved drugs.

PHOTOSENSITIZATION TYPES AND MECHANISMS

Normally ineffective levels UVR or visible irradiation of skin containing a specific radiation-absorbing molecule, or **chromophore**, may result in abnormal biological effects.

A wide range of such chromophores exist and may be classified as systemic or topical and endogenous or exogenous (Table 12.1). *Endogenous* photosensitizing agents are normal skin constituents generally present in abnormally high concentrations, usually because of a disturbance in tissue enzymatic function. On the other hand, *exogenous* agents are chemicals or drugs absorbed either into the skin by topical contact or by a systemic route such as oral or parenteral. Potential agents of this sort are primarily drugs (Table 12.2), but also include sunscreens, dyestuffs, plant materials and environmental contaminants.

The absorption of radiant energy by a photosensitizing chromophore within the skin may raise its electronic state from ground level

Table 12.1　General classification of photo-sensitizers

Endogenous
Abnormal metabolites: uroporphyrin, coproporphyrin
Normal constituents: protoporphyrin, kynurenic acid, tryptophan

Exogenous
Drugs: antibiotics, tranquillizers, antidepressants, anti-inflammatories, diuretics, antiarrhythmics, antihypertensives
Plant materials: furocoumarins, α-terthienyl, polyacetylenes
Dyestuffs: thiazides, methylene blue, toluidine blue, xanthenes, fluorescein, eosin, erythrosin, rose bengal, anthraquine-based dyes, Disperse Blue 35, benzanthrone
Polycyclic hydrocarbons: pitch, coal tars, anthracene, acridine, fluoranthrene
Perfumes and cosmetics: bergamot oil containing 5-methoxypsoralen, musk ambrette, 6-methylcoumarin
Sunscreens, inks: para-aminobenzoic acid, benzophenones, benzoylmethanes, cinnamates
Tattoos: cadmium sulphide
Miscellaneous: cyclamate sweetener, blankophore fabric whitener, quinoxaline-n-dioxide

to an excited short-lived state, the so-called **singlet state**, by electronic rearrangement; this may then undergo further transformation into a more biologically active, longer lived species, the **triplet state**, which may interact directly with biological systems or indirectly through interaction with oxygen. Most photo-sensitized reactions are in fact so-called oxygen-dependent type I effects through electron or hydrogen transfer, producing photo-sensitized substrate radicals. Such agents then react directly with cellular oxygen or else lead to damage to biological structures by super-oxide, peroxide or hydroxyl products. In type II reactions, lipid, nucleic acids and proteins may be directly damaged following the formation instead of reactive singlet-state oxygen.

Thus, whatever the source or means of access to the skin, a chromophore, following interaction with UVR or visible radiation, may become sufficiently reactive to induce a change in that biological system. However, because of the complexity of such interactions, the variability in damage mechanisms and clinical changes produced by photosensitizers

Table 12.2　Potential photosensitizing drugs

Antibiotics	Fluoroquinolones
	Nalidixic acid
	Tetracyclines
	Sulphonamides
Antifungals	Griseofulvin
Diuretics and cardiovascular agents	Thiazides
	Frusemide
	Amiodarone
	Quinidine
Non-steroidal anti-inflammatory drugs	Naproxen
	Tiaprofenic acid
	Piroxicam
	Azapropazone
	Benoxaprofen (now discontinued)
Psoralens	
Psychoactive drugs	Phenothiazines, for example chlorpromazine, thioridazine
	Protriptyline
Retinoids	Isotretinoin
	Etretinate
	Acitretin

is huge, as reflected by the wide variety of apparently different pathogenic mechanisms such as phototoxicity, photoallergy and pseudoporphyria (Table 12.3) and the broad range of clinical presentations, even within one mechanism, such as phototoxicity.

SYSTEMIC PHOTOSENSITIZATION

Drug–radiation interaction effects may not only be confined to acute damage to cutaneous structures, a range of other, relatively unexplored events also being possible (Plate 20). Thus, there may conceivably be systemic toxicity from toxic photoproducts generated within the skin and then released into the circulation and the photobiological study of chlordiazepoxide effects in rats has revealed that the combination of irradiation and drug (but neither alone) may result in significant liver damage (Bakri *et al.*, 1985). However, little is yet known of such drug effects in man.

Table 12.3 Mechanisms and manifestations of drug- and chemical-induced photosensitivity

Phototoxicity
Pseudoporphyria
Photoallergy
Lupus erythematosus
Lichenoid reactions
Pellagra

Further, skin cancer, another endpoint of phototoxic damage from chemicals and drugs, urgently needs to be investigated by laboratory study, while yet another area of interest is the possible loss of therapeutic efficacy by a photolabile drug circulating in the skin of a sunbather or sunbed user. It is not yet known whether such issues are real or merely theoretical or laboratory phenomena.

PHOTOTOXICITY

The commonest photosensitization mechanism seen is without doubt phototoxicity, which occurs in any subject if sufficient cutaneous photosensitizer is exposed to enough causal irradiation. Although photototoxicity is often described as an exaggerated sunburn reaction, it is clear that each photosensitizer has its own characteristic clinical features (Table 12.4) and it is likely that the photochemical uniqueness of an individual agent relates not only to its chemical structure but also its anatomical point of skin localization. Thus, immediate urticarial reactions involve mast cells and are likely to be dermal in origin, while an exaggerated sunburn effect (Table 12.4) seems likely to arise from the epidermis.

Other presentations include that seen with the psoralen photosensitization of phytophotodermatitis caused by fruits, vegetables and

Table 12.4 Major patterns of cutaneous phototoxicity

Skin reactions	*Photosensitizers*
Prickling or burning during exposure; immediate erythema; oedema or urticaria with higher doses; sometimes delayed erythema or hyperpigmentation	Coal tar; pitch; anthraquinone-based dyestuffs; benoxaprofen; amiodarone; chlorpromazine
Exaggerated sunburn	Fluoroquinolone antibiotics; chlorpromazine; amiodarone; thiazide diuretics; quinine; demethylchlortetracycline and other tetracyclines
Late-onset erythema; blisters with slightly higher doses; hyperpigmentation only with low doses	Psoralens; phytophotodermatitis; berloque dermatitis
Increased skin fragility with blisters from trauma (pseudoporphyria)	Nalidixic acid; frusemide; tetracycline; naproxen; amiodarone

weeds (Drever and Hunter, 1970; Freeman *et al.*, 1984), in which psoralen-containing sap comes into contact with the skin, either directly or by being splattered up by a rotary mower or strimmer device. Subsequent exposure to UVA (315–400 nm) wavelengths then results in the development of erythema at the contact sites some 24 hours later, this reaching a maximum at about 48–72 hours, often with blister development. Thereafter, during the healing phase, an intense melanin pigmentation usually develops and persists for many months (Johnson, 1993).

A number of phototoxic drugs are also capable of so-called pseudoporphyria induction (Table 12.4), in which, rather than acute skin photosensitization, the major feature is chronic skin fragility with blistering and sometimes later milia formation following mild trauma. The proposed initial diagnosis is usually one of hepatic cutaneous porphyria, but normal porphyrin studies and a careful drug history instead reveal the true cause. The same problem is also occasionally seen without drugs in chronic renal failure patients, for uncertain reasons.

New phototoxic agents continue to be reported in the systemic drug group and this decade has seen the emergence of a new group of such drugs, the fluoroquinolone antibiotics.

IN VITRO PHOTOTOXIC ASSESSMENT

To define the exact phototoxic potential of a systemic agent requires careful study design. Although a range of *in vitro* test systems (Arlett *et al.*, 1995; Maguire and Kaidbey, 1982) now exist, it is still unclear which, if any, should be adopted as routine screens for phototoxicity. The value of such systems is to predict which drugs and to what degree new agents are photosensitizing. The problem is to answer the key questions. First, is a drug phototoxic at therapeutic dose levels and if so, how does it compare with other members of the same drug group? Next, what is the

wavelength dependency for the reaction and what is its mechanism? Finally, what are its effects *in vivo* in a clinical study?

While the findings from *in vitro* models provide important insights, direct application to the *in vivo* situation is often precluded by the following complexities:

1. the metabolism of the initial photosensitizer may lead to the production of other photoactive agents;
2. the radiation reaching a potential photosensitizer may depend on its cellular location;
3. the photosensitizer or its photoactive metabolites may become bound to subcellular structures so as to alter its photochemistry.

IN VIVO HUMAN VOLUNTEER STUDIES

Too often in the past, the phototoxic potential of a drug has only emerged as a feature of its postmarketing surveillance. However, with the combination of new *in vitro* and *in vivo* techniques, it has now become feasible in most cases to predict such phototoxic potential long before the drug's release into the market place. In addition, despite the continuing absence of clear regulatory guidelines, it is now generally possible to design a study capable of generating objective data on the likely clinical features relating to a phototoxic drug and their severity, wavelength dependency, relationship to irradiation dose and duration. Such a study should be of sufficient power to give the required information, be conducted blind, contain both positive as well as placebo comparators and have a measure of volunteer compliance. Within such a technique, baseline minimal erythema dose (MED) phototesting of normal volunteers should be conducted with a broad-spectrum light source, either a filtered solar simulator or a monochromator opened up to give broad wavebands chosen to represent the different UVR and visible components of the solar spectrum and the testing then repeated with the volunteers taking the drug at a time of stable pharmacokinetics. If significant photosensitivity is detected in any individual, the phototesting should then be repeated to enable assessment of the time scale for a return to baseline after cessation of drug exposure.

By comparison of the on-drug MEDs with the baseline median values, a phototoxic factor can be established as:

$$\text{Phototoxic factor} = \frac{\text{baseline } MED}{\text{on-drug MED}}$$

for each waveband tested. An indication of the exposure time to artificial or solar irradiation necessary for the induction of erythema can then be obtained by convolution of the action spectrum for such erythema into the emission spectrum of the solar or other source. Ultimately, of course, the relative importance of a particular wavelength in inducing erythema will depend on whether it is present in the radiation to which the patient is likely to be exposed, such as for example window glass-transmitted sunlight or UVA sunbed radiation.

Such objective data have only been produced in recent times, but it remains unfortunate that too few such studies, which are predominantly pharmaceutically funded, reach publication, apparently because they seem to be perceived as of only regulatory interest.

It should be emphasized that *in vitro* and *in vivo* drug and chemical photosensitization studies pick up only phototoxicity. Mechanisms that involve a sensitized immune system such as photoallergy or drug-induced lupus erythematosus, or those essentially of an idiosyncratic nature such as pseudoporphyria, some rare types of phototoxicity and drug-induced pellagra continue to be largely detected by post-marketing surveillance techniques.

Many drugs have been reported to cause photosensitivity (DeLeo, 1992), some of the commoner offenders being listed in Table 12.2. Although it is the major cause of exogenous cutaneous photosensitization (Ljunggren and Bjellerup, 1986), the exact incidence of drug photosensitivity is unknown. In addition, there are major differences in reported incidences for individual drugs, such as 16–25% for chlorpromazine (Ayd, 1956; Calnan *et al.*, 1962) and 1–26% for tetracycline (Orentreich *et al.*, 1961), probably relating to local variations in patient sunlight exposure, skin type and drug dosage. Furthermore, while some agents produce predictably frequent photosensitization, such as for example amiodarone and chlorpromazine, others such as the thiazides and quinine which appear to be idiosyncratic, only arise in a minority of those taking the drug. Thus, the Committee on Safety of Medicines adverse reaction reporting system lists approximately 250 drugs as possible photosensitizers, yet only a minority appear to cause frequent trouble and only a few of these have been studied in detail to define their true photosensitizing role.

FLUOROQUINOLONE ANTIBIOTICS

Nalidixic acid, the first member of this group, has long been known as a photosensitizer (Bilsland and Douglas, 1990; Burry and Crosby, 1996; Ramsay and Obreshkova, 1974), but has relatively restricted clinical therapeutic activity as compared with the more recently synthesized fluoroquinolones. Thus, these newer agents, characterized by a fluorine substitution at molecular position 4, have longer half-lives and a greater degree and breadth of antibacterial activity.

Rather than the pseudoporphyria reaction, namely skin fragility and blistering of the exposed sites in the presence of normal porphyrin values, as seen on occasions with nalidixic acid (Buchbinder *et al.*, 1962), the newer fluoroquinolones may cause a photosensitivity characterized by skin redness, blistering and subsequent peeling of the exposed areas, described as an exaggerated sunburn reaction (Plate 21) (Ferguson, 1995). On occasions, however, there may instead be photo-onycholysis, in which the nail plate separates from the nail bed as a consequence of the phototoxicity (Baran and Brun, 1986; Gonzalez and Henwood, 1989).

Earlier marketed fluoroquinolones, such as ciprofloxacin (Jensen *et al.*, 1987; Jungst and Mohr, 1987), norfloxacin (Ferguson and Johnson, 1993) and enoxacin (Izu *et al.*, 1992; Kawabe *et al.*, 1989; Petri and Tronnier, 1986), are all phototoxic but the clinical reactions appear mild and their incidence low (< 2.4%) (Schiefe *et al.*, 1993). As a group, they were therefore initially labelled as weak photosensitizers, capable of producing a reaction only when the drug dosage and levels of insolation were high (Ferguson and Johnson, 1992). It has since become clear, however, that other members of the group have a much greater phototoxic potential, clinical reactions not only occurring with a higher incidence (fleroxacin 10–15% (Bowie *et al.*, 1989; Kawabe *et al.*, 1989), lomefloxacin 4–10% (Food and Drug Administration, 1993; Lopitaux *et al.*, 1985), pefloxacin (Christ and Lehnert, 1990) and sparfloxacin (Mizutani *et al.*, 1995)) but also with an apparently greater severity (Cohen and Bergstresser, 1994; Correia and Delgado, 1994; Kuramaji and Shono, 1992). Thus, on at least one occasion, severe phototoxicity has been a major contributing factor in halting the development programme of a new fluoroquinolone.

Patients with low levels of skin pigmentation are known to be most susceptible to psoralen phototoxic effects (Bech-Thomsen *et al.*, 1994) and in the absence of data to the contrary, it seems reasonable to make the assumption that fluoroquinolone photosensitization will follow the same pattern. In addition, while fluoroquinolones are in general taken for short periods, on occasions prolonged courses are taken at high doses, particularly, for example, in cystic fibrosis, and this patient group has indeed reported a very high incidence of phototoxicity of greater than 50% (Burdge *et al.*, 1995; Jensen *et al.*, 1987).

Further, although fluoroquinolone photosensitivity is in general caused by UVA (315–400 nm) irradiation, there may be exceptions to this and the experimental drug BAY 3118 produced clear evidence of reactivity to visible wavelengths (400±30 nm) (data on file).

The identification of the wavelengths responsible for fluoroquinolone photosensitization is of more than academic interest. Thus, knowledge that the UVA region is involved allows preventive advice, indicating that it is important to protect the skin from not only direct but also window glass-transmitted sunlight, from sunbed exposure and from high-altitude, reflected sunlight, for example, when skiing. Such information also reinforces the need for a broad-spectrum sunblock rather than agents that protect only in the UVB region.

Knowledge that a photosensitization response is phototoxic in origin may also be of some value, since with a short drug half-life, fluoroquinolone photosensitivity may perhaps be reduced by evening dosing, thereby leading to lower skin levels at the time of potential maximum insolation (Lowe *et al.*, 1994; Young *et al.*, 1994).

PHOTOCARCINOGENESIS

A recent concern of as yet unknown clinical significance has been the published finding of fluoroquinolone-associated photocarcinogenesis in mice (Johnson *et al.*, 1997; Klecak *et al.*, 1997; Urbach, 1997). The data suggest that particularly fleroxacin and lomefloxacin but also other phototoxic members of the group are mouse skin phototumorigens. Thus, as few as five subacute phototoxic episodes appear to induce mouse epidermal tumours within six weeks (Johnson *et al.*, 1997), but although an increased tumour risk in humans from psoralen phototoxicity was predicted by such a murine study, it does seem that the albino mouse model is particularly sensitive in this respect.

SULPHONAMIDES

The importance of sulphonamide photosensitivity in clinical practice has reduced with the decline in their use. However, a notable exception may occur with the sulphapyridine released from sulphasalazine, this sulphonamide component potentially being significantly absorbed from the intestine of patients with inflammatory bowel disease (Nielsen, 1982). Photosensitization reactions associated with the drug are of a painful burning, often blistering, UVA-dependent type.

TETRACYCLINES

Cutaneous photosensitivity associated with the tetracyclines used in current medical practice is now rarely reported (Bjellerup, 1986). However, occasionally doxycycline can produce a 24-hour delayed erythema-type skin reaction (Layton and Cunliffe, 1992; Orentreich *et al.*, 1961), while minocycline, although only rarely associated with an inflammatory skin response, is capable of leading to a persistent blue-grey pigmentation of the exposed skin (Okada *et al.*, 1989), which does nevertheless gradually resolve following drug cessation; a recent study also suggests that laser therapy may be rapidly effective in clearance of this problem (Knoell *et al.*, 1996). In the past, substantial photosensitivity has also been associated with demethylchlortetracycline in particular, but this agent is now only used in bone growth studies. Finally, although the majority of tetracycline photosensitization cases present with classic delayed erythemal photosensitivity, some patients may instead rarely experience pseudoporphyria (Epstein *et al.*, 1976).

NON-STEROIDAL ANTI-INFLAMMATORY AGENTS

Despite their otherwise anti-inflammatory actions, this group of drugs are the most commonly incriminated phototoxic agents, although this of itself may not be a true reflection of their photosensitizing ability for they are extensively used in clinical practice. Nevertheless, benoxaprofen, withdrawn in 1982, was associated with a high incidence of broad-spectrum phototoxicity characterized by the occurrence of an immediate unpleasant burning sensation, as well as with urticaria on phototesting followed by an erythema that persisted for 48 hours (Ferguson *et al.*, 1982); exposed site milia and photo-onycholysis were also reported. In addition, a particular problem of both clinical and regulatory interest was the alleged occurrence of persistent photosensitivity by many former users, a claim later apparently refuted by careful phototest study (Frain-Bell, 1982).

In current practice, mild to moderate photosensitivity reactions are associated with the use particularly of phenylpropionic acid derivatives such as ketoprofen, tiaprofenic acid and naproxen.

On the other hand the response seen with the enolic acid derivative piroxicam occurs in only a small percentage of patients yet can be severe, as seen in Plate 22, where a female inpatient demonstrates a blistering phototoxic response following irradiation with the window glass-transmitted UVA wavelengths from sunlight. Further, Kochevar and colleagues (1986) have demonstrated a metabolite of piroxicam to be phototoxic both *in vitro* and *in vivo*, thus raising the possibility that cutaneous photosensitivity may occur only in individuals in whom this metabolite is preferentially formed or retained within the skin. However, recent studies have also suggested another possibility, namely the possible production of a photometabolite, also perhaps handled in idiosyncratic fashion (Miranda *et al.*, 1991).

AMIODARONE

This agent, which is prescribed as a cardiac anti-dysrhythmic, has a wide range of adverse effects – it consequently tends to be used only as a drug of last resort. Phototoxicity consists of an immediate burning, prickling sensation coupled with erythema that is biphasic, re-emerging by 24 hours; the problem is common, with an incidence of 40–60% of those taking the drug (Chalmers *et al.*, 1982). As expected, the effects are dose related, as well as being UVA and visible wavelength dependent; in addition, the drug has a long half-life and can thus persist within the skin for many months. A further unusual feature seen in a minority of patients is an unsightly golden-brown or slate-grey pigmentation resulting from an amiodarone metabolite complex within the skin. After drug cessation, pigmentation and susceptibility to erythema may then continue for months or even years, although in many patients drug continuation may be the only option. In such cases, a desensitization course with narrowband TL-01 phototherapy has been helpful (Collins and Ferguson, 1995) and should be considered if broad-spectrum sunscreens and clothing photoprotection prove unsatisfactory.

PHENOTHIAZINES

Chlorpromazine was first reported as capable of photosensitization by Epstein *et al.* (1957), with an incidence of 16–25%. Direct sunlight or its window glass-transmitted UVA wavelengths can induce an immediate unpleasant sensation and erythema of exposed sites; if severe, cutaneous blistering is possible (Plate 23). In addition, as for amiodarone, a golden or slate-grey pigmentation may occasionally arise, an effect which need not be preceded by clinical phototoxicity and, unlike with psoralen, only occurs in a few subjects taking the drug.

Chlorpromazine phototoxicity may not necessarily be due to the chlorpromazine itself, for extensive processing of the drug creates downstream metabolites, some of which are more phototoxic *in vitro* than the mother compound (Ljunggren and Moller, 1977). Thus, variable metabolic processing may contribute to the differing phototoxic susceptibilities between subjects.

Finally, following the discovery of chlorpromazine-photosensitized DNA cleavage, there has been interest in the agent as a potential photomutagen but clinical evidence for such an effect is scant.

DIURETICS

As thiazides are closely chemically related to the sulphonamides, they might well be expected to induce phototoxicity and, indeed, for chlorthiazide and hydrochlorthiazide, this has been commonly reported. A wide range of morphologies for the reaction have also been described, ranging from dermatitis (Robinson *et al.*, 1985) to erythema (Addo *et al.*, 1987), a lichen planus-like response (Harber *et al.*, 1959) and a lupus erythematosus (LE)-type reaction (Reed *et al.*, 1985), thus suggesting that the drugs may have a complex range of photosensitization mechanisms.

The phototoxic type of response with thiazide appears idiosyncratic and is not clearly understood, but seems to have a broad waveband dependency, namely UVB and A (Addo *et al.*, 1987). On the other hand, patients with the lupus-like picture show the immunological features of LE, with positive circulating anti-Ro and -La antibodies (Fine, 1989).

When a patient develops severe photosensitivity with a thiazide, it may not always be possible to stop diuretic use, but since bumetanide has a lower phototoxic potential (Lowe *et al.*, 1989), it may be used instead with a reduced likelihood of photosensitization.

Finally, the diuretic frusemide can precipitate a pseudoporphyria reaction with bullae and fragility in a few subjects following UVA exposure (Burry and Lawrence, 1976) and may also occasionally need to be replaced.

RETINOIDS

Systemic retinoids may induce phototoxic responses, *in vitro* and *in vivo* studies

(Ferguson and Johnson, 1986, 1989) having revealed an idiosyncratic problem with severe responses on occasion (Plate 24). Drug cessation or dosage reduction and UVB and A photoprotection should be used, while as with other possible photosensitizers, advance warning to users about such prophylactic measures should be routine.

PHOTOALLERGY

This significant if uncommon phenomenon continues to be of particular clinical and scientific interest, the terms **photoallergy** and **phototoxicity** having been introduced early by Stephan Epstein in 1939 to distinguish between the different possible skin reactions after the intradermal injection of sulphanilamide followed by sunlight exposure. Thus, in addition to the early phototoxic reaction seen in most subjects, a few also developed an exposed-site dermatitis response ten days later. He noted the similarity of the reaction to that of contact allergic dermatitis and suggested an allergen had been created by the combination of sunlight exposure and the drug.

Subsequent reports noted contact photoallergy with the use of phenothiazines, especially chlorpromazine, 3,4′,5′,5-tetrachlorsalicylanilide (TCSA) in soaps as a bacteriostat, 3,4′5-tribromosalicylanilide, bithionol, hexachlorophene, bromochlorsalicylanilide (Multifungin), Fentichlor and 4-chloro-2-hydroxybenzoic acid-N-n-butylamide (Jadit). Herman and Sams (1972) also noted the occurrence of similar reactions. However, such photoallergic contact dermatitis decreased dramatically after the removal of halogenated phenolic compounds from toiletries (Smith and Epstein, 1977), although it has apparently occasionally recurred with the use of quinoxaline-n-dioxide (Quindoxin), a foodstock animal growth promoter, the fragrance material musk ambrette, also crossreactive with other musk compounds, and 6-methylcoumarin (Raugi *et al.*, 1979; Wojnarowska and Calnan, 1986) (Table 12.5).

The photoallergic potentials of TCSA, chlorpromazine, sulphanilamide and musk ambrette have all been confirmed in experimental studies (Granstein *et al.*, 1983; Maguire and Kaidbey, 1982; Takigawa and Miyachi, 1982). In addition, the precise mechanism for the occurrence of photoallergy with tolbutamide, sulphanilamide and chlorpromazine is considered to be delayed-type hypersensitivity reaction of the contact allergic type, probably to a photoproduct of the mother drug (Burckhardt, 1948; Maguire and Kaidbey, 1983).

PERSISTENT LIGHT REACTION (PLR)

This often loosely used term describes a continuing state of eczematous photosensitivity following an initial photoallergic response, despite avoidance of the original photoallergen. Initially reported following photosensitization by substances such as TCSA, the term has since been applied as an attempted mechanistic explanation of the chronic actinic dermatitis photosensitivity dermatitis/actinic reticuloid) syndrome despite a frequent lack of convincing evidence for photoallergy by the photopatch test investigation.

Until more evidence is forthcoming not only on the possible mechanisms for such an effect but also the identification of candidate chemicals, it seems prudent to reserve judgement on the existence and role of PLR as an explanation for the chronic photodermatitis/actinic reticuloid state seen in middle-aged and elderly males.

SYSTEMIC CHEMICALS OR DRUGS REPORTED AS PHOTOALLERGENS

Throughout the relevant literature, there are sporadic reports of photoallergic reactions to agents taken systemically. While in such instances the diagnosis is usually made on the morphology of the skin eruption, a few cases also have evidence of positive photopatch test results, although rarely with

Table 12.5 Major reported topical photoallergens

Sulphonamides/sulphonylureas	Sulphanilamide; tolbutamide; carbutamide; chlorpropamide
Phenothiazines	Promethazine; chlorpromazine
Halogenated phenols	3,3',4',5-Tetrachlorosalicylanilide (TCSA); 3,4',5 tribromosalicylanilide (TBS); 3,4,4'-tribromocarbanilide (TCC); hexachlorophene; bithionol; Fentichlor; 4-chloro-2-hydroxybenzoic acid-N-n-butylamide (Jadit)
Quinoxaline-n-dioxide	
Furocoumarins	8-Methoxypsoralen; 5-methoxyangelicin: 6-methoxyangelicin (Sphondin)
Fragrances	6-Methylcoumarin; musk ambrette
Sunscreens	Para-aminobenzoic acid (PABA); PABA derivatives; dibenzoylmethanes; benzophenones

adequate irradiation or contact control site data. Thus, whether such responses truly represent photoallergy or instead phototoxicity or irritancy so as to produce a low-grade erythema is a continuing source of uncertainty. Further information is needed, but it is clear in the meantime that standardization of the method of photopatch testing is essential to facilitate the future interpretation of reports.

Photoallergy occurs at a low concentration of drug or chemical and is difficult to avoid once established. Consequently, industry has tended to search for alternative agents and most photoallergens in time become obsolete. However, a recent group to emerge have been the UVB- and A-absorbing sunscreening chemicals which, as for drug phototoxicity, appear to be activated mostly by the UVA wavelengths.

SUNSCREENS

Sunscreens are extensively used to protect the skin from the harmful effects of UVR and in recent years, a great increase has occurred in their use not only for the prevention of sunburn in normal subjects but also in the form of cosmetics and toiletries in part to reduce the process of photoageing and photocarcinogenesis. Such preparations can be classified into two major groups, namely physical and chemical agents. Thus, physical sunscreens such as zinc oxide and titanium dioxide reduce the amount of ultraviolet and visible radiation entering the skin by means of reflection and scattering, while chemical sunscreens act instead by absorbing this radiation. The higher the chemical concentration in absorbent screens, the more effective is the absorption, but unfortunately such a higher concentration may also produce a greater contact and photocontact sensitization rate, a problem only rarely seen with physical screens and their excipients.

Nevertheless, the incidence of contact allergy and photoallergy to sunscreens appears low (De Groot *et al.*, 1987; Goncalo *et al.*, 1995) with photoallergy less common than direct contact reactions, but there is concern about the possibility of significant underreporting particularly as no efficient postmarketing surveillance systems exist to record such reactions. In addition, since photoallergy testing is not conducted in all centres, some reactions may simply be put down to contact allergy, so perhaps leading to significant under-recording of true photoallergic events.

SPECIFIC SUNSCREEN AGENTS CAPABLE OF CAUSING PHOTOALLERGY

Para-amino benzoic acid (PABA)

This agent has been extensively used as a sunscreen for many years and in common with many agents developed later, was initially thought to be a poor photoallergic sensitizer; however, in recent times this opinion has been reversed (Dromgoole and Maibach, 1990).

As a consequence, worldwide use of this compound has now declined, with its replacement by PABA derivatives and other chemically related alternatives now giving protection also extending into the UVA region.

Benzophenones

Mexenone and oxybenzone (Plate 25) are benzophenones used extensively in sunscreen products, both of which have been reported as capable of inducing photoallergic reactions, thus somewhat limiting their use. As for most other photoallergens, the UVA wavelengths are predominant in producing the oxybenzone photocontact reaction (Collins and Ferguson, 1994).

Dibenzoylmethanes

In Europe since 1980, the dibenzoylmethanes, Avobenzone and Eusolex 8020, have both been widely used as UVA sunscreens and reported as capable of causing photoallergy, with the latter having the more frequent reports (Goncalo *et al.*, 1995).

Although photoallergy to the camphor derivatives, the salicylates and the cinnamates appears less common, it must be stressed that the increasing use of these agents, along with the more widespread use of standardized photopatch testing procedures, may in future indicate more clearly their true potential for photosensitization.

PHOTOPATCH TESTING

Differences exist worldwide in the practice and interpretation of photopatch testing. In 1996, the British Photodermatology Group therefore met to determine a list of the currently most relevant photoallergens and to provide advice concerning an optimal standardized technique (British Photodermatology Group, 1997). Thus, although the wavelength dependence of photoallergy is known for only a few allergens (Cripps and Enta, 1970; Freeman *et al.*, 1970; Giovinazzo *et al.*, 1981), it is thought that for the majority it lies in the UVA (315–400 nm) region. For practical use, therefore, it is suggested that lamps routinely used for PUVA are also suitable for photopatch testing and that a radiation dose that would not produce a reaction in normal subjects (i.e. $5 \, J/cm^2$, be used as a routine. By the choice of such a low irradiation dose, phototoxic reactions can be avoided (DeLeo *et al.*, 1992; Hölzle *et al.*, 1991), which should thus enable photoallergic responses to emerge from what has previously been a mass of false-positive reactions (DeLeo *et al.*, 1992; Leow *et al.*, 1994; Thune *et al.*, 1988).

As with the technique of patch testing, mid upper back skin adjacent to the paravertebral area should be used, the photoallergens being applied in duplicate. Any of three protocols in current use may then be followed. In accordance with one such method, both sets of photoallergens are removed at 24 hours and the responses read. One set is then irradiated with the UVA source while the other is kept covered, after which reading may be conducted over the following 72 hours whenever possible. As with ordinary patch testing, strongly positive photoallergic reactions can readily be distinguished from mild irritant responses and it is generally only in the middle ground that problems arise. Further, in patients with severe abnormal photosensitivity, for example in chronic actinic dermatitis, evaluation will be required prior to testing, for in such patients even a 5 J/cm^2 irradiation may spoil the investigation by producing a strongly positive, irradiation-only control.

As many of the agents currently regularly tested no longer feature in the environment, it seems sensible that they should no longer be used and only photoallergens of clinical relevance investigated. On this basis, therefore, an updated series has been produced which concentrates on sunscreen agents, musk ambrette and any other topical product of possible relevance for the individual patient (Table 12.6).

THE MANAGEMENT OF PHOTOSENSITIZATION REACTIONS

Drug- and chemical-induced photosensitive skin reactions can be anticipated with the use of a wide range of substances. In addition, we now have a substantial amount of information available concerning phototoxic drug wavelength dependencies, times for the skin to return to normal after the stopping of such drugs and drug and radiation dose–response relationships. As a result there are now considerable data concerning possible preventive precautions available to patients about to take a photoactive drug.

However, much more work is still required to understand the clinical significance of other phototoxic drug-related phenomena such as photodegradation, systemic photoproduct toxicity and photocarcinogenesis. In addition, at a mechanistic level, we also need to understand more about the processes involved in idiosyncratic photosensitivity responses and about the immunologically mediated reactions. Only then will we have achieved a reasonable understanding of the complex problem of chemical and drug photosensitivity.

REFERENCES

Addo, H.A., Ferguson, J. and Frain-Bell, W. (1987) Thiazide-induced photosensitivity: a study of 33 subjects. *British Journal of Dermatology*, **116**, 749–60.

Arlett, C., Earl, L., Ferguson, J. *et al.* (1995) British Photodermatology Group Workshop. Predictive *in vitro* methods for identifying photosensitizing drugs: a report. *British Journal of Dermatology*, **132**, 271–4.

Ayd, J.F. Jr (1956) The dermatologic and systemic manifestations of chlorpromazine hypersensitivity. Their clinical significance and management. *Journal of Nervous and Mental Disorders*, **124**, 84–7.

Bakri, A., Beijersbergen van Henegouwen, G. and Chanal, J.L. (1985) Involvement of the N$_4$-oxide group in the phototoxicity of chlordiazepoxide in the rat. *Photodermatology*, **2**, 205–12.

Baran, R. and Brun, P. (1986) Photo-onycholysis induced by the fluoroquinolones pefloxacine and oxfloxacine. *Dermatologica*, **173**, 185–8.

Bech-Thomsen, N., Angelo H.R. and Wulf, H.C. (1991) Skin pigmentation as a predictor of

Table 12.6   A proposed standard series of photocontact allergens (British Photodermatology Group, 1997)

Para-aminobenzoic acid (PABA) (5%, 10%)
Octyl dimethyl PABA (Padimate O, Eusolex 6007, Escalol 507) (2%, 10%)
2-Ethylhexy p-methoxycinnamate (Parsol MCX) (2%, 10%)
2-Hydroxy-4-methoxybenzophenone (oxybenzone, benzophenone 3, Eusolex 4360) (2%, 10%)
4-Tert-butyl-4-methoxy dibenzoylmethane (Parsol 1789) (2%, 10%)
Musk ambrette (1%, 5%)
Patient's own product(s) (diluted as appropriate)

minimal phototoxic dose after oral methoxsalen. *Archives of Dermatology*, **130**, 464–8.

Bilsland, D. and Douglas, W.S. (1990) Sunbed pseudoporphyria induced by nalidixic acid. *British Journal of Dermatology*, **123**, 547.

Bjellerup, M. (1986) Tetracycline phototoxicity – an experimental and clinical study. Thesis, Lund University, Malmo, Sweden.

Bowie, W.R., Willetts, V. and Jewesson, P.J. (1989) Adverse reactions in a dose-ranging study with a new long-acting fluoroquinolone, fleroxacin. *Antimicrobial Agents and Chemotherapy*, **33**, 1778–82.

British Photodermatology Group (1997) Workshop report – photopatch testing. Methods and indications. *British Journal of Dermatology*, **136**, 371–6.

Buchbinder, M., Webb, J.C., Anderson, L.V. and McCabe, W.R. (1962) Laboratory studies and clinical pharmacology of nalidixic acid (WIN 18,320). *Antimicrobial Agents and Chemotherapy*, **2**, 308–17.

Burckhardt, W. (1948) Photoallergische Ekzeme durch Sulfanilamidsalben. *Dermatologica*, **96**, 280.

Burdge, D.R., Nakielna, E.M. and Rabin, H.R. (1995) Photosensitivity associated with ciprofloxacin use in adult patients with cystic fibrosis. *Antimicrobial Agents and Chemotherapy*, **39**, 793.

Burry, J.N. and Crosby, R.W.L. (1966) A case of phototoxicity to nalidixic acid. *Medical Journal of Australia*, **2**, 698.

Burry, J.N. and Lawrence, J.R. (1976) Phototoxic blisters from high frusemide dosage. *British Journal of Dermatology*, **94**, 495–9.

Calnan, C.D., Frain-Bell, W. and Cuthbert, J.W. (1962) Occupational dermatitis from chlorpromazine. *Transactions of St John's Hospital Dermatological Society*, **47**, 49–74.

Charlmers, R.T.G., Muston, H.L., Srinivas, V. and Bennett D.H. (1982) High incidence of amiodarone-induced photosensitivity in North-West England. *British Medical Journal*, **285**, 341.

Christ, W. and Lehnert, T. (1990) Toxicity of the quinolones, in *The New Generation of Quinolones*, (eds C. Siporin *et al.*), Marcel Dekker, New York, pp. 165–87.

Cohen, J.B. and Bergstresser, P.R. (1994) Inadvertent phototoxicity from home tanning equipment. *Archives of Dermatology*, **130**, 804–6.

Collins, P. and Ferguson, J. (1994) Photoallergic contact dermatitis to oxybenzone. *British Journal of Dermatology*, **131**, 124–9.

Collins, P. and Ferguson, J. (1995) Narrow-band (TL-01) phototherapy: an effective preventative

treatment for the photodermatoses. *British Journal of Dermatology*, **132**, 956–63.

Correia, O. and Delgado, L. (1994) Bullous photodermatosis after lomefloxacin. *Archives of Dermatology*, **130**, 808–9.

Cripps, D.J. and Enta, T. (1970) Absorption and action spectra studies on bithionol and halogenated salicylanilides. *British Journal of Dermatology*, **82**, 230–42.

De Groot, A.C., Van Der Walle, H.B., Jagtman, B.A. and Weyland, J.W. (1987) Contact allergy to 4-isopropyl-dibenzoylmethane and 3-(4'-methylbenzylidene) camphor in the sunscreen Eusolex 8021. *Contact Dermatitis*, **16**, 249–65.

DeLeo, V.A. (1992) *Topics in Clinical Dermatology – Photosensitivity*, Igaku Shoin, New York, p. 61.

DeLeo, V.A., Suarez, S.M. and Maso, M.J. (1992) Photoallergic contact dermatitis. Results of photopatch testing in New York, 1985 to 1990. *Archives of Dermatology*, **128**, 1513–18.

Drever, J.C. and Hunter, J.A.A. (1970) Giant hogweed dermatitis. *Scottish Medical Journal*, **15**, 315–19.

Dromgoole, S.H. and Maibach, H.I. (1990) Contact sensitization and photocontact sensitization of sunscreening agents, in *Sunscreens: Development, Evaluation, and Regulatory Aspects*, (eds N.J. Lowe and N.A. Shaath), Marcel Dekker, New York, pp. 313–40.

Epstein, F.H., Brunsting, L.A., Peterson, M.C. *et al.* (1957) A study of photosensitivity occurring with chlorpromazine therapy. *Journal of Investigative Dermatology*, **28**, 329–38.

Epstein, J.H., Tuffanelli, D.L., Seibert, J.S. and Epstein, W.L. (1976) Porphyria-like cutaneous changes induced by tetracycline hydrochloride photosensitization. *Archives of Dermatology*, **112**, 661–6.

Epstein, S. (1939) Photoallergy and primary phototoxicity to sulfanilamide. *Journal of Investigative Dermatology*, **2**, 43–51.

Ferguson, J. (1995) Fluoroquinolone photosensitization: a review of clinical and laboratory studies. *Photochemistry and Photobiology*, **62**, 954–8.

Ferguson, J. and Johnson, B.E. (1986) Photosensitivity due to retinoids: clinical and laboratory studies. *British Journal of Dermatology*, **115**, 275–83.

Ferguson, J. and Johnson, B.E. (1989) Retinoid associated phototoxicity and photosensitivity. *Pharmacology and Therapeutics*, **40**, 123–35.

Ferguson, J. and Johnson, B.E. (1993) Clinical and laboratory studies of the photosensitizing potential of norfloxacin, a 4-quinolone broad-spectrum antibiotic. *British Journal of Dermatology*, **128**, 285–95.

Ferguson, J. and Johnson, B.E. (1992) Recently developed photosensitizing agents, in *Biological Responses to Ultraviolet A Radiation*, (ed. F. Urbach), Valdemar Publishing, Overland Park, pp. 107–19.

Ferguson, J., Addo, H.A., McGill, P.E. *et al.* (1982) A study of benoxaprofen-induced phototoxicity. *British Journal of Dermatology*, **107**, 429–42.

Fine, R.M. (1989) Subacute cutaneous lupus erythematosus associated with hydrochlorothiazide therapy. *International Journal of Dermatology*, **28**, 375–6.

Food and Drug Administration (1993) FDA Committee urges stronger warnings on Maxaquin. *Script*, **1810**, 32–3.

Frain-Bell, W. (1982) Photosensitivity dermatitis and actinic reticuloid. *Seminars in Dermatology*, **1**, 161–8.

Freeman, K., Hubbard, S.H.C. and Warin, A.P. (1984) Strimmer rash. *Contact Dermatitis*, **10**, 117–18.

Freeman, R.G., Hudson, H.T., Carnes, R. and Knox, J.M. (1970) Salicylanilide photosensitivity. *Journal of Investigative Dermatology*, **54**, 145–9.

Giovinazzo, V.J., Ichikawa, H., Kochevar, I.E. *et al.* (1981) Photoallergic contact dermatitis to musk ambrette: action spectra in guinea pigs and man. *Photochemistry and Photobiology*, **33**, 773–7.

Goncalo, M., Ruas, E., Figueiredo, A. and Goncalo, S. (1995) Contact and photocontact sensitivity to sunscreens. *Contact Dermatitis*, **33**, 278–80.

Gonzalez, J.P. and Henwood, J.M. (1989) Pefloxacin: a review of its antibacterial activity, pharmacokinetic properties and therapeutic use. *Drugs*, **37**, 628–68.

Granstein, R.D., Morison, W.L. and Kripke, M.L. (1983) The role of UVB radiation in the induction and elicitation of photocontact hypersensitivity to TCSA in the mouse. *Journal of Investigative Dermatology*, **80**, 158–62.

Harber, L.C., Lashinsky, A.M. and Baer, R.L. (1959) Skin manifestations of photosensitivity to chlorothiazide and hydrochlorothiazide. *Journal of Investigative Dermatology*, **33**, 83–4.

Herman, P.S. and Sams, W.M. Jr (1972) *Soap Photodermatitis: Photosensitivity to Halogenated Salicylanilides*, C. C. Thomas, Springfield, Illinois.

Hölzle, E., Neumann, N., Hausen, B. *et al.* (1991) Photopatch testing: the 5-year experience of the German, Austrian and Swiss photopatch test group. *Journal of the American Academy of Dermatology*, **25**, 59–68.

Izu, R., Gardeazabal, J., Gonzalez, M. *et al.* (1992) Enoxacin-induced photosensitivity: study of two cases. *Photodermatology, Photoimmunology and Photomedicine*, **9**, 86–8.

Jensen, T., Pedersen, S.S., Nielsen, C.H., Holby, N. and Koch, C. (1987) The efficacy and safety of ciprofloxacin and ofloxacin in chronic *Pseudomonas aeruginosa* infection in cystic fibrosis. *Journal of Antimicrobial Chemotherapy*, **20**, 585–94.

Johnson, B.E. (1993) The naturally occurring psoralens and other plant photosensitizers and their mode of action, in *Plants and the Skin*, (ed. C.R. Lovell), Blackwell Scientific Publications, London, pp. 66–78.

Johnson, B.E., Gibbs, N.K. and Ferguson, J. (1997) Quinolone antibiotic with potential to photosensitize skin tumorigenesis. *Journal of Photochemistry and Photobiology (B: Biology)*, **37**, 171–3.

Jungst, G. and Mohr, R. (1987) Side effects of ofloxacin in clinical trials and in postmarketing surveillance. *Drugs*, **34** (suppl 1), 144–9.

Kawabe, Y., Mizuno, N. and Sakakibara, S. (1989) Photoallergic reaction caused by enoxacin. *Photodermatology*, **6**, 58–60.

Klecak, G., Urbach, F. and Urwyler, H. (1997) Fluoroquinolone antibacterials enhance UVA-induced skin tumours. *Journal of Photochemistry and Photobiology (B: Biology)*, **37**, 174–81.

Knoell, K.A., Milgraum, S.S. and Kutenplon, M. (1996) Q-switched ruby laser treatment of minocycline-induced cutaneous hyperpigmentation. *Archives of Dermatology*, **132**, 1251–3.

Kochevar, I.E., Morison, W.L., Lamm, T.L. *et al.* (1986) Possible mechanisms of piroxicam induced photosensitivity. *Archives of Dermatology*, **122**, 1283–7.

Kuramaji, Y. and Shono, M. (1992) Scarified photopatch testing in lomefloxacin photosensitivity. *Contact Dermatitis*, **26**, 5–10.

Layton, A.M. and Cunliffe, W.J. (1992) Photosensitive eruptions to doxycycline – a dose related phenomenon. *British Journal of Dermatology*, **127** (suppl 30), 31.

Leow, Y.H., Wong, W.K., Ng, S.K. *et al.* (1994) Two years experience of photopatch testing in Singapore. *Contact Dermatitis*, **31**, 181–205.

Ljunggren, B. and Bjellerup, M. (1986) Systemic drug photosensitivity. *Photodermatology*, **3**, 26–35.

Ljunggren, B. and Moller, H. (1977) Phenothiazine phototoxicity: an experimental study on chlorpromazine and its metabolites. *Journal of Investigative Dermatology*, **68**, 313–17.

Lopitaux, R., Hermet, R., Sirot, J., Filiu, P. and Terver, S. (1985) Tolérance de la perfloxacine au cours du traitement d'une série d'infections ostéo-articulaires. *Thérapie*, **40**, 349–52.

Lowe, G., Walker, E.M., Johnson, B.E. and Ferguson, J. (1989) Thiazide-induced photosensitivity, the use of bumetanide as alternative therapy: *in vitro* and *in vivo* studies. *British Journal of Dermatology*, **121** (suppl), 58.

Lowe, N.J., Fakouhi, T.D., Stern, R.S. *et al.* (1994) Photoreactions with a fluoroquinolone antimicrobial: evening versus morning dosing. *Clinical Pharmacology and Therapeutics*, **56**, 587–91.

Maguire, H.C. Jr and Kaidbey, K. (1982) Experimental photoallergic contact dermatitis: a mouse model. *Journal of Investigative Dermatology*, **79**, 147–52.

Maguire, H.C. Jr and Kaidbey, K. (1983) Studies in experimental photoallergy. in *The effect of ultraviolet radiation on the immune system*. (ed.) Parrish, J.A., Johnson & Johnson Baby Products Co., Skillman, New Jersey, pp. 181–92.

Makinen, M., Forbes, P.D. and Stenbäck, F. (1997) Quinolone antibacterials: a new class of photochemical carcinogens. *Journal of Photochemistry and Photobiology (B: Biology)*, **37**, 182–7.

Miranda, M.A., Vargaws, F. and Serrano, G. (1991) Photodegradation of piroxicam under aerobic conditions. The photochemical keys of the piroxicam enigma. *Journal of Photochemistry and Photobiology (B: Biology)*, **8**, 199–202.

Mitzutani, K., Tokuta, Y., Iwamoto, Y. and Takigawa, M. (1995) Photosensitivity dermatitis induced by sparfloxacin. *Rinsho-Hifuku*, **49**, 113–18.

Nielsen, O.H. (1982) Sulphasalazine intolerance: retrospective survey of the reasons for discontinuing treatment with sulphasalazine in patients with chronic inflammatory bowel disease. *Scandinavian Journal of Gastroenterology*, **17**, 389–93.

Okada, N., Moriya, K., Nishida, K. *et al.* (1989) Skin pigmentation associated with minocycline therapy. *British Journal of Dermatology*, **121**, 247–54.

Orentreich, A., Harber, L.C. and Tromovitch, T.A. (1961) Photosensitivity and photo-onycholysis due to demethylchlortetracyline. *Archives of Dermatology*, **83**, 730–7.

Petri, H. and Tronnier, H. (1986) Efficacy of enoxacin in the treatment of bacterial infections of the skin with regards to photosensitization. *Infection*, **14** (suppl 3), 213–16.

Ramsay, C.A. and Obreshkova, E. (1974) Photosensitivity from nalidixic acid. *British Journal of Dermatology*, **91**, 523–8.

Raugi, G.J., Storrs, J. and Larsen, W.G. (1979) Photoallergic contact dermatitis to men's perfumes. *Contact Dermatitis*, **5**, 251.

Reed, B.R., Huff, J., Jones, S.K. *et al.* (1985) Subacute cutaneous lupus erythematosus associated with hydrochlorothiazide therapy. *Annals of Internal Medicine*, **103**, 49–51.

Robinson, H.N., Morison, W.L. and Hood, A.F. (1985) Thiazide diuretic therapy and chronic photosensitivity. *Archives of Dermatology*, **121**, 522–4.

Schiefe, R.T., Cramer, W.R. and Decker, E.L. (1993) Photosensitizing potential of ofloxacin. *International Journal of Dermatology*, **32**, 413–16.

Smith, S.Z. and Epstein, J.H. (1977) Photocontact dermatitis to halogenated salicylanilides and related compounds. *Archives of Dermatology*, **113**, 1372–4.

Takigawa, M. and Miyachi, Y. (1982) Mechanisms of contact photosensitivity in mice. I. T cell regulation of contact photosensitivity to tetrachlorsalicylanilide under genetic restrictions of the major histocompatibility complex. *Journal of Investigative Dermatology*, **78**, 108–15.

Thune, P., Jansen, C., Wennersten, G. *et al.* (1988) The Scandinavian multi-center photopatch study 1980–1985: final report. *Photodermatology*, **5**, 261–9.

Urbach, F. (1997) Phototoxicity and possible enhancement of photocarcinogenesis by fluorinated quinolone antibiotics. *Journal of Photochemistry and Photobiology (B: Biology)*, **37**, 169–70.

Wojnarowska, I. and Calnan, C.D. (1986) Contact and photocontact allergy to musk ambrette. *British Journal of Dermatology*, **114**, 667.

Young, A.R., Fakouhi, D., Roniker, B. *et al.* (1994) Wavelength dependency of skin photosensitization by lomefloxacin. *Photochemistry, Photobiology and Photomedicine*, **59** (special issue), 60S.

George H. Elder

INTRODUCTION

The cutaneous porphyrias are a group of disorders of haem biosynthesis in which the skin is photosensitized by porphyrins. Günther, in his 1911 classification of the porphyrias (then called haematoporphyrias), recognized two distinct types of illness associated with increased porphyrin excretion. Haematoporphyria acuta was characterized by acute neurovisceral attacks without skin lesions, while haematoporphyrias congenita and chronica were skin disorders distinguished mainly by the age at which they start and characterized by the occurrence of fragile skin, bullae and erosions in areas exposed to light. Fifty years later, Magnus *et al.* (1961) added a third type of illness when they showed that the increased formation of protoporphyrin, a porphyrin too lipophilic to be excreted in urine, causes acute photosensitivity without skin fragility or usually bullae.

The seven main types of porphyria now recognized are listed in Table 13.1. The clinical features may be identical in more than one type and more than one type has been reported in the same individual (Freeseman *et al.*, 1997; Nordmann and Deybach, 1990). Skin lesions occur in five of the main porphyrias and these cutaneous porphyrias and their variants are the subject of this chapter.

Most cutaneous porphyrias are inherited, although identical skin lesions, also caused

by photosensitization by porphyrins, have been reported in other, often acquired disorders. These include porphyrin-producing hepatic tumours (O'Reilly *et al.*, 1988), Alagille syndrome and other defects of porphyrin excretion (Mallon *et al.*, 1995; Poh-Fitzpatrick *et al.*, 1990) and idiopathic sideroblastic anaemia (Lim *et al.*, 1992).

BIOCHEMISTRY

BIOCHEMISTRY AND METABOLISM

Haem is synthesized from succinyl CoA and glycine by a series of irreversible reactions that take place in all human cells except mature erythrocytes (Kappas *et al.*, 1995) (Fig. 13.1). The substrates of the reactions that convert porphobilinogen (PBG) to protoporphyrin IX are unstable and rapidly autoxidize to a variety of porphyrins if they accumulate in tissues or body fluids. About 80–85% of the haem produced in this process each day is used in the formation of haemoglobin; most of the rest is incorporated into hepatic haemoproteins, particularly microsomal cytochrome P450s which metabolize a wide range of drugs, foreign chemicals and endogenous compounds.

The genes for all the enzymes of human haem biosynthesis have now been characterized (Table 13.2) (Grandchamp *et al.*, 1995; Kappas *et al.*, 1995; Roberts *et al.*, 1995). All, except those for the rate-controlling enzyme aminolaevulinic acid (ALA) synthase (ALAS), being encoded by a single gene, two of which,

Photodermatology. Edited by J.L.M. Hawk. Published in 1998 by Chapman & Hall, London. ISBN 0 412 72460 X.

Table 13.1   The main types of porphyria

Disorder	Acute attacks	Bullae, fragile skin	Acute photosensitivity	Inheritance
ALA dehydratase porphyria (ADP)	+	−	−	Autosomal recessive
Acute intermittent porphyria (AIP)	+	−	−	Autosomal dominant
Congenital erythropoietic porphyria (CEP)	−	+	−	Autosomal recessive
Porphyria cutanea tarda (PCT)	−	+	−	Complex [1]
Hereditary coproporphyria (HCP)	+	+	−	Autosomal dominant
Variegate porphyria (VP)	+	+	−	Autosomal dominant
Erythropoietic protoporphyria (EPP)	−	−	+	Autosomal dominant

[1] See p. 000.

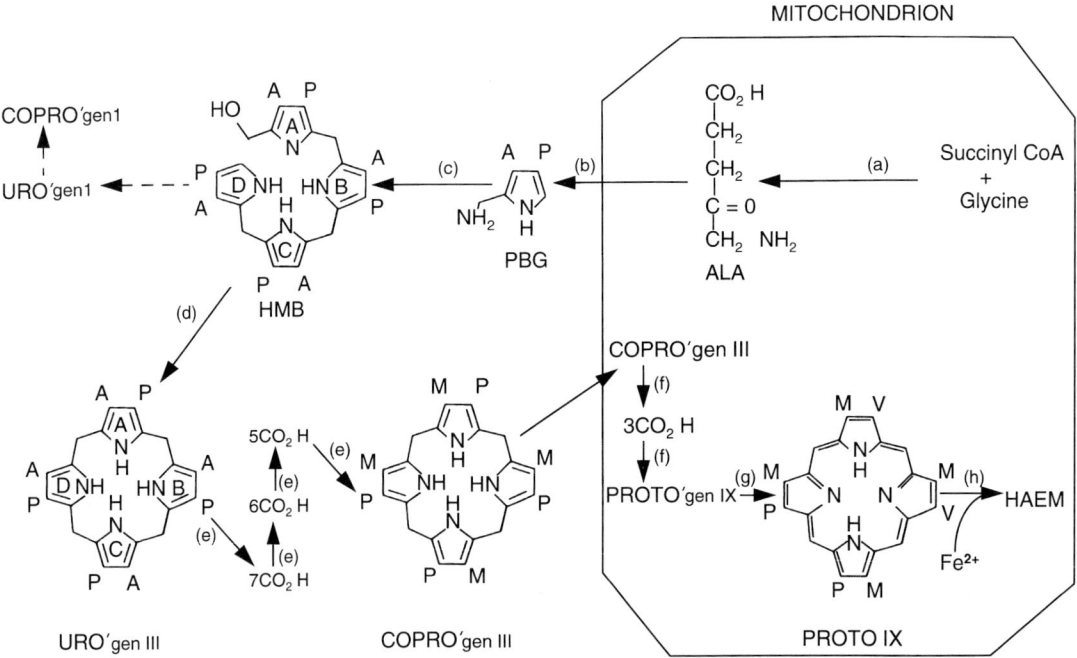

Figure 13.1   The pathway of haem biosynthesis. ALA, 5-aminolaevulinate; PBG, porphobilinogen; HMB, hydroxymethylbilane; URO′gen, COPRO′gen, PROTO′gen, PROTO, uroporphyrinogen, coproporphyrinogen, protoporphyrinogen and protoporphyrin. Enzymes are ALA synthase (a), ALA dehydratase (b), PBG deaminase (c), uroporphyrinogen III synthase (d), uroporphyrinogen decarboxylase (e), coproporphyrinogen oxidase (f), protoporphyrinogen oxidase (g) and ferrochelatase (h). A, P, M and V denote acetic acid, propionic acid, methyl and vinyl side chains.

(Table 13.1) undergo tissue-specific expression and processing. The overall rate of biosynthesis is regulated by different mechanisms in erythroid and liver tissue (Table 13.2) (May *et al.*, 1995; Ponka, 1997). In the liver, synthesis of the ALA synthase, encoded by the ALAS-1 gene, is inhibited by haem through complex mechanisms acting at transcriptional, translational and post-translational levels (May *et al.*, 1995). Activity is readily increased by compounds that induce cytochrome P450 synthesis or otherwise

Table 13.2 Genes for enzymes of human haem biosynthesis

Enzyme	Gene symbol	Size (kb)	No. of exons	Chromosomal location	Tissue expression
5-Aminolaevulinate synthase	ALAS-1	–	–	3p21.1	Ubiquitous
	ALAS-2	22	11	Xp11.21	Erythroid
5-Aminolaevulinate dehydratase[1]	ALAD	13	13	9q34	Ubiquitous, erythroid[3]
Porphobilinogen deaminase[2]	HMBS	10	15	11q24.1–24.2	Ubiquitous, erythroid[4]
Uroporphyrinogen III synthase	UROS	45	9	10q25.2–26.3	Ubiquitous
Uroporphyrinogen decarboxylase	UROD	3	10	1p34	Ubiquitous
Coproporphyrinogen oxidase	CPX	14	7	3q12	Ubiquitous
Protoporphyrinogen oxidase	PPOX	5	13	1q21–23	Ubiquitous
Ferrochelatase	FECH	45	11	18q21.3	Ubiquitous

Alternative names are [1] porphobilinogen synthase; [2] hydroxymethylbilane synthase; [3] separate ubiquitous and erythroid mRNAs; [4] separate erythroid and ubiquitous isoenzymes

decrease the regulatory haem pool in the liver. In contrast, erythroid cell ALA synthase activity is resistant to induction by most drugs but increased by tissue-specific enhancement of transcription during erythroid differentiation and influenced by the availability of iron (Ponka, 1997).

In normal circumstances, the close co-ordination of ALA formation and haem synthesis prevents significant loss of precursors from the pathway, their total daily excretion representing less than 2% of ALA production. Hydrophilic compounds such as ALA, PBG uroporphyrin and heptacarboxylic porphyrin are preferentially excreted in the urine. As hydrophobicity increases with progression down the biosynthetic pathway, the biliary route gradually predominates; coproporphyrin being excreted by both routes with preferential biliary excretion of the series I isomer and protoporphyrin being fully biliary. There is also some enterohepatic circulation of coproporphyrin and protoporphyrin. Cholestasis diverts coproporphyrin from the bile to the urine and decreases faecal porphyrin excretion. Finally, faecal protoporphyrin is not derived solely from biliary excretion, a variable amount, along with some related dicarboxylic porphyrins, being formed in the gut by bacteria from dietary haem and other sources.

PATHOLOGY

BIOCHEMICAL GENETICS

Each of the porphyrias results from the partial deficiency of an enzyme of haem biosynthesis (Kappas *et al.*, 1995; Nordmann and Deybach, 1990) (Table 13.3). In the autosomal dominant group, enzyme activity is generally decreased to about half normal, consistent with little or no expression of activity from the mutant allele and unimpaired expression from the normal. In addition, activities may be further reduced in clinically overt erythropoietic protoporphyria (EPP) and in the autosomal dominant form of porphyria cutanea tarda (PCT), for which possible explanations are discussed later. Decreased enzyme activity is compensated for by an increase in substrate concentration that is usually sufficient to maintain required rates of haem synthesis. This increase is secondary to enhanced ALAS activity from negative feedback regulation by haem. This substrate concentration increase varies widely between tissues (see Table 13.1) and, particularly in the autosomal dominant porphyrias, between individuals. Thus, at half-normal activity, it may be undetectable in one individual and yet in another, even in the same family, lead to sufficient porphyrin overproduction to cause photosensitization.

Table 13.3   Enzyme defects in the cutaneous porphyrias

Enzyme		Disorder	Enzyme activity (% mean control)	Main site of overproduction of porphyrin(ogen)s
Uroporphyrinogen III synthase	CEP		2–20	Erythroid cells
Uroporphyrinogen decarboxylase	(i)	PCT (sporadic)	16–47[1]	Hepatocytes
	(ii)	PCT (familial)	29–58[2], 41–57[3]	Hepatocytes
	(iii)	HEP	3–28	Hepatocytes
Coproporphyrinogen oxidase	(i)	HCP	48–53	Hepatocytes
	(ii)	Homozygous HCP	10	Hepatocytes
Protoporphyrinogen oxidase	(i)	VP	43–59	Hepatocytes
	(ii)	Homozygous VP	<10	Hepatocytes
Ferrochelatase	EPP		28 ± 8	Erythroid cells

HEP: hepatoerythropoietic porphyria; other abbreviations as in Table 13.1
[1] liver only; [2] liver; [3] erythrocytes

In the autosomal recessive porphyrias, enzyme activities are decreased to a greater extent and haem precursor overproduction is thus more sustained and less variable.

The patterns of haem precursor overproduction that characterize each cutaneous porphyria (Table 13.4) reflect accumulation of the substrate of the defective enzyme together with, during acute neurovisceral attacks of variegate porphyria (VP) and hereditary coproporphyria (HCP), the superimposed consequences of secondarily limited haem synthesis at the PBG deaminase stage (Meissner, 1993).

PHOTOBIOLOGY OF PORPHYRINS

The ability of porphyrins to photosensitize the human skin was first demonstrated directly in 1912 by Meyer-Betz, who injected himself with haematoporphyrin. More recently, such photosensitization has also been recognized as a consequence of the use of porphyrins or ALA for the photodynamic therapy of cancer.

Injury of the skin by porphyrins requires their accumulation in the dermis, irradiation at wavelengths around 400 nm and oxygen (Magnus, 1980; Spikes, 1984). The electronic spectra of porphyrins show a strong absorption (so-called Soret peak) in the 400 nm region, a wavelength at which light penetrates well to the deeper layers of the dermis. Although plasma porphyrin concentrations are always increased in photosensitized patients, there is no simple correlation between these and the presence of skin lesions; other factors such as the type of porphyrin, extent of uptake into the dermis, intensity of light exposure and the degree of natural photoprotection being important. Indeed, in chronic renal failure, plasma porphyrin concentrations may be increased eightfold without being associated with photodamage (Poh-Fitzpatrick et al., 1982).

Absorption of radiation energy by a porphyrin converts it to a singlet excited state which either (and more usually) decays rapidly to the ground state with emission of red light (fluorescence) or else undergoes intersystem crossing to the triplet state, which has a relatively long half-life in the several hundred microseconds range. Porphyrins in the triplet state react with molecular oxygen by energy transfer to give singlet oxygen or, less efficiently, by electron transfer to form the superoxide anion. In addition, they may react directly with other compounds, thus initiating free radical reactions. However, singlet oxygen is probably the main product and mediator of skin photodamage in the porphyrias.

Table 13.4 The cutaneous porphyrias: patterns of overproduction of haem precursors

Disorder	Urine PBG/ALA	Urine Porphyrins	Faecal porphyrins	Erythrocyte porphyrins	Plasma porphyrins
Congenital erythropoietic porphyria	Not increased	Uro I, copro I	Copro I	Zn- and free proto, copro I, uro I	Uro I, copro I
Porphyria cutanea tarda	Not increased	Uro I and III, hepta III[1]	Isocopro, hepta[1]	Not increased	Uro, hepta
Hereditary coproporphyria	PBG> ALA[2]	Copro III (Uro from PBG)	Copro III	Not increased	Copro III
Variegate porphyria	PBG> ALA[2]	Copro III (Uro from PBG)	Proto IX>copro III, porphyrin-peptide conjugates (X-porphyrin)	Not increased	Porphyrin-protein conjugates
Erythropoietic protoporphyria	Not increased	Not increased	Proto IX (60% of patients)	Proto IX (free)	Proto IX

[1] Hexa- and pentacarboxylic porphyrins are increased to a smaller extent
[2] PBG and ALA are increased during an acute neurovisceral attack but may be normal when only skin lesions are present

The distribution and targets of photo-damage are determined to some extent by the physicochemical properties of the porphyrin photosensitizer, protoporphyrin having particular affinity for membrane lipid, for example in endothelial cell and lysosomal membranes, while the hydrophilic uro and coproporphyrins preferentially accumulate in the lower epidermis and cells of the basement membrane zone. Such differences seem likely to explain the clinical distinction between the skin reactions of EPP and the bullous porphyrias. At the molecular level, porphyrin-catalysed photodynamic reactions cause damage to proteins, lipids and DNA (Spikes, 1984), may activate complement (Lim *et al.*, 1984), degramulate mast cells (Glover *et al.*, 1990) and enhance degradation of the dermis and basement membrane by metallo-proteinases (Hermann *et al.*, 1996).

HISTOPATHOLOGY OF THE SKIN

The histopathological changes in exposed skin are qualitatively similar in all the cutaneous porphyrias (Epstein *et al.*, 1973; Wolff *et al.*, 1982), the characteristic, consistent feature being the presence of amorphous, hyaline material (Plate 26), positive to periodic acid-Schiff (PAS) stain, in and around the walls of upper dermal and small blood vessels and often at the dermoepidermal junction. Electron microscopy shows this to consist of reduplicated and partially fragmented basement membrane and finely fibrillar material permeating and surrounding the vessel walls but sharply demarcated from the surrounding tissue (Ryan and Madill, 1968). Such deposits are generally more prominent in EPP, where they form irregular cuffs around small vessels, than in the bullous porphyrias, where they are instead restricted to the vessel walls and their immediate vicinity. The clinical presence of bullae results from splits in the lamina lucida of the basement membrane (Dabski and Beutner, 1991), collagen fibres and basement membrane fragments being

attached to the epidermal roof, while dermal papillae stiffened by hyaline deposits project into the floor, giving a so-called 'festooned' appearance. There is virtually no inflammatory infiltrate, but proteolytic enzymes released from damaged keratinocytes may instead be responsible for secondary connective tissue damage.

Electron microscopic, histochemical and immunological findings suggest that the amorphous hyaline material is derived from the walls and contents of blood vessels. Direct immunofluorescence shows deposits of IgG, some IgM, fibrinogen and complement around the vessels and at the dermoepidermal junction, while the thickened, reduplicated basement membranes contain type IV collagen and other structural components of normal basement membrane (Wick *et al.*, 1979). In the acute photosensitivity flare of EPP, the vascular endothelial cell is apparently the primary site of damage (Schnait *et al.*, 1975), while the hyaline deposits in the chronic lesions of this and other porphyrias appear to represent a cumulative, reparative response to repeated episodes of such injury with local leakage of vascular contents.

The sclerodermoid lesions of the bullous porphyrias, on the other hand, resemble those of true scleroderma, often occurring in areas that are not exposed to light; these may well result from uroporphyrin-stimulated collagen formation by fibroblasts in the dark (Varigos *et al.*, 1982).

THE BULLOUS PORPHYRIAS

PORPHYRIA CUTANEA TARDA AND RELATED DISORDERS

Cases that would now be recognized as either PCT or VP were included together by Günther in his 1911 porphyria classification as 'haematoporphyria chronica'. When Waldenstrom reclassified the disorders in 1937, he renamed this group 'porphyria cutanea tarda', but did not distinguish between PCT and VP which were then unrecognized as separate entities. In 1957, however, Waldenstrom, recognizing the work of Dean and Barnes in South Africa on the disease that was later (1959) named VP and following Watson's distinction in the United States between the purely cutaneous PCT and 'mixed porphyria' (later VP), divided 'porphyria cutanea tarda' into the two groups 'symptomatica' and 'hereditaria'. The first group is now known simply as PCT, the second as VP.

PCT, the commonest of all porphyrias, results from the decreased activity of the enzyme uroporphyrinogen decarboxylase (URO-D) in the liver. In contrast to other porphyrias, however, it is not a single monogenic disorder with a simple pattern of inheritance. Most cases appear to be provoked in susceptible individuals by various common agents, notably alcohol, hepatitis C virus (HCV) and oestrogens, which in normal circumstances do not cause porphyria. Estimates of the prevalence of PCT range from 1 in 25 000 for North America to over 1 in 5000 for Czechoslovakia. In the United Kingdom, however, the incidence is about 2–5 per million population per year (Elder, 1998).

Classification

PCT may be divided into three types by the measurement of URO-D in erythrocytes and by family studies. About 80% of patients have sporadic or type I PCT (Elder, 1998; Held *et al.*, 1989), with no family history of the disease and normal erythrocyte URO-D activity, the enzyme deficiency being restricted to the liver. Most of the others have familial or type II PCT, URO-D activity being decreased to half normal in both erythrocytes and other tissues by an inherited, autosomal dominant defect. Less than 10% of type II individuals develop symptoms. The remainder of patients have the third type of PCT (type III), which is biochemically indistinguishable from type I but occurs in more than one member of a family.

In addition, toxic forms of PCT have followed exposure to chemicals that decrease hepatic URO-D activity, a large outbreak occurring in the late 1950s following the consumption in South-Eastern Turkey of grain contaminated with hexachlorobenzene (Cripps *et al.*, 1984), while other cases have been reported after industrial accidents releasing 2,3,5,7-tetrachlorodibenzo-*p*-dioxin (TCDD) (Pazderova *et al.*, 1981).

Clinical features

Skin lesions

Skin lesions of sun-exposed skin, particularly the backs of the hands and the face, are the only consistent clinical feature of PCT. The commonest are increased mechanical fragility, superficial erosions from trivial trauma, subepidermal bullae, hypertrichosis and pigmentation. The tense bullae are not surrounded by inflammation (Plate 27) and are usually filled with clear fluid, although haemorrhagic blisters are possible. Erosions and collapsed bullae then become crusted and heal slowly to leave atrophic scars, milia and areas of hypo- and hyperpigmentation; the scarring is worsened by secondary infection but even minor photomutilation is uncommon, except rarely in those who work outside in sunny climates. The fragility is present in virtually all patients and its absence provides strong evidence against a bullous porphyria. The hyperpigmentation, often patchy and mainly of the face and hands, and hypertrichosis are, however, less frequent, although long, dark, lanugo-type hair, particularly of the frontotemporal region, the upper cheeks and extending to the eyebrows, may be prominent. Less common lesions still, seen particularly in long-standing cases, include sclerodermatous changes, which may affect covered areas of the thorax in addition to light-exposed skin, scarring alopecia, ageing changes, onycholysis and conjunctival damage. These features are not, however, diagnostic for PCT. Clinically and histologically indistinguishable skin lesions occur in all the bullous porphyrias (see Table 13.1), while similar skin fragility, erosions and blisters, without porphyrin overproduction, may also be produced by drugs ('pseudoporphyria') (see Chapter 00) and the prolonged use of sunbeds. Finally, a form of blistering sometimes associated with long-term haemodialysis may also be difficult to distinguish from PCT.

Most patients with PCT present in middle age (Table 13.5) with blisters and erosions, but hypertrichosis, particularly of the face in women, may sometimes be the dominant feature (Plate 28); acute photosensitivity is very uncommon. Type II PCT presents at a younger age than the other types, but there is such wide overlap that only onset before the age of 20 strongly suggests its presence. Otherwise the three types are clinically indistinguishable in the absence of a family history, which is present in less than 7% of patients (Table 13.5). Occasionally, PCT may be first identified during physical examination for some other disorder, usually chronic liver disease.

Precipitating factors

PCT is often the first clinical sign of hepatocyte injury provoked by one or more of a number of factors that appear important in its pathogenesis (Table 13.5), at least one being present in most patients irrespective of the type of PCT (Siersema *et al.*, 1995). Most male patients consume at least 40 g ethanol per day, of whom the majority show some evidence of liver cell damage (Bruguera, 1986). In addition, the association between PCT and the use of natural or synthetic oestrogens for oral contraception, postmenopausal symptoms or prostatic carcinoma is also well established (Grossman *et al.*, 1979), while the occasional onset of the disorder during pregnancy may also be an oestrogen effect, although iron supplementation may also contribute.

The role of hepatotropic viruses in the precipitation of PCT has been recognized more recently (Fargion *et al.*, 1992), reported

Table 13.5 Porphyria cutanea tarda: aetiological factors

Country	Sex	No. of patients	Age at onset (years)	Alcohol abuse[1]	Oestrogens	Anti-HCV antibodies	Cys282Tyr mutation in HFE gene	Family history of PCT
USA	M	17	7–76 (44)	11	2			1
	F	23	26–66 (47)	6	14			1
Italy	M	70	61.5 ± 8.2	28		56		
	F	4	62.1 ± 8.1					
Spain	M	86	–	58		70		5
	F	9	–	17		5		
Germany	M	66	59 ± 14	36	24	8		6
	F	40						
UK	M	43	25–72			10	40[2]	5
	F	39	6–79					

Numbers, unless otherwise indicated, denote numbers of patients
[1] Greater than 40–60 g/day
[2] 19 homozygotes, 7 C282Y/H63D compound heterozygotes and 14 heterozygotes
Data from Elder (1998) and references therein and Elder and Worwood (1988).

prevalences of HCV antibodies ranging from 79% to 8% (Elder, 1998); these tend to be higher in Southern Europe and the United States than in Northern Europe and are broadly related to the level of endemicity in the local population. Risk factors for HCV infection are, however, present in less than 25% of PCT patients. The prevalences in type I and type II PCT are similar. Other hepatotropic viruses have also been implicated in PCT pathogenesis, some series having shown a small increase in hepatitis B prevalence (Navas *et al.*, 1995), while hepatitis A may also precipitate symptoms (Coburn *et al.*, 1985). PCT may also complicate the later stages of HIV infection (Castanet *et al.*, 1994), an association which appears to be independent of HCV and other infections.

Abnormalities of iron metabolism are common in PCT. At least 80% of patients have some degree of hepatic siderosis and hepatic non-haem iron concentrations and total-body iron stores are increased in about 65% of patients (Lundvall *et al.*, 1970). This overload is mild to moderate in most patients, less than 20% having grade 4 siderosis, iron stores in excess of 4 g or a transferrin saturation of 62% or greater (Edwards *et al.*, 1989; Fargion *et al.*, 1996), while clinically overt haemochromatosis is unusual. The cause of the overload is uncertain, although the high prevalence of PCT among black South Africans has been attributed to consumption of alcoholic beverages with a high iron content (Sweeney, 1986) and similar dietary factors may perhaps also operate elsewhere. Inheritance of one or more haemochromatosis genes is also an important cause (Edwards *et al.*, 1989), about 45% of patients in the United Kingdom being heterozygotes or homozygotes for the putative haemochromatosis mutation Cys282Tyr in the HFE gene (Elder and Worwood, 1998).

Associated conditions

Most patients with PCT have some degree of liver cell damage, even young women with disease precipitated by oestrogens (Sweeney, 1986). However, clinical evidence of liver disease is unusual apart from abnormal biochemical tests of liver function, although all patients have markedly increased hepatic porphyrin concentrations with uroporphyrin crystals in the hepatocytes (Fakan and Chlumska, 1987); needle biopsy samples fluorescing red in UVA light. Apart from this and siderosis, the most frequent histopathological abnormalities are mild fatty infiltration, focal necrosis and inflammation of fibrotic portal tracts (Bruguera, 1986); cirrhosis is, however, present in less than 15% of cases but appears to carry a greater risk of hepatocellular carcinoma than other types of cirrhosis. The risk is increased by a long symptomatic period (ten years or more), decreased by early effective treatment and not solely related to HCV or hepatitis B infection (Siersema *et al.*, 1992). In spite of apparent variation in the prevalence of aetiological factors, the pathology of the liver is similar in most series. Whether porphyrin accumulation contributes to either the initiation of hepatocyte damage or its progression is controversial.

PCT has been reported in association with a wide range of other conditions, many of which affect the liver or alter iron metabolism. These include chronic renal failure treated by long-term haemodialysis, systemic lupus erythematosus, haematological malignancies, sideroblastic anaemia, thalassaemia and non-insulin dependent diabetes mellitus (Kappas *et al.*, 1995).

Laboratory investigation

Abnormalities of porphyrin metabolism

The diagnosis of PCT is established in adults by the demonstration of overproduction of uroporphyrin and other acetic acid-substituted porphyrins derived from the substrates of the URO-D reaction (see Figure 13.1, Table 13.4 and Appendix D). Urinary PBG excretion is normal. In children, the measurement of erythrocyte URO-D and protoporphyrin concentrations distinguishes PCT from hepatoerythropoietic porphyria (HEP).

VP, drug-induced pseudoporphyria and the bullous dermatosis of chronic renal failure are the most important differential diagnoses of PCT; plasma or faecal porphyrin determination being essential to differentiate VP since its urinary porphyrin pattern may occasionally be similar to that of PCT (Day *et al.*, 1982). In pseudo porphyria, porphyrin metabolism is normal. In patients with renal failure undergoing long-term haemodialysis, PCT is best identified by faecal porphyrin analysis, plasma uroporphyrin concentrations, although usually higher in overt PCT, being increased in both conditions (Poh-Fitzpatrick *et al.*, 1982). The adult-onset form of CEP also resembles PCT clinically but is readily distinguished by laboratory investigation (Table 13.4).

Other laboratory investigations

The serum ferritin concentration and transferrin saturation may be increased and reflect iron overload; iron deficiency in an untreated patient with a bullous porphyria, however, provides very strong evidence against PCT. About 50% of patients have abnormal biochemical tests of liver function, particularly transaminase levels, while all patients should be screened for hepatitis B and C, haemochromatosis and, when appropriate, HIV infection. Full investigation of any underlying liver disease, including any suspected hepatocellular carcinoma, may also be indicated in individual cases.

Pathogenesis

Individuals with PCT appear to be predisposed by inheritance to develop URO-D deficiency as a response to hepatocyte injury by alcohol, HCV, and other common agents. Recent research has given some indication of

the factors that may determine this predisposition (Elder, 1998).

Uroporphyrinogen decarboxylase

Biochemical and genetic studies indicate that there is no liver-specific inherited defect in the structure or expression of URO-D in sporadic PCT (Garey *et al.*, 1993). In familial PCT, 11 disease-specific mutations of the URO-D gene have been reported (Elder, 1998). All but two were restricted to a single family indicating that this disease, like other porphyrias, is likely to show extensive allelic heterogeneity. These mutations markedly decrease or abolish enzyme activity and immunoreactivity, the residual URO-D at half-normal concentration being encoded by the normal allele.

Inactivation of hepatic URO-D

Clinical expression of PCT appears to result from progressive inactivation of structurally normal URO-D in the liver so that activities fall to around 20% or less of normal; levels at which there is sufficient overproduction of porphyrins to produce photosensitization. Although better documented in sporadic PCT, this process probably also occurs in familial PCT although less inactivation is likely to be required because the starting concentration of enzyme is lower. The inactivation process is iron dependent, inhibits catalytic activity without decreasing the concentration of enzyme protein and is reversible (Elder and Roberts, 1995). Iron itself does not directly inhibit human URO-D (de Verneuil *et al.*, 1983).

In experimental uroporphyria in rodents, a model for PCT, inactivation of URO-D is accelerated by induction of a cytochrome P450 of the CYPIA subfamily, probably CYPIA2, iron overload and increased supply of ALA (Constantin *et al.*, 1996). CYPIA2 catalyses the NADPH-dependent oxidation of uroporphyrinogen to uroporphyrin (Lambrecht *et al.*, 1992), a reaction which, in the presence of iron, may also produce an unidentified, uroporphyrinogen-derived inhibitor of URO-D (De Matteis, 1988).

Susceptibility genes for PCT

Both the predisposition to PCT in humans and the susceptibility to experimental uroporphyria in mice appear to be determined at least in part by inherited factors (Constantin *et al.*, 1996). The Cys282Tyr mutation in the HFE gene has been identified as a susceptibility factor for sporadic and familial PCT (Elder and Worwood, 1998). Other genes whose products influence the rate of inactivation of URO-D may also predispose to PCT. Candidates include genes controlling other aspects of iron metabolism, hepatic ALA formation and CYPIA induction.

Treatment

PCT responds to two specific treatments ineffective in other cutaneous porphyrias, namely depletion of body iron stores (Rocchi *et al.*, 1986a) and low-dose oral chloroquine (Ashton *et al.*, 1981; Kordac *et al.*, 1989), which produce prolonged clinical and biochemical remission in most patients irrespective of the type of PCT.

Iron depletion is effective even in patients with no evidence of iron overload and appears to act by reversing the inactivation of URO-D (Elder *et al.*, 1985); replacement of iron then leads to relapse. To achieve this, one unit of blood is removed by venesection every one or two weeks until the transferrin saturation approaches 15% or the haemoglobin falls to 11–12 g/dl; serum ferritin measurements can also be used to monitor treatment (Rocchi *et al.*, 1986b), but the endpoint may be more difficult to determine because of co-existing liver disease. The aim of the therapy is to reduce iron stores to just below normal, and this effect should be monitored, porphyrin measurements being less relevant. Removal of 2.5–7.0 l of blood is usually required and may

clearly precede any clinical improvement or substantial decrease in porphyrin excretion. Full remission, however, which may then last for years, is usual within about six months.

Chloroquine complexes with uroporphyrin and promotes its release from the liver, possibly by stimulating exocytosis; it may also inhibit porphyrin formation (Kordac *et al.*, 1989). Oral chloroquine (125 mg twice weekly for adults) often produces clinical improvement by about four months but should be continued until urinary uroporphyrin excretion decreases to 100 nmol/day, which may take ten months or more (Ashton *et al.*, 1981). It should be noted that antimalarial doses of chloroquine provoke acute hepatotoxicity and marked uroporphyrinuria in PCT, reactions which may occasionally be the first sign of the disease, while even at the low doses recommended, initial minor increases in serum transaminase activities are common.

Desferrioxamine infusion may sometimes be useful if venesection and chloroquine are both contraindicated (Rocchi *et al.*, 1986b).

PCT complicating chronic haemodialysis may be difficult to treat. Venesection and chloroquine are contraindicated and standard dialysis procedures do not remove porphyrins. However, reduction of hepatic iron stores by treatment with erythropoietin is often effective (Sarkell and Patterson, 1993), even without supplementation by venesection.

Both venesection and oral chloroquine are similarly effective for PCT and may be combined if response to either is poor. Venesection will prevent iron-induced liver damage in homozygotes for the haemochromatosis gene and ensure compliance, but may be unsafe in ischaemic heart disease, difficult to perform or poorly tolerated. On the other hand, possible drawbacks to chloroquine treatment are poor compliance and potential hepatotoxicity, although liver morphology has remained largely unaltered and the progress of any underlying liver disease has not appeared to be accelerated (Chlumska *et al.*, 1980; Kordac *et al.*, 1989).

Patients should also abstain from alcohol and any oestrogen preparations should be withdrawn unless there are strong indications for their continued use. These measures alone may on occasion lead to clinical remission, but specific treatment is advisable if skin lesions cause any disability. Hypertrichosis, however, resolves slowly and may need physical removal. On the other hand, attacks of acute porphyria do not occur in PCT and patients do not need to avoid the drugs and anaesthetic agents that provoke acute porphyria. Finally, associated conditions should be managed as in the absence of PCT, their nature and severity probably being the main determinants of prognosis.

The usefulness of the measurement of erythrocyte URO-D as an aid to the management of PCT is debatable, the type of PCT not altering the treatment of an individual patient. Further, the benefit of identifying latent type II PCT in families and advising affected individuals to avoid alcohol and oestrogens remains unproven and needs to be balanced against the possible disadvantageous psychological effects of identifying a genetic defect.

Conditions related to porphyria cutanea tarda

Hepatoerythropoietic porphyria

HEP is a rare cutaneous porphyria caused by severe URO-D deficiency. About 30 patients have been reported, all, apart from one adult-onset case, having developed skin lesions in early childhood (Hift *et al.*, 1993a; Moran-Jimenez *et al.*, 1996). The most severely affected patients resemble those with CEP, while others may have a relatively mild PCT-like disease. Non-cutaneous manifestations are unusual, but two patients had a haemolytic anaemia withhepatosplenomegaly (Smith, 1986) and one developed a left-sided hemiparesis (Parsons *et al.*, 1994).

The porphyrin excretion pattern of HEP resembles that of PCT, but the erythrocyte protoporphyrin concentration is also increased, mainly as its zinc chelate. In addition, erythrocyte URO-D measurements range from 3% to 25% of normal and thus provide unequivocal differentiation from PCT.

Because the parents of patients with HEP are biochemically indistinguishable from those having latent type II PCT, HEP has been regarded as the homozygous counterpart of this disorder. However, the relationship between the two conditions has now been explored by mutational analysis (Roberts *et al.*, 1995). Patients with HEP are homoallelic or heteroallelic for URO-D gene mutations with variable effects on catalytic activity. Nine such mutations have now been identified in HEP (Elder, 1998), the most frequent, Gly281Glu, being found in Spain and North Africa and associated with the early onset of severe skin lesions. This mutation may cause overt PCT in heterozygotes, although with very low clinical penetrance, but other, milder mutations may never cause the disease and thus be truly autosomal recessive.

AUTOSOMAL DOMINANT ACUTE PORPHYRIAS AND RELATED CONDITIONS

Skin lesions clinically and histologically indistinguishable from those of PCT may occur in VP (Timonen *et al.*, 1990), HCP and their rare homozygous counterparts. VP frequently presents as a purely cutaneous condition, which may be mistaken for PCT, and HCP usually as an acute porphyria, but with minor skin lesions in about one third of cases (Kappas *et al.*, 1995). Skin lesions are uncommon in HCP in the absence of acute porphyria but may occasionally occur alone secondary to cholestasis (Hawk *et al.*, 1978). However, with an estimated prevalence of two per million of the population, HCP is much less common than VP and will therefore not be described further here.

Variegate porphyria

Variegate porphyria results from decreased protoporphyrinogen oxidase (PPOX) activity and is inherited in an autosomal dominant pattern with low clinical penetrance, about 80% of affected individuals being asymptomatic. The condition emerged as a distinct clinical entity largely through the work of Dean and Barnes in South Africa during the 1940s and 1950s (Dean, 1971). About 1 in 300, or 10–20 000, of the South African Afrikaans-speaking population are sufferers, having inherited the condition from an orphan girl who emigrated to the Cape of Good Hope from Holland and married one of the first Dutch settlers in 1688 (Dean, 1971). Elsewhere, however, the prevalence is much lower, being 1.3 per 100 000 in Finland (Mustajoki, 1980) and probably similar in other parts of Western Europe.

Clinical features

Symptoms usually start after the age of 20, onset before puberty being very rare. In South Africa and the United Kingdom patients present with skin lesions alone (58–73%), with an acute attack of porphyria alone (12–19%) or with both features combined (15–23%) (Eales *et al.*, 1980; Elder *et al.*, 1997). In Finland, however, although a similar proportion have skin lesions (75%), these are usually not sufficiently severe for medical advice to be sought and patients thus present with acute porphyria (Mustajoki, 1980); this difference has been attributed to relatively low light intensity. Acute attacks, but not skin lesions, are commoner in women (Eales *et al.*, 1980), while asymptomatic relatives may have mild skin fragility that has hitherto been regarded as normal within the family. In addition, VP, as for acute intermittent porphyria, may be associated with an increased risk of hepatocellular carcinoma (Kappas *et al.*, 1995).

The clinical features of an acute attack of VP are indistinguishable from those of acute intermittent porphyria (Elder *et al.*, 1997; Kappas *et al.*, 1995), most patients presenting with severe acute abdominal pain, often accompanied by pain in the back and lower limbs. Mental confusion is also common and there may be convulsions, often associated with hyponatraemia. A predominantly motor peripheral neuropathy may then follow the abdominal pain onset and progress to complete paralysis. The pain usually resolves within two weeks, but recovery from the neuropathy is slow and related to the required length of axonal regeneration. Progress in the management of acute porphyrias has decreased the risk of death therefrom (Mustajoki and Nordmann, 1993), but a severe attack remains a life-threatening emergency. Attacks may be provoked by drugs, particularly barbiturates, anticonvulsants and progestogens, and by alcohol, severe calorie restriction, infection or mental stress (Kappas *et al.*, 1995); in at least 30% of patients, however, there is no identifiable precipitant. In VP, acute attacks usually occur only once or occasionally; disabling repeated attacks, often in women and sometimes regularly premenstrual are much less common than in acute intermittent porphyria.

Laboratory investigation

In clinically overt VP, the plasma always contains a unique porphyrin-protein complex with a fluorescence emission peak at 624–626 nm (Poh-Fitzpatrick, 1980), unequivocally establishing the diagnosis provided the erythrocyte free protoporphyrin concentration is not increased. Other abnormalities also reflect decreased PPOX activity and the propensity of the resultant excess protoporphyrinogen to react covalently with proteins and peptides (see Table 13.4). Thus, protoporphyrin, coproporphyrin III and hydrophilic porphyrin-peptide conjugate concentrations are increased in the faeces, except rarely when intercurrent cholestasis blocks biliary excretion. PBG and ALA excretion increase during the onset phase of an acute attack but may return to normal as symptoms resolve; concentrations may, however, be normal or increased to only a small extent when only skin lesions are present. The laboratory diagnosis of VP and methods for the detection of latent disease in asymptomatic relatives are described in Appendix D.

Molecular genetics

Current investigations suggest that VP, like other autosomal dominant porphyrias, is heterogeneous at the DNA level, over 30 mutations causing the condition having now been identified in the PPOX gene. One mutation (Arg59Trp) is present in most South African patients, which is consistent with a high prevalence of the disease as the result of a founder effect (Meissner *et al.*, 1996). Elsewhere, however, particular mutations tend to be shared by only up to 10% of the population.

Treatment and management

The skin lesions of VP are often mild with a fluctuating course and spontaneous remissions. However, drugs and other compounds, including alcohol, that are known to provoke acute porphyria should be withdrawn, as should any potentially cholestatic compounds. In addition, avoidance of sunlight, for example by using light cotton gloves, may provide relief, as may reflectant sunscreens; β-carotene is not usually effective. Treatment of any skin lesions is symptomatic, but acute attacks are managed as for the other acute porphyrias (Elder *et al.*, 1997; Mustajoki and Nordmann, 1993).

The families of patients with overt VP should be screened for latent disease and all individuals found to have the condition, latent or overt, advised to avoid drugs known to provoke acute porphyria and to take only those considered safe; a list of these medications should be provided. Lists are available from specialist centres and patient support

groups. Such individuals should also be made aware that alcohol and low-calorie diets may precipitate acute porphyria and be strongly advised to become teetotal and to wear some form of warning jewellery in case emergencies arise in which drugs are needed. Otherwise, they should be encouraged to lead normal lives, pregnancy and elective surgery, for example, carrying little risk provided the diagnosis is known in advance. They should also be informed of the separate risks of producing affected (1 in 2) and symptomatic (about 1 in 10) offspring.

Homozygous variants

Homozygous variegate porphyria

At least 12 families containing one or more siblings with homozygous VP have been reported since the condition was first described in 1984. PCT-like skin lesions have appeared in all patients before the age of two years (Hift *et al.*, 1993b), the lesions often being mild, while hypertrichosis has been the dominant feature in some (Plate 29). Other features are not always present but include growth and mental retardation, clinodactyly, flexion deformities of the fingers, convulsions and nystagmus (Hift *et al.*, 1993b), but not as yet acute attacks of porphyria. A family history of overt VP is unusual. Homozygous VP differs biochemically from ordinary VP only in that PPOX activities are much lower, at less than 20% of normal, and as in all other homozygous porphyrias, erythrocyte protoporphyrin concentrations are increased. Parents of affected children may be consanguineous and their PPOX activities are generally 50–70% of normal; in addition, they may have other biochemical features of latent VP. Molecular analysis has shown homozygosity or compound heterozygosity for PPOX mutations, one South African patient having the Arg59Trp mutation on one allele and a mutation with less effect on PPOX activity on the other (Meissner *et al.*, 1996).

Homozygous hereditary coproporphyria

Homozygous HCP has been reported in one patient, a girl who presented at age four years with growth retardation, hypertrichosis and pigmentation and later had attacks of acute porphyria (Grandchamp *et al.*, 1977, 1995).

Harderoporphyria

This rare condition is characterized by markedly decreased coproporphyrinogen oxidase activity with increased faecal excretion of harderoporphyrin, a tricarboxylic intermediate of the reaction catalyzed by this enzyme; both abnormalities are caused by a specific mutation of the coproporphyrinogen oxidase gene (Lamoril *et al.*, 1998). Five such patients have been reported from three families (Lamoril *et al.*, 1998; Doss *et al.*, 1984; Grandchamp *et al.*, 1977), all with neonatal hyperbilirubinaemia and haemolysis, and, in two infants, subepidermal porphyric bullae. Mild photosensitivity and compensated haemolytic anaemia persist into adult life. Symptomatic heterozygotes have not been reported and the condition may well be truly an autosomal recessive disorder distinct from HCP.

CONGENITAL ERYTHROPOIETIC PORPHYRIA

Congenital erythropoietic porphyria (CEP), or Günther's disease, the rarest and most severe of the cutaneous porphyrias, results from a deficiency of uroporphyrinogen III synthase (see Fig. 13.1 and Table 13.3). The disease was first described by Schultz in 1874 and extensively studied by Günther and Garrod in the early decades of this century, being one of two additional conditions included in the second (1923) edition of the latter's *The Inborn Errors of Metabolism* after its autosomal recessive inheritance had been recognized. A patient with the disorder, Matthias Petry,

acted as a source of natural porphyrins for Hans Fischer's Nobel prize-winning work on tetrapyrrole chemistry. CEP occurs worldwide and its prevalence in the United Kingdom is about 2 in every 3 million live births.

Clinical features

Most patients present in early infancy (Fritsch *et al.*, 1997; Kappas *et al.*, 1995; Nordmann and Deybach, 1986), blisters on the light-exposed skin, occasionally following phototherapy for hyperbilirubinaemia, and reddish-brown staining of the napkin by urinary porphyrins being common early signs. Porphyrins also accumulate in amniotic fluid throughout pregnancy and the mother may thus sometimes notice brown discoloration of the fluid at the onset of labour. The skin lesions resemble those of PCT but are more severe and as patients age, progressive damage leads to photomutilation with erosion of the terminal phalanges, onycholysis, destruction of the ears, nose and eyelids and scarring alopecia (Plate 30). Facial hypertrichosis and patchy pigmentation are also common, while keratoconjunctivitis and other lesions caused by the scleral accumulation of porphyrin may sometimes lead to blindness.

Haemolytic anaemia and splenomegaly are common in CEP, the severity of the anaemia varying from fully compensated to severe and a small proportion of patients becoming transfusion dependent. There may also be marked fluctuations in the severity of the anaemia during the course of the illness, while splenomegaly may lead to thrombocytopenia with marked bruising; in addition, thrombocytopenia and leucopenia may occasionally be present at birth. Rarely, the anaemia is severe enough to lead to hydrops fetalis with death *in utero* or soon after birth (Verstraeten *et al.*, 1993).

Porphyrin in CEP accumulates in growing bones and discolours the skeleton, although the only manifestation visible during life is erythrodontia, namely brown teeth that fluoresce red in ultraviolet light. Other skeletal abnormalities include the compression and collapse of vertebrae, pathological fractures, decreased bone density and osteolytic lesions secondary to erosion by the hyperplastic bone marrow. In some patients, vitamin D metabolism may be impaired by the strict avoidance of sunlight.

The spectrum of severity of CEP ranges from fatal hydrops fetalis through severe disease starting in infancy, the commonest type, to milder forms presenting in later childhood or adult life. In adult-onset CEP the skin lesions may be no more severe than in PCT or even so slight as to be overlooked and patients may therefore present instead with thrombocytopenia secondary to hypersplenism (Murphy *et al.*, 1995) or with apparent haematuria because of their red urine. The prognosis for patients with infantile-onset CEP has been somewhat improved by modern supportive care but remains difficult to predict and although death during childhood is unusual, most patients reported in the past have died before age 40.

Laboratory investigation

Biochemical abnormalities

The hallmark of CEP is massive overproduction of isomer type I porphyrins (see Table 13.4 and Appendix D), the urine often being coloured red by the very high concentrations. Although uroporphyrin I is usually the main component, exceptional cases of severe disease in infancy associated with coproporphyrin I predominance have also been reported (Huang *et al.*, 1996). Erythrocytes contain both uroporphyrin I and coproporphyrin I, while protoporphyrin may also be increased as in other haemolytic anaemias. Erythrocyte uroporphyrinogen III synthase activity is markedly decreased, with little difference between the severe and mild forms (Nordmann and Deybach, 1994).

Haematological abnormalities

Although the degree of anaemia varies, most patients show some evidence of haemolysis with a normochromic, normocytic anaemia, reticulocytosis and increased urobilinogen excretion (Fritsch *et al.*, 1997; Kappas *et al.*, 1995; Nordmann and Deybach, 1982). In addition, the bone marrow shows normoblastic hyperplasia, most of the normoblasts showing persistent red fluorescence, mainly localized to the nucleus, under UV light and these fluorescent normoblasts, but not the non-fluorescent ones, are mor-phologically abnormal, with haem-containing inclusion bodies in their nuclei. Other haematological abnormalities are less well documented but as previously indicated, thrombocytopenia and other features of hypersplenism may be present, while leucopenia appears to be uncommon, even in severely affected children.

Molecular pathology and genetics

The bone marrow is the main source of porphyrin overproduction in CEP, studies of patients treated by bone marrow transplantation suggesting that less than 1% of the excess uroporphyrin comes from other tissues (Zix-Kieffer *et al.*, 1996). The haemolysis and increased ineffective erythropoiesis characteristic of the condition lead to an increased rate of erythroid haem synthesis and the compensatory changes required to achieve this in the face of markedly decreased uroporphyrinogen III synthase activity are reflected in overproduction of porphyrins, usually to a much greater extent than in other types of porphyria. Porphyrin enters the plasma by leakage from the circulating red cells, which lose porphyrin as they age, by the destruction of red cells in the spleen and as a consequence of the ineffective erythropoiesis.

The mechanism of the decreased survival of erythroid cells is uncertain (Nordmann and Deybach, 1982). However, it is known that porphyrin-containing cells readily photo-haemolyse *in vitro* and, possibly, in the superficial circulation, but this is unlikely to be the main explanation as the haemolysis is not necessarily related to light exposure, also occurring *in utero* and within the bone marrow. Instead, the metabolic abnormality appears to lead to an intrinsic membrane defect (Kappas *et al.*, 1995) but if this is caused by porphyrin, it must be related to the accumulation of hydrophilic forms, such as uroporphyrin, since haemolysis is not a feature of EPP where the lipophilic protoporphyrin predominates.

Molecular genetics

The phenotypic variability of CEP is reflected by heterogeneity at the DNA level, 18 mutations having been reported in the uroporphyrinogen III synthase gene that causes CEP in homozygotes or compound heterozygotes (Fontanellas *et al.*, 1996). However, one mutation (Cys73Arg) which decreases enzyme activity by more than 98% (Xu *et al.*, 1995) is present on about 50% of alleles in patients of European ancestry, all the others being restricted to just one or a few families (Fontanellas *et al.*, 1996). Of patients with this mutation, homozygotes have severe, infantile-onset disease, while disease severity in compound heterozygotes is influenced by the nature of the mutation on the other allele. Mutations that have less effect on catalytic activity tend to be associated with milder disease and some have been identified only in late-onset CEP (Fontanellas *et al.*, 1996; Xu *et al.*, 1995).

Treatment and prognosis

Infantile-onset CEP is a socially disabling disease, severe damage to the skin only being mitigated by the strict avoidance of sunlight including, for example, personal shielding with suitable light-filtering film (Huang *et al.*,

1996) and by good skin care with the prompt treatment of secondary infection. Reflectant sunscreens may be useful as an adjunct to these physical measures but are not usually sufficient by themselves, while β-carotene rarely provides significant protection.

Attempts at decreasing porphyrin over-production have focused on the suppression of erythropoiesis or interruption of the enterohepatic circulation. Hypertransfusion, for example, perhaps supplemented with hydroxyurea (Guarini *et al.*, 1994) or intravenous haematin (Rank *et al.*, 1990), may temporarily decrease porphyrin formation, but its long-term use is difficult. Further, initial reports that the trapping of porphyrins in the bowel by orally administered activated charcoal may lead to clinical and biochemical improvement have not been substantiated (Minder *et al.*, 1994).

Haemolytic anaemia may require repeated blood transfusions with desferrioxamine therapy to prevent iron overload, while for patients who become transfusion dependent, splenectomy may decrease the need for transfusion, but usually with only temporary effect. Thus, allogeneic bone marrow transplantation would now seem to be the treatment of choice for children with severe disease, provided, however, that bone marrow or umbilical cord blood is available from an HLA-compatible sibling donor (Zix-Kieffer *et al.*, 1996). In addition, future selection of patients for transplantation may be helped by better understanding of genotype/phenotype correlations, while for patients for whom there is no suitable donor, gene transfer therapy remains a potential alternative (Moreau-Gaudry *et al.*, 1996).

Prenatal diagnosis is available for CEP by measurement of uroporphyrin I levels in amniotic fluid, uroporphyrinogen III synthase activity in amniotic cells and, when the causative mutations have been identified in a previous sibling, by DNA mutation analysis (Ged *et al.*, 1996).

PORPHYRIA AND ACUTE PHOTOSENSITIVITY

ERYTHROPOIETIC PROTOPORPHYRIA

Erythropoietic protoporphyria (EPP) is a life-long, inherited disorder characterized by acute photosensitivity caused by the increased production of protoporphyrin IX secondary to decreased ferrochelatase enzyme activity (see Table 13.3) (DeLeo *et al.*, 1976; Todd, 1994). It was first defined as a porphyria in 1961 by Magnus *et al.*, although cases with similar clinical features had been reported previously (Kosenow and Treibs, 1953). EPP occurs in all races and has an estimated prevalence in Western Europe in the range of 1 in 75 000 (Went and Klasen, 1984) to 1 in 130 000 (Murphy *et al.*, 1985).

Clinical features

Symptoms and physical examination

Patients present with acute cutaneous photosensitivity normally starting in early childhood between the ages of one and six years, although their disorder may not be recognized as EPP until much later. Onset of symptoms during adult life is also possible, but very rare (Henderson *et al.*, 1995). Thus, the risk that children within affected families will develop symptoms falls steeply after five years and becomes negligible after the age of 14 (DeLeo *et al.*, 1976). Recent series show no difference in prevalence between the sexes.

An intense burning, pricking, itching sensation usually begins within 5–30 minutes (very rarely, several hours) of exposure to sunlight, the face and hands being most frequently affected. The symptoms then persist for several hours or occasionally days as an intensely painful burning sensation not relieved by darkness or covering of the skin, young children often becoming very distressed and sometimes crying for hours; patients characteristically seek relief by plunging their hands into cold water or dampening their skin with wet towels. The skin may look normal throughout although there is often erythema from early on and later oedematous swelling with crusting, while petechiae, vesicles, acute photo-onycholysis and urticaria are less common features; the lesions may sometimes be exacerbated by excoriation. The redness and swelling then often subside within a few hours, only rarely persisting for more than a few days, and very often there is nothing abnormal to see by the time the patient reaches the doctor, such that the whole episode may be dismissed as severe sunburn, particularly as a family history of EPP is absent in up to 55% of patients (Went and Klasen, 1984). Conversely, when a family history is present, anxious parents may need to be reassured that sunburn is not the first sign of EPP. Disease symptoms tend to be more severe during spring and summer, absent during the winter and sometimes improved during pregnancy (Went and Klasen, 1984), while overall severity may fluctuate over long periods of time in the same patient and vary markedly between patients, those who tan easily in particular often being less severely affected.

Recurrent episodes of photosensitivity may lead to chronic skin changes but these are often minor and may be hard to detect. Shallow linear scars over the bridge of the nose, small pit-like scars elsewhere on the face and some puckering around the mouth are characteristic (Plate 31), while the skin may also become thickened and waxy, especially over the knuckles, and appear prematurely aged; however, skin fragility with subepidermal bullae is not a feature of EPP except rarely after very excessive exposure.

Hepatobiliary disease

Progressive hepatic failure is an uncommon but serious complication of EPP (Bloomer, 1988), jaundice, sometimes associated with right-sided upper abdominal pain, often being the first symptom. Deterioration is then usually rapid, although removal of any aggravating factors such as alcohol intake (Bonkovsky and Schned, 1986) may delay progress; spontaneous recovery is very unusual (Van Wijk *et al.*, 1988). The liver damage is initiated by the accumulation and subsequent crystallization of protoporphyrin in hepatocytes, which leads as a result to cell damage, cholestasis with further retention of protoporphyrin and eventually cirrhosis (Bloomer, 1988); liver failure may then occur at any age, although most patients have been older than 30. Reports of the incidence of hepatic disease vary and biochemical tests of liver function are abnormal in 3–35% of patients; however, not all of these show protoporphyrin deposition or hepatocellular necrosis and fibrosis (Bloomer, 1988; DeLeo *et al.*, 1976; Doss and Frank, 1989). Nevertheless, over 30 patients in whom liver disease has either been fatal or required transplantation have been reported (De Torres *et al.*, 1996; Todd, 1994) and combination of the figures from retrospective published series (Todd, 1994) suggests that the complication affects about 2–5% of patients.

EPP may also increase the risk of cholelithiasis, gallstones from EPP patients containing protoporphyrin (DeLeo *et al.*, 1976) and their formation very likely being promoted by the high concentration of this compound in the bile of many patients (Morton *et al.*, 1988).

Anaemia

About 25% of EPP patients have a mild, hypochromic, microcytic anaemia (DeLeo *et al.*, 1976), some also with biochemical evidence of iron deficiency (Rademakers *et al.*, 1993). In addition, iron is deposited in the mitochondria of erythroblasts irrespective of the iron status of the patient and may lead to the formation of ring sideroblasts (Rademakers *et al.*, 1993). These changes have been attributed to the impairment of erythropoiesis by ferrochelatase deficiency.

Laboratory investigation

The diagnosis of EPP is established by the demonstration of increased free protoporphyrin in erythrocytes and plasma (see Table 13.4 and Appendix D), the protoporphyrin in other conditions in which total erythrocyte porphyrin is increased being present mainly as its zinc chelate and retained within the cell. These latter conditions include iron deficiency, lead poisoning and various anaemias. Distinction between the two forms of protoporphyrin and measurement of the plasma porphyrin are essential if diagnostic errors are to be avoided (see Appendix D). Erythrocyte protoporphyrin measurements using cord or peripheral blood from infants from affected families may point to the future development of EPP if unequivocally increased (Badcock and Szep, 1996), but such data should be interpreted with caution as there is little information on how the risk of later symptoms relates to presymptomatic findings. Finally, minor increases in free protoporphyrin are found in some asymptomatic adult relatives of EPP patients, as are increased numbers of fluorocytes (Went and Klasen, 1984), thus suggesting ferrochelatase deficiency.

Other porphyrin measurements are not required for the diagnosis of EPP, although faecal protoporphyrin excretion is increased in about 60% of patients (DeLeo *et al.*, 1976; Doss and Frank, 1989) (see Table 13.4). Urinary porphyrin excretion is normal in uncomplicated EPP, although patients with liver disease may develop coproporphyrinuria secondary to impaired biliary excretion.

Molecular pathology and inheritance

Although ferrochelatase activity is decreased in all tissues, erythroid cells are the main site of overproduction of protoporphyrin in EPP (Bloomer, 1988; Samuel *et al.*, 1988); concentrations are higher in late normoblasts and reticulocytes, before falling rapidly as the cells age and protoporphyrin diffuses into the plasma to bind to albumin and haemopexin. Most of this protoporphyrin is excreted in the bile, although an undetermined proportion undergoes enterohepatic circulation first (Bloomer, 1988). Hepatic accumulation of protoporphyrin probably results from the liver's inability to excrete the load presented to it; as excretory function deteriorates, accumulation accelerates.

The inheritance of EPP is complex. In most families, ferrochelatase deficiency is inherited in an autosomal dominant manner although the majority of affected individuals are not photosensitive; thus, from a study of 91 families, Went and Klasen (1984) estimated that only 2–3% of the offspring of affected individuals are likely to develop symptoms. Ferrochelatase activities in affected individuals who are asymptomatic are close to half normal, as would be expected if the gene allelic to the mutant gene was functioning normally, while in those with overt EPP, they are significantly lower at 10–30% of normal (Nordmann and Deybach, 1990). Such observations suggest that the co-inheritance of two defective ferrochelatase genes may be required for the clinical expression of EPP (Gouya et al., 1996; Norris et al., 1990; Went and Klasen, 1984). Twenty-five mutations that abolish or markedly reduce catalytic activity have now been identified in the ferrochelatase gene, most restricted to one or a few families, suggesting extensive allelic heterogeneity (Elder, 1988). Inheritance of one of these mutations in con-junction with a normal other allele decreases activity to half normal, whereas for symptoms to occur, inheritance of a second 'low-expression' allele also appears necessary (Went and Klasen, 1984). An allele of this type, which expresses low levels (about 50% of normal) of structurally normal mRNA for ferrochelatase, has recently been identified (Gouya et al., 1996) and the widespread occurrence in the population of this or a similar low-expression allele may explain the association found recently between a common polymorphism in

the ferrochelatase gene and clinically overt EPP (Poh-Fitzpatrick et al., 1997).

Some EPP families also show an autosomal recessive pattern of inheritance (Lamoril et al., 1991; Goerz et al., 1996; Sarkany et al., 1994), symptomatic individuals being homozygotes or compound heterozygotes for mutations that alter the structure of cDNA for ferrochelatase, thus having lower ferrochelatase activities than most other EPP patients. More extensive molecular analysis of EPP is now required to determine whether mutations identified in families of this type may also cause overt disease in association with the so-called 'low-expression' allele mentioned above. In addition, it has been suggested that inheritance of two disabling mutations may predispose to the liver disease of EPP (Sarkany et al., 1995), but no clear relationship between genotype and phenotype has yet been demonstrated.

Treatment and management of families

Photosensitivity

Avoidance of sunlight prevents photosensitivity but has social consequences that may be unacceptable. Patients may, however, develop a distinctive style of clothing that provides sunlight protection, although this is not usually easy for children of school age. Although absorbent sunscreens, whether designed for UVB or UVA protection, are largely ineffective as they do not normally block UVA and visible light, reflectant screens containing zinc oxide or titanium dioxide may be helpful if not too cosmetically unacceptable because of their white appearance; this can, however, be improved by the addition of a pigment such as iron oxide (Kaye et al., 1991). Producing a photoprotective tan by the application of UVA visible radiation-absorbing dihydroxyacetone or by gradually increasing exposure to sunlight may also be helpful in a few patients, while desensitization of the skin by psoralen photochemotherapy (PUVA) (Parrish et al.,

1982) or narrow-band UVB phototherapy (Collins and Ferguson, 1995) in the spring has been reported to provide some relief in many patients.

Oral β-carotene, which acts as a singlet oxygen quencher, was introduced as a treatment for EPP by Mathews-Roth *et al.*, in 1970, the recommended dose ranging from 30–90 mg/day for children to 100–300 mg/day for adults (Mathews-Roth, 1984; Roelandts, 1995), adjusted to maintain a plasma concentration of 6–8 mg/l. An initial trial for three months is recommended with treatment discontinuation thereafter if ineffective and it is important to use pure, synthetic β-carotene in order to ensure dosage. Uncontrolled series suggest that this regimen provides at least some photoprotection in over 75% of patients (Mathews-Roth, 1986), the only controlled trial, which showed no difference between the β-carotene and placebo groups, having been carried out at a lower dose (Corbett *et al.*, 1977). A few patients experience gastrointestinal discomfort, but β-carotene otherwise has few side effects apart from a yellowish discoloration of the skin. The related carotenoid, canthaxanthin, alone or in combination with β-carotene, has also been used to treat EPP, but canthaxanthin may crystallize in the retina and although this may well be harmless, is probably best avoided. Recently, oral cysteine has also been advocated as a treatment for EPP (Mathews-Roth *et al.*, 1994) but larger controlled trials with objective monitoring by monochromator phototesting are required to confirm any effectiveness; N-acetylcysteine has also been recommended, but seems ineffective (Todd, 1994). Finally, since phototoxic tissue injury from operating theatre lights is a possible hazard of surgery in EPP patients, protection in the form of appropriate light filters and other precautions should be provided (Todd and Burrows, 1992).

Since most of the protoporphyrin in EPP comes from erythroid cells, the disorder should be further treatable by allogeneic bone marrow transplantation or in the future by gene transfer therapy via haemopoietic stem cells (Moreau-Gaudry *et al.*, 1996), after ablation of the recipient's marrow. However, such procedures are likely to remain unacceptably hazardous for all except patients at risk of severe liver disease. Thus, until they can be accurately selected beforehand, further progress in this direction is unlikely to be made.

Prediction and treatment of liver disease

At present, there is no reliable method for predicting hepatic failure in EPP, although as liver function deteriorates, erythrocyte and plasma porphyrin concentrations increase, coproporphyrinuria appears and there is a relative decrease in faecal protoporphyrin excretion (Bloomer, 1988; Doss and Frank, 1989). However, porphyrin measurements appear to have little predictive value. It has been suggested that patients with very high faecal protoporphyrin excretion (Bloomer, 1988) or autosomal recessive disease (Sarkany *et al.*, 1994) may be particularly at risk. Nevertheless, all patients should have at least annual biochemical tests of liver function, persistent abnormalities being investigated by liver biopsy and further treatment considered if even mild hepatocellular necrosis and fibrosis are present.

Initially treatment of EPP liver disease is aimed at slowing the hepatic accumulation of protoporphyrin either by interruption of its enterohepatic circulation with cholestyramine, the most widely used if not satisfactorily evaluated treatment, or as a short-term measure by suppression of erythropoiesis by hypertransfusion or intravenous haematin (Bloomer, 1988; Todd, 1994); the correction of any iron deficiency may also reduce protoporphyrin levels in some patients but have the reverse effect in others (Bloomer, 1988; McClements *et al.*, 1992). Once liver failure develops, however, liver transplantation becomes the only treatment, special precautions being needed to prevent potentially fatal patient organ photonecrosis during the operation (Johnson and Fusaro, 1992). Specific postoperative complications include severe polyneuropathy, resembling that seen in the acute porphyrias (Herbert *et al.*, 1991) and the accumulation of protoporphyrin in the transplanted liver (Meerman *et al.*, 1993).

Genetic counselling

Went and Klasen (1984) estimated a 2–3% risk of clinical EPP for the children of affected parents, but recent evidence that the mode of inheritance of EPP is heterogeneous suggests that this figure is unlikely to be applicable to all families. Investigation for ferrochelatase deficiency by enzymatic or DNA methods is complex but may be helpful when parents are particularly anxious, perhaps because there is a family history of liver disease. However, outside autosomal recessive families, ferrochelatase deficiency does not reliably predict symptoms, although it increases the risk that an individual will develop overt EPP to about 10–20% (Went and Klasen, 1984), while co-inheritance of a haplotype associated with the 'low-expression' allele further increases this risk (Poh-Fitzpatrick *et al.*, 1997).

CONDITIONS RELATED TO
ERYTHROPOIETIC PROTOPORPHYRIA

Sideroblastic anaemia with photosensitivity

The abnormalities of haem biosynthesis that occur in the sideroblastic anaemias are rarely associated with cutaneous photosensitivity. However, four patients who developed EPP-like photosensitivity in association with idiopathic sideroblastic anaemia between the ages of 41 and 71 years (Lim *et al.*, 1992), all with increased erythrocyte and plasma protoporphyrin concentrations, have been reported. In addition, a 73-year-old man with sideroblastic anaemia and the biochemical abnormalities of

EPP without photosensitivity has been described (Lim *et al.*, 1992). The explanation for this rare association is uncertain, but chromosomal abnormalities are common in the bone marrow in sideroblastic anaemia and partial deletions of chromosome 18q, where the ferrochelatase gene is located (see Table 13.2), were present in the bone marrow of two of the three patients investigated cytogenetically. Thus, predominance in the bone marrow of erythroid cells in which this gene is deleted may largely explain this rare complication of sideroblastic anaemia.

REFERENCES

Ashton, R.E., Hawk, J.L.M. and Magnus, I.A. (1981) Low-dose oral chloroquine in the treatment of porphyria cutanea tarda. *British Journal of Dermatology*, **111**, 609–13.

Badcock, N.R. and Szep, D.A. (1996) Diagnosis of erythropoietic protoporphyria using cord blood. *Annals of Clinical Biochemistry*, **33**, 73–4.

Bloomer, J.R. (1988) The liver in protoporphyria. *Hepatology*, **8**, 402–7.

Bonkovsky, H.L. and Schned, A.R. (1986) Fatal liver failure in protoporphyria: synergism between ethanol excess and the genetic defect. *Gastroenterology*, **90**, 191–201.

Bruguera, M. (1986) Liver involvement in porphyria. *Seminars in Dermatology*, **5**, 178–85.

Castanet, J., Lacour, J.P., Bodokh, I. *et al.* (1994) Porphyria cutanea tarda in association with human immunodeficiency virus infection: is it related to hepatitis C virus infection? *Archives of Dermatology*, **130**, 664–5.

Chlumska, A., Chlumsky, J. and Malina, L. (1980) Liver changes in porphyria cutanea tarda patients treated with chloroquine. *British Journal of Dermatology*, **102**, 261–6.

Coburn, P.R., Coleman, J.C., Cream, J.J. *et al.* (1985) Porphyria cutanea tarda and porphyria variegata unmasked by viral hepatitis. *Clinical and Experimental Dermatology*, **10**, 169–73.

Collins, P. and Ferguson, J. (1995) Narrow-band UVB (TL-01) phototherapy: an effective preventative treatment for the photodermatoses. *British Journal of Dermatology*, **132**, 956–63.

Constantin, D., Francis, J.E., Akhtar, A. *et al.* (1996) Uroporphyria induced by 5-aminolevulinic acid in *Ahr^d* SWR mice. *Biochemical Pharmacology*, **52**, 1407–13.

Corbett, M.F., Herxheimer, A., Magnus, I.A. *et al.* (1977) The longterm treatment with beta-carotene in erythropoietic protoporphyria: a controlled trial. *British Journal of Dermatology*, **97**, 655–62.

Cripps, D.J., Peters, H.A., Gocmen, A. *et al.* (1984) Porphyria turcica due to hexachlorobenzene – a 20 to 30 year follow-up study on 204 patients. *British Journal of Dermatology*, **111**, 413–22.

Dabski, C. and Beutner, E.H. (1991) Studies of laminin and type IV collagen in blisters of porphyria cutanea tarda and drug-induced pseudoporphyria. *Journal of the American Academy of Dermatology*, **25**, 28–32.

Day, R.S., Eales, L. and Meissner, D. (1982) Coexistent variegate porphyria and porphyria cutanea tarda. *New England Journal of Medicine*, **307**, 36–41.

Dean, G. (1971) *The Porphyrias*, Pitman Medical, London.

DeLeo, V.A., Poh-Fitzpatrick, M., Mathews-Roth, M. *et al.* (1976) Erythropoietic protoporphyria: 10 years experience. *American Journal of Medicine*, **60**, 8–22.

De Matteis, F. (1988) Role of iron in the hydrogen peroxide-dependent oxidation of hexahydroporphyrins (porphyrinogens): a possible mechanism for the exacerbation by iron of hepatic uroporphyria. *Molecular Pharmacology*, **33**, 463–9.

De Torres, I., Demetris, A.J. and Randhawa, P.S. (1996) Recurrent hepatic allograft injury in erythropoietic protoporphyria. *Transplantation*, **61**, 1412.

De Verneuil, H., Sassa, S. and Kappas, A. (1983) Purification and properties of uroporphyrinogen decarboxylase from human erythrocytes. *Journal of Biological Chemistry*, **258**, 2450–60.

Doss, M.O. and Frank, M. (1989) Hepatobiliary implications and complications in protoporphyria, a 20-year study. *Clinical Biochemistry*, **22**, 223–30.

Doss, M., Von Tiepermann, R. and Kepp, W. (1984) Harderoporphyrin coproporphyria. *Lancet*, **1**, 292.

Eales, L., Day, R.S. and Blekkenhorst, G.H. (1980) The clinical and biochemical features of variegate porphyria: an analysis of 300 cases studied at Groote Schuur Hospital, Cape Town. *International Journal of Biochemistry*, **12**, 837–54.

Edwards, C.Q., Griffen, L.M., Goldgar, D.E. *et al.* (1989) HLA-linked hemochromatosis alleles in sporadic porphyria cutanea tarda. *Gastroenterology*, **98**, 972–81.

Elder, G.H. (1988) Genetic defects in the porphyrias: types and significance. *Clinics in Dermatology*, **16**, 225–34.

Elder, G.H. (1997) Porphyria cutanea tarda. *Seminars in Liver Disease*, **18**, 67–76.

Elder, G.H. and Roberts, A.G. (1995) Uroporphyrinogen decarboxylase. *Journal of Bioenergetics and Biomembranes*, **27**, 207–14.

Elder, G.H. and Worwood, M. (1998) Mutations in the hemochromatosis (HFE) gene, porphyria cutanea tarda and iron overload. *Hepatology*, **27**, 289–91.

Elder, G.H., Urquhart, A.J., De Salamanca, R. *et al.* (1985) Immunoreactive uroporphyrinogen decarboxylase in the liver in porphyria cutanea tarda. *Lancet*, **1**, 229–32.

Elder, G.H., Hift, R. and Meissner, P.N. (1997) The acute porphyrias. *Lancet*, **349**, 1613–17.

Epstein, J.H., Tuffanelli, D.L. and Epstein, W.L. (1973) Cutaneous changes in the porphyrias – a microscopic study. *Archives of Dermatology*, **107**, 689–98.

Fakan, F. and Chlumska, A. (1987) Demonstration of needle-shaped hepatic inclusions in porphyria cutanea tarda using the ferric ferricyanide reduction test. *Virchows Archives A*, **411**, 365–8.

Fargion, S., Piperno, A., Cappellini, M.D. *et al.* (1992) Hepatitis C virus and porphyria cutanea tarda: evidence of a strong association. *Hepatology*, **16**, 1322–6.

Fargion, S., Fracanzani, A.L., Romano, R. *et al.* (1996) Genetic hemochromatosis in Italian patients with porphyria cutanea tarda: possible explanation for iron overload. *Journal of Hepatology*, **24**, 564–9.

Fontanellas, A. Bensidhoum, M., De Salamanca, R.E. *et al.* (1996) A systematic analysis of the mutations of the uroporphyrinogen III synthase gene in congenital erythropoietic porphyria. *European Journal of Human Genetics*, **4**, 274–82.

Freeseman, A.G., Hofweber, K. and Doss, M.O. (1997) Co-existence of deficiency of uroporphyrinogen III synthase and decarboxylase in a patient with congenital erythropoietic porphyria and his family. *European Journal of Clinical Chemistry and Clinical Biochemistry*, **35**, 35–9.

Fritsch, C., Bolsen, K., Ruzicka, T. and Goerz, G. (1997) Congenital erythropoietic porphyria. *Journal of the American Academy of Dermatology*, **36**, 594–610.

Garey, J.R., Franklin, K.F., Brown, A.D. *et al.* (1993) Analysis of uroporphyrinogen decarboxylase complementary DNAs in sporadic porphyria cutanea tarda. *Gastroenterology*, **105**, 165–9.

Ged, C., Moreau-Gaudry, F., Taine, L. *et al.* (1996) Prenatal diagnosis in congenital erythropoietic porphyria by metabolite measurement and DNA mutation analysis. *Prenatal Diagnosis*, 16, 83–6.

Glover, R.A., Bailey, C.S., Barrett, K.E. *et al.* (1996) Histamine release from rodent and human mast cells induced by protoporphyrin and ultraviolet light: studies of the mechanism of mast-cell activation in erythropoietic protoporphyria. *British Journal of Dermatology*, 134, 880–5.

Goerz, G., Bunselmeyer, S., Bolsen, K. *et al.* (1996) Ferrochelatase activities in patients with erythropoietic protoporphyria and their families. *British Journal of Dermatology*, 134, 880–5.

Gouya, L., Deybach, J-C., Lamoril, J. *et al.* (1996) Modulation of the phenotype in dominant erythropoietic protoporphyria by a low expression of the normal ferrochelatase allele. *American Journal of Human Genetics*, 58, 292–9.

Grandchamp, B., Phung, N. and Nordmann, Y. (1977) Homozygous case of hereditary coproporphyria. *Lancet*, 2, 1348–9.

Grandchamp, B., Lamoril, J. and Puy, H. (1995) Molecular abnormalities of coproporphyrinogen oxidase in patients with hereditary coproporphyria. *Journal of Bioenergetics and Biomembranes*, 27, 215–20.

Grossman, M.E., Bickers, D.R., Poh-Fitzpatrick, M.B. *et al.* (1979) Porphyria cutanea tarda. Clinical features and laboratory findings in 40 patients. *American Journal of Medicine*, 67, 277.

Guarini, L., Piomelli, S. and Poh-Fitzpatrick, M.B. (1994) Hydroxyurea in congenital erythropoietic porphyria. *New England Journal of Medicine*, 331, 1091–2.

Hawk, J.L.M., Magnus, I.A., Elder, G.H. *et al.* (1978) Deficiency of hepatic coproporphyrinogen oxidase in hereditary coproporphyria. *Journal of the Royal Society of Medicine*, 71, 775–7.

Held, J.L., Sassa, S., Kappas, A. *et al.* (1989) Erythrocyte uroporphyrinogen decarboxylase activity in porphyria cutanea tarda: a study of 40 consecutive patients. *Journal of Investigative Dermatology*, 93, 332–4.

Henderson, C.A., Jones, S., Elder, G. *et al.* (1995) Erythropoietic protoporphyria presenting in an adult. *Journal of the Royal Society of Medicine*, 88, 476P–77P.

Herbert, A., Corbin, D., Williams, A. *et al.* (1991) Erythropoietic protoporphyria: unusual skin and neurological problems after liver transplantation. *Gastroenterology*, 100, 1753–7.

Hermann, G., Wlaschek, M., Bolsen, K. *et al.* (1996) Photosensitization of uroporphyrin augments the ultraviolet A-induced synthesis of matrix metalloproteinases in human dermal fibroblasts. *Journal of Investigative Dermatology*, 107, 398–403.

Hift, R., Meissner, P.N., Todd, G. *et al.* (1993a) Hepatoerythropoietic porphyria precipitated by viral hepatitis. *Gut*, 34, 1632–4.

Hift, R., Meissner, P.N., Todd, G. *et al.* (1993b) Homozygous variegate porphyria: an evolving clinical syndrome. *Postgraduate Medical Journal*, 69, 781–6.

Huang, J., Zaider, E., Roth, P. *et al.* (1996) Congenital erythropoietic porphyria: clinical, biochemical, and enzymatic profile of a severely affected infant. *Journal of the American Academy of Dermatology*, 34, 924–7.

Johnson, J.A. and Fusaro, R.M. (1990) Liver transplantation in patients with erythropoietic protoporphyria. *Gastroenterology*, 98, 1726–7.

Johnson, J.A. and Fusaro, R.M. (1992) Broad-spectrum photoprotection: the roles of tinted auto windows, sunscreens and browning agents in the diagnosis and treatment of photosensitivity. *Dermatology*, 185, 237–41.

Kappas, A., Sassa, S., Galbraith, R.A. *et al* (1995) The porphyrias, in *The Molecular and Metabolic Basis of Inherited Disease*, 7th edn (eds C.R. Scriver, A.L. Beaudet, W.S. Sly *et al.*), McGraw-Hill, New York, pp. 2103–59.

Kaye, E.T., Levin, J.A., Blank, I.H. *et al.* (1991) Efficiency of opaque photoprotective agents in the visible light range. *Archives of Dermatology*. 127, 351–5.

Kordac, V., Jirsa, M., Kotal, P. *et al.* (1989) Agents affecting porphyrin formation and secretion: implications for porphyria cutanea tarda. *Seminars in Hematology*, 26, 16–23.

Kosenow, W. and Treibs, A. (1953) Lichtuberempfindlickeit and porphyrinamie. *Zeitschrift Kinderheilbind*, 73, 82.

Lambrecht, R.W., Sinclair, P.R., Gorman, N. *et al.* (1992) Uroporphyrinogen oxidation catalyzed by reconstituted cytochrome P450IA2. *Archives of Biochemistry and Biophysics*, 254, 504–10.

Lamoril, J., Puy, H., Gouya, L. *et al.* (1998) Neonatal haemolytic anaemia due to inherited harderoporphyria: clinical characteristics and molecular basis. *Blood*, 91, 1–6.

Lim, H.W., Poh-Fitzpatrick, M.B. and Gigli, I. (1984) Activation of the complement system in patients with porphyrias after irradiation *in vivo*. *Journal of Clinical Investigation*, 74, 1961–5.

Lim, H.W., Cooper, D., Sassa, S. *et al.* (1992) Photosensitivity, abnormal porphyrin profile and sideroblastic anemia. *Journal of the American Academy of Dermatology*, **27**, 287–92.

Lundvall, O., Weinfeld, A. and Lundin, P. (1970) Iron storage in porphyria cutanea tarda. *Acta Medica Scandinavica*, **188**, 37–53.

Magnus, I.A. (1980) Cutaneous porphyrias. *Clinical Haematology*, **9**, 273–302.

Magnus, I.A., Jarrett, A., Prankerd, T.A.J. *et al.* (1961) Erythropoietic protoporphyria: a new porphyria syndrome with solar urticaria due to protoporphyrinaemia. *Lancet*, **2**, 448–51.

Mallon, E., Wojnarowska, F., Hope, P. *et al.* (1995) Neonatal bullous eruption as a result of transient porphyrinaemia in a premature infant with hemolytic disease of the newborn. *Journal of the American Academy of Dermatology*, **33**, 333–6.

Mathews-Roth, M.M. (1984) Treatment of erythropoietic protoporphyria with beta-carotene. *Photodermatology*, **1**, 318–21.

Mathews-Roth, M.M. (1986) Beta-carotene therapy for erythropoietic protoporphyria and other photosensitivity diseases. *Biochimie*, **68**, 875–84.

Mathews-Roth, M.M., Pathak, M.A., Fitzpatrick, T.B. *et al.* (1970) Beta-carotene as a photoprotective agent in erythropoietic protoporphyria. *New England Journal of Medicine*, **282**, 1231–4.

Mathews-Roth, M.M., Rosner, B., Benfell, K. and Roberts, J.E. (1994) A double-blind study of cysteine photoprotection in erythropoietic protoporphyria. *Photodermatology, Photoimmunology and Photo-medicine*, **10**, 244–8.

May, B.K., Dogra, S.C., Sadlon, T.J. *et al.* (1995) Molecular regulation of haem biosynthesis in higher vertebrates. *Progress in Nucleic Acids Research and Molecular Biology*, **51**, 1–51.

McClements, B.M., Bingham, A., Callender, M.E. *et al.* (1992) Erythropoietic protoporphyria and iron therapy. *British Journal of Dermatology*, **127**, 534–7.

Meerman, L., Karrenbeld, A., Van Hattum, J. *et al.* (1993) Recurrence of ultrastructural liver cell damage after liver transplantation for erythropoietic protoporphyria. *Gastroenterology*, **104**, A952.

Meissner, P.N., Adams, R. and Kirsch, R. (1993) Allosteric inhibition of human lymphoblast and purified porphobilinogen deaminase by protoporphyrinogen and coproporphyrinogen: a possible mechanism for the acute attack of variegate porphyria. *Journal of Clinical Investigation*, **91**, 1436–44.

Meissner, P.N., Dailey, T.A. and Hift, R.J. *et al.* (1996) A R59W mutation in human protoporphyrinogen oxidase results in decreased enzyme activity and is prevalent in South Africans with variegate porphyria. *Nature Genetics*, **13**, 95–7.

Minder, E.I., Schneider-Yin, X. and Moll, F. (1994) Lack of effect of oral charcoal in congenital erythropoietic porphyria. *New England Journal of Medicine*, **331**, 1092–3.

Moran-Jimenez, M.J., Ged, C., Romana, M. *et al.* (1996) Uroporphyrinogen decarboxylase complete gene sequence and molecular study of three families with hepatoerythropoietic porphyria. *American Journal of Human Genetics*, **58**, 712–21.

Moreau-Gaudry, F., Ged, C. and De Verneuil, H. (1996) Gene therapy for erythropoietic porphyria. *Gene Therapy*, **3**, 843–4.

Morton, K.O., Schneider, F., Weimer, M.K. *et al.* (1988) Hepatic and bile porphyrins in patients with protoporphyria and liver failure. *Gastroenterology*, **94**, 1488–92.

Murphy, A., Gibson, G., Elder, G.H. *et al.* (1995) Adult-onset congenital erythropoietic porphyria. *Journal of the Royal Society of Medicine*, **88**, 357P–58P.

Murphy, G.M., Hawk, J.L.M., Corbett, M.F. *et al.* (1985) The U.K. erythropoietic protoporphyria register: a progress report. *British Journal of Dermatology*, **113**, 11.

Mustajoki, P. (1980) Variegate porphyria. *Quarterly Journal of Medicine*, **49**, 191–203.

Mustajoki, P. and Nordmann, Y. (1993) Early administration of heme arginate for acute porphyric attacks. *Archives of Internal Medicine*, **153**, 2004–8.

Navas, S., Bosch, P., Castillo, I. *et al.* (1995) Porphyria cutanea tarda and hepatitis C virus and B virus infection: a retrospective study. *Hepatology*, **21**, 279–84.

Nordmann, Y. and Deybach, J.C. (1986) Congenital erythropoietic porphyria. *Seminars in Dermatology*, **5**, 106–14.

Nordmann, Y. and Deybach, J.C. (1990) Human hereditary porphyrias, in *Biosynthesis of Heme and Chlorophylls*, (ed. H.A. Dailey), McGraw-Hill, New York, pp. 491–542.

Norris, P.G., Nunn, A.V., Hawk, J.L.M. *et al.* (1990) Genetic heterogeneity in erythropoietic protoporphyria: a study of the enzymatic defect in nine affected families. *Journal of Investigative Dermatology*, **95**, 260–3.

O'Reilly, K., Snape, J. and Moore, M.R. (1988) Porphyria cutanea tarda resulting from primary hepatocellular carcinoma. *Clinical and Experimental Dermatology*, **13**, 44–8.

Parrish, J.A., Le Vine, M.J., Morison, W.L. *et al.* (1979) Comparison of PUVA and beta-carotene in the treatment of polymorphous light eruption. *British Journal of Dermatology*, **100**, 187–91.

Parsons, J.L., Sahn, E.E., Holden, K.R. *et al.* (1994) Neurologic disease in a child with hepatoery-thropoietic porphyria. *Pediatric Dermatology*, **11**, 216–21.

Pazderova-Vejlupkova, J., Nemcova, M., Pickova, J. *et al.* (1981) The development and prognosis of chronic intoxication by tetrachlorodibenzo-p-dioxin in men. *Archives of Environmental Health*, **36**, 5–11.

Poh-Fitzpatrick, M.B. (1980) A plasma porphyrin fluorescence marker for variegate porphyria. *Archives of Dermatology*, **116**, 543–7.

Poh-Fitzpatrick, M.B., Sosin, A.E. and Bemis, J. (1982) Porphyrin levels in plasma and erythro-cytes of chronic hemodialysis patients. *Journal of the American Academy of Dermatology*, **7**, 100–4.

Poh-Fitzpatrick, M.B., Zadier, E., Sciales, C. *et al.* (1990) Cutaneous photosensitivity and copro-porphyrin abnormalities in the Alagille syndrome. *Gastroenterology*, **99**, 831–5.

Poh-Fitzpatrick, M.B., Piomelli, S., Deybach, J.C. *et al.* (1997) Erythropoietic protoporphyria: a triallelic inheritance model. *Journal of Investigative Dermatology*, **108**, 598.

Ponka, P. (1997) Tissue-specific regulation of iron metabolism and heme synthesis: distinct control mechanisms in erythroid cells. *Blood*, **89**, 1–25.

Rademakers, L.H.P.M., Koningsberger, J.C., Sorber, C.W.J. *et al.* (1993) Accumulation of iron in erythroblasts of patients with erythropoietic protoporphyria. *European Journal of Clinical Investigation*, **23**, 130–8.

Rank, J.M., Straba, J.G., Weimer, M.K. *et al.* (1990) Hematin therapy in late onset congenital erythropoietic porphyria. *British Journal of Haematology*, **75**, 617–22.

Roberts, A.G., Whatley, S.D., Daniels, J. *et al.* (1995) Partial characterization and assignment of the gene for protoporphyrinogen oxidase and varie-gate porphyria to human chromosome 1q23. *Human Molecular Genetics*, **4**, 2387.

Rocchi, E., Gibertini, P., Cassanelli, M. *et al.* (1986a) Iron removal therapy in porphyria cutanea tarda: phlebotomy versus slow subcutaneous desfer-rioxamine infusion. *British Journal of Dermatology*, **114**, 621–9.

Rocchi, E., Gibertini, P., Cassanelli, M. *et al.* (1986b) Serum ferritin in the assessment of liver iron overload and iron removal therapy in porphyria cutanea tarda. *Journal of Laboratory and Clinical Medicine*, **107**, 36–42.

Roelandts, R. (1995) Photo(chemo)therapy and general management of erythropoietic protopor-phyria. *Dermatology*, **190**, 330–1.

Ryan, E.A. and Madill, G.T. (1968) Electron microscopy of the skin in erythropoietic proto-porphyria. *British Journal of Dermatology*, **80**, 561.

Samuel, D., Boboc, B., Bernau, J. *et al.* (1988) Liver transplantation for protoporphyria: evidence for the predominant role of the erythropoietic tissue in protoporphyrin overproduction. *Gastroenterology*, **95**, 816–19.

Sarkany, R.P.E., Alexander, G.J.M.A. and Cox, T.M. (1994) Recessive inheritance of erythropoietic protoporphyria with liver failure. *Lancet*, **343**, 1394–6.

Sarkell, B. and Patterson, J.W. (1993) Treatment of porphyria cutanea tarda of end-stage renal disease with erythropoietin. *Journal of the American Academy of Dermatology*, **29**, 499–500.

Schnait, F.G., Wolff, K. and Konrad, K. (1975) Erythropoietic protoporphyria – submicroscopic events during the acute photosensitivity flare. *British Journal of Dermatology*, **92**, 545.

Siersema, P.D., ten Kate, F.J.W., Mulder, P.G.H. *et al.* (1992) Hepatocellular carcinoma in porphyria cutanea tarda: frequency and factors related to its occurrence. *Liver*, **12**, 56–61.

Siersema, P.D., Rademakers, L.H.P., Cleton, M.I. *et al.* (1995) The difference in liver pathology between sporadic and familial forms of porphyria cutanea tarda – the role of iron. *Journal of Hepatology*, **23**, 259–67.

Smith, S.G. (1986) Hepatoerythropoietic porphyria. *Seminars in Dermatology*, **5**, 125–37.

Spikes, J.D. (1984) Photobiology of porphyrins, in *Porphyrin Localization and Treatment of Tumors*, (eds D.R. Doiron and C.J. Gomer), Liss, New York, pp. 19–39.

Sweeney, G.D. (1986) Porphyria cutanea tarda, or the uroporphyrinogen decarboxylase deficiency diseases. *Clinical Biochemistry*, **19**, 3–14.

Timonen, K., Niemi, K-M., Mustajoki, P. *et al.* (1990) Skin changes in variegate porphyria. *Archives of Dermatological Research*, **282**, 108–14.

Todd, D.J. (1994) Erythropoietic protoporphyria. *British Journal of Dermatology*, **131**, 751–66.

Todd, D.J. and Burrows, D. (1992) Predictable hazards of erythropoietic protoporphyria. *Clinical and Experimental Dermatology*, **17**, 141.

Van Wijk, H.J., Van Hattum, J., Baart De La Faille, H. *et al.* (1988) Blood exchange and transfusion therapy for acute cholestasis in protoporphyria. *Digestive Disorders and Science*, **33**, 1621–5.

Varigos, G., Schiltz, J.R. and Bickers, D.R. (1982) Uroporphyrin I stimulation of collagen biosyn-thesis in human skin fibroblasts. *Journal of Clinical Investigation*, **69**, 129–35.

Verstraeten, L., Regemorter, N.V., Pardon, A. *et al.* (1993) Biochemical diagnosis of a fatal case of Günther's disease in a newborn with hydrops foetalis. *European Journal of Clinical Chemistry and Clinical Biochemistry*, **31**, 121–8.

Went, L.N. and Klasen, E.C. (1984) Genetic aspects of erythropoietic protoporphyria. *Annals of Human Genetics*, **48**, 105–17.

Wick, G., Hönigsmann, H. and Timpl, R. (1979) Immunofluorescence demonstration of type IV collagen and a noncollagenous glycoprotein in thickened vascular basal membranes in protoporphyria. *Journal of Investigative Dermatology*, **73**, 335–8.

Wolff, K., Hönigsmann, H., Rauschmeier, W. *et al.* (1982) Microscopic and fine structural aspects of porphyrias. *Acta Dermatovenereologica (Stockholm)*, **100** (suppl), 17–28.

Xu, W., Warner, C.A. and Desnick, R.J. (1995) Congenital erythropoietic porphyria: identification and expression of ten mutations in the uroporphyrinogen III synthase gene. *Journal of Clinical Investigation*, **95**, 905–12.

Zix-Kieffer, I., Langer, B., Eyer, D. *et al.* (1996) Successful cord blood stem cell transplantation for congenital erythropoietic porphyria (Günther's disease). *Bone Marrow Transplantation*, **18**, 217–20.

Warwick L. Morison, Laura E. Towne and Barbara Honig

The photoaggravated dermatoses are disorders induced or exacerbated by exposure to ultraviolet radiation (UVR) from sunlight or artificial sources and are a diverse group of often unknown aetiology; photosensitivity typically occurs in only a subset of the patients affected. Several of the disorders are thought to occur through autoimmune mechanisms, such as, for example, lupus erythematosus (LE), dermatomyositis (DM), pemphigus and bullous pemphigoid (BP), while a number of inflammatory dermatoses which under some circumstances are exacerbated by sunlight are also mentioned.

LUPUS ERYTHEMATOSUS

LE is a chronic inflammatory disorder which can involve multiple organ systems and is best considered as a continuum of disease types. Patients with discoid LE (DLE) have disease that is primarily confined to the skin, while those with systemic disease (SLE) demonstrate multisystem involvement with marked immunological abnormalities; skin involvement is present in 60–70% of SLE patients. Genetic factors, viruses, environmental stimuli and immunological abnormalities are all factors contributing to the aetiology of LE, while photosensitivity is common, although the precise photobiological mechanisms have not been fully elucidated.

Photodermatology. Edited by J.L.M. Hawk. Published in 1998 by Chapman & Hall, London. ISBN 0 412 72460 X.

Cutaneous lesions of LE are found mainly on sun-exposed areas (Plate 32) such as the dorsum of the nose and the malar eminences. Ultraviolet exposure induces new lesions in previously normal-appearing skin in only a small subset of these patients (Morison, 1983), but may exacerbate existing lesions in nearly all DLE and approximately 30% of SLE patients. In addition, the systemic manifestations of SLE have also been reported to be potentially adversely affected by UVR.

Patients with LE may exhibit serum antibodies against cytoplasmic and nuclear components. Thus, indirect immunofluorescence (IMF) screening tests for serum antinuclear antibodies (ANA) are positive in virtually all patients with SLE, but negative or only faintly positive in those with DLE. In addition, serum antibodies to double-stranded DNA (dsDNA) are thought to be specific for SLE but are quite rare in DLE, while anti-Ro cytoplasmic antibody has a strong association with photosensitivity (Provost and Reichlin, 1981).

The lupus band test is a direct IMF study used to evaluate clinically involved as well as normal-appearing skin, a positive test demonstrating deposition of immunoglobulin (Ig) and complement at the basement membrane zone (BMZ). The deposits most commonly found are IgG, traces of IgM and components of the classic and alternate complement pathways. In patients with DLE, the test is negative in normal but positive in lesional skin, while patients with SLE are positive in almost all sun-exposed normal and 50% of non-exposed normal skin.

The first clear demonstrations of abnormal cutaneous responses to UVR in patients with LE occurred in the 1960s and early 1970s (Baer and Harber, 1965; Cripps and Rankin, 1973; Epstein *et al.*, 1965; Everett and Olson, 1996; Freeman *et al.*, 1969), when it was noted that artificial irradiation of skin produced clinical lesions, the prolongation of delayed erythema and an enhanced erythema in selected patients. In one particular study, five of nine patients with photosensitivity and LE developed follicular papules or plaques after repeated UVB (280–315 nm) exposure (Epstein *et al.*, 1965), while another patient with subacute SLE demonstrated a decreased minimal erythema dose (MED) to UVB with an abnormal persistence of erythema (Baer and Harber, 1965). Cripps and Rankin (1973) then showed that at 300 nm there may be a slightly decreased MED and persistent erythema in patients with disseminated DLE, while a positive lupus band test and histological LE developed at sites of exposure in some of these patients after many weeks. Kind *et al.* (1987) further demonstrated sensitivity to both UVA (315–400 nm) and UVB radiation in over 40 LE patients, while histologically, UVA-exposed lesions showed a deep and superficial perivascular lymphocytic infiltrate with neutrophils in the vessel walls. UVB exposed lesions, on the other hand, demonstrated a similar perivascular infiltrate but also typical epidermal changes.

Photosensitivity secondary to less classic or less often considered UVR sources has also been reported. In 1992, 13 of 30 photosensitive SLE patients surveyed reported flares of their disease in response to exposure to standard fluorescent lights (Rihner and McGrath, 1992), symptoms reported having included rash, fatigue, joint pain, headache and nausea. Radiometric measurements by the authors suggested a significant emission of both UVB and UVA by standard fluorescent lamps, although it was noted that acrylic diffusers covering such lamps block most of this emission. In 1995, a case report was also presented of photoexacerbation secondary to UVA emission from a photocopier (Klein *et al.*, 1995) affecting a 34-year-old woman with a history of SLE who worked as a photocopy technician. After discontinuation of her employment, her skin manifestations markedly improved. Radiometric measurements of several photocopiers was conducted and the UVA emission noted to range between the relatively low values of 0.04 and 0.38 mW/cm^2, while UVB emission was non-existent. The patient also underwent phototesting which resulted in the development of erythematous annular plaques at both the UVA and UVB exposure sites, punch biopsy of these sites being consistent with LE; photopatch tests were negative.

It is thus clear that multiple studies have documented the exacerbation of LE skin lesions after UVR exposure, but the precise mechanisms of such photoexacerbation are poorly understood. However, there are several intriguing immunological theories which have been put forward and these are discussed.

Exposure of DNA to UVR results in the formation of photoproducts called UV-DNA, which are antigenic and stimulate the formation of antibodies in animals; these antibodies react specifically with UV-DNA and native DNA (nDNA) (Levine *et al.*, 1966). In general, however, DNA is a weak antigen, pure nDNA and denatured DNA not typically inducing antibody formation, and there is evidence that the antigenic determinants in UV-DNA may be UVR-induced thymine dimers (Levine *et al.*, 1966; Natali and Tan, 1971; Tan, 1968). Conformational changes in DNA secondary structure, however, may also play a role (Wakizaka and Okuhara, 1979).

UV-DNA has been identified by an immunofluorescent antibody technique in both mouse (Tan and Stoughton, 1969a) and human (Tan and Stoughton, 1969b) skin after UV irradiation. However, no UV-DNA is found at non-irradiated sites, while removal of the stratum corneum before irradiation results in more. UV-DNA can also be detected in hairless mouse epidermal cells for 24 hours after UVC exposure, but is not found at 48 hours (Jarzabek-Chorzelska *et al.*, 1976). Further, serum from mice previously exposed to UVR inhibits the activity of UV-DNA antibodies for up to 15 hours after exposure (Tan, 1971), suggesting a photoproduct is released from the skin into the circulation, while UV exposure in mice with circulating UV-DNA antibody produces immunofluorescent immunoglobulin and complement deposition in skin in a pattern similar to that seen in LE patients (Natakum and Tan, 1973). Additionally, if irradiated DNA is given to an animal preimmunized to it, glomerular immune complexes may subsequently be demonstrated (Natali and Tan, 1972), a course of events which may help explain the pathophysiology of immune complex-mediated LE nephritis.

All these findings suggest that circulating UV-DNA antibodies may play an important role in the pathogenesis of LE skin lesions, such UV-DNA perhaps being formed in the skin following irradiation and released into the circulation. The photoproduct may then stimulate the production of UV-DNA antibody, which may later react with similar lesions in the skin, fix complement and induce the inflammatory response. Thus, UV-induced cellular DNA alterations may lead to immune complex formation in cutaneous LE lesions (Biesecker *et al.*, 1972), thereby resulting in disease exacerbation and a positive lupus band test.

SLE patients may also perhaps have a partial defect in DNA repair following UV irradiation (Beighlie and Teplitz, 1975; Cleaver, 1970; Emerit and Michelson, 1981; Zarmansky *et al.*, 1985), studies having demonstrated UVC-irradiated lymphocytes from patients with SLE to incorporate less tritiated thymidine than normal lymphocytes (Beighlie and Teplitz, 1975). However, in other studies, fibroblasts from LE skin

biopsies have shown normal repair synthesis (Cleaver, 1970). There have also been reports of increased spontaneous chromosomal aberrations in the lymphocytes of patients with SLE and of a photoactive, chromosome-damaging agent in the serum of such patients; this agent is thought to be enhanced by exposure to 360–400 nm radiation and to be an unstable hydroperoxide originating in lymphocytes (Emerit and Michelson, 1981). Thus, defective UV-DNA repair could perhaps contribute to the SLE process by allowing UV-altered DNA to persist long enough for antibody production to occur.

Alterations to intracellular and surface macromolecules other than DNA may also be induced by UVR, UVA and UVB irradiation, for example affecting both RNA and protein synthesis. Thus, many photosensitive SLE patients express anti-Ro/SSA ribonucleoprotein antibodies (Mond *et al.*, 1989; Synkowski *et al.*, 1982) and there is *in vitro* evidence that UVR exposure enhances Ro antigen expression on cultured keratinocytes, thus providing a target for the anti-Ro antibodies (Le Feber *et al.*, 1984). In addition, a 1994 study demonstrated that UVB irradiation of epidermal keratinocytes resulted in an increased expression of calreticulin (Kawashima *et al.*, 1994), a high-affinity calcium-binding protein and constituent of the Ro/SSA complex, while along with Ro/SSA, two recent studies have looked at other soluble intracellular antigens such as SSB and SM (Dorgolan *et al.*, 1992; Jones, 1992), the majority of SLE patients in one demonstrating an increased expression of such antigens on the keratinocyte cell membrane in response to exposure in just ten minutes midday summer sunlight. The antigen expression was thought to be mainly due to UVB, but a contribution from UVA could not be completely ruled out. One group then went on to confirm that UVB induced the cell surface antigen expression not by increased passive antigen leakage to the cell membrane but by increased protein synthesis, while further study indicated that the expression occurred predominantly on some but not all sublethally injured cells. Furthermore, the number of injured cells did not significantly increase with increasing doses of UVB but rather the number of such cells expressing antigen, while interestingly, UVA in this study did not induce the expression of antigen although it did cause a similar degree of cell injury. Thus, the above findings all suggest that cutaneous cellular exposure, in particular to UVB radiation, may enhance the expression of certain cell surface antigens to provide a target for antibodies; the resulting antigen–antibody complex might then initiate disease by antibody-directed cell cytotoxicity.

In addition to the above antigenic alterations, UVR may act to exacerbate LE by yet other mechanisms, the irradiation of mice with broad-spectrum UVR inhibiting delayed-type hypersensitivity, local graft-versus-host reactions, contact hypersensitivity responses, the rejection of UVR-induced tumours and Langerhans cell activity, while also inducing the formation of antigen-specific suppressor T lymphocytes (Kripke and Morison, 1985). Thus, both local and system immunological alteration is possible following UVR exposure.

Potent cutaneous immunological mediators are also released or stimulated by UVR exposure, non-lethal *in vivo* and *in vitro* UV irradiation inducing interleukin-1 (IL-1) production by epidermal cells and monocytes respectively (Ansel *et al.*, 1983, 1984) and UV-irradiated mouse serum also demonstrating increased IL-1 activity (Gahring *et al.*, 1984). Since this substance is known to be involved in amplifying inflammatory responses, its UV-induced cutaneous and systemic production in LE may perhaps further stimulate an already hyperactive humoral immune system.

DERMATOMYOSITIS

DM is a chronic inflammatory disease characterized by both a myopathy and skin mani-

festations; muscle involvement without skin changes is also possible, in which case the disorder is called polymyositis. The aetiology is unknown, but a so-called autoimmune pathogenesis has long been considered likely.

Patients generally present with progressive, bilateral, principally proximal muscle weakness. Skin lesions are also almost always present at the time of presentation and most commonly include a heliotrope erythema of particularly the eyelids and surrounding skin, so-called Gottron's papules, usually of the extensor surfaces of the limbs near the joints, nailfold hypertrophy with telangiectasia and an irregular, often streaky macular erythema of especially sun-exposed skin.

Laboratory findings in DM include in particular elevations in circulating muscle enzyme concentrations, an abnormal electromyogram and abnormal muscle biopsy findings. Circulating autoantibodies have also been identified and in associated connective tissue overlap syndromes, the anti-DNA, anti-ribonucleoprotein (RNP) and anti-Ro antibodies appear to predominate, while the presence of the anti-tRNA synthetase enzyme correlates with the presence of extramuscular disease. Finally, the HLA-DR3 phenotype is overrepresented in both black and Caucasian patients.

Although DM has long been accepted as a photoaggravated dermatosis, the incidence and nature of this photosensitivity have been poorly documented. Estimates of between 37% and 50% have been made, but the studies documenting these numbers have been small. For example, one study considered ten patients suffering from DM (Cheong *et al.*, 1994), three of whom reported the photoaggravation of existing cutaneous lesions, while two reported an abnormal transient erythema after 30 minutes' sunlight exposure in the summer. Two also demonstrated a reduced minimal erythemal dose with monochromatic irradiation testing (one at 307.5 nm and the other at 340 nm and 360 nm), while one of the six who agreed to low-dose solar-simulated (IR) radiation of unaffected skin developed a lesion within 24 hours at the irradiation site with the clinical and IMF characteristics of DM; this then persisted for three weeks.

In contrast to LE, little has been written about the mechanism of photosensitivity in DM. However, the most frequently cited hypothesis is that UVR may induce the production of antigenic substances which then initiate a harmful immunological response. For example, the first case report of DM occurring during PUVA therapy was published in 1994 (Sinoway *et al.*, 1994), the patient being a 35-year-old woman with biopsy-proven psoriasis who developed the clinical and laboratory findings of DM after two months' treatment. In this instance, it was hypothesized that psoralen-DNA photoproducts may be immunogenic and that such antigen production, combined with the recognized PUVA-induced suppression of CD8+ T-cell immunological activity, may thereby result in autoantibody formation and the expression of DM. However, studies looking carefully at the precise mechanism of photosensitivity in DM are lacking.

PEMPHIGUS

Pemphigus is a chronic, relapsing, sometimes fatal, bullous disease characterized by the presence of intraepidermal acantholytic blisters, circulating intercellular antibodies and the deposition of immunoglobulin and complement between epidermal cells, IgG being found in nearly all affected patients, although IgA and IgM have also been noted.

One form of the disease, a localized variety known as pemphigus erythematosus or sometimes pemphigus foliaceus, may in some patients be induced or exacerbated by sunlight. In addition, it has been shown that exposure of the previously exposed normal skin of such patients to a MED of UVB radiation is able to induce acantholysis in some instances (Cram and Winkelmann, 1965; Jacobs, 1965), while in others exposure to multiples of the MED was required. A positive Nikolsky's sign typical of the disease could also be demonstrated at the test sites 24 hours after exposure (Cram and Winkelmann, 1965), a response blocked by prior chloroquine phosphate but not systemic corticosteroids. On the other hand, chemical irritation, maceration, occlusion, friction and heat exposure of the skin in the patients did not produce acantholysis.

The classic form of pemphigus, namely pemphigus vulgaris, has not historically been thought to be associated with sunlight sensitivity. UVR applied to the normal skin of such patients, however, has been shown in some instances to produce the characteristic histological and immunohistochemical changes of the disease (Cram and Fukuyama, 1972). Thus, five hours after exposure, deposits of IgG and complement were detected, while at 24 hours this deposition had increased and microscopic acantholysis had become detectable. Thus, a chronological and quantitative relationship apparently exists between the presence of immunoglobulin and complement and the development of acantholysis (Cram and Fukuyama, 1972). In one study, two patients were given systemic corticosteroids and subsequently phototested; bound immunoglobulins were detected in the 0- and 24-hour skin specimens of only one of the patients and neither patient demonstrated bound complement or microscopic acantholysis. This suggests, in this instance, that there may after all be a suppressive effect of corticosteroids on the induction of lesions by UV exposure in patients with pemphigus vulgaris.

The effect of UV irradiation in an *in vitro* organ culture model for pemphigus has also been studied (Gschnait *et al.*, 1978) and in contrast with the *in vivo* situation, no increase in acantholytic activity or immunoglobulin binding after UV irradiation was seen. The investigators thus hypothesized that the circulatory system of the skin may play a role in photoinduction of acantholysis, one possible explanation being that an organ culture lacks complement. In other words, pemphigus antibodies are unable to fix complement *in vitro*, but probably do *in vivo*.

From the foregoing, it is apparent that UVR exposure can induce or exacerbate pemphigus, perhaps inducing the expression of pemphigus antigens in damaged skin, contributing to the formation of other cross-reacting antigens or causing a breakdown of the dermoepidermal barrier (Inderbitzen and Katz, 1971). Further studies are necessary to clarify these matters.

BULLOUS PEMPHIGOID

BP is characterized by the formation of subepidermal blisters. BP antigen has been localized to the basal keratinocyte and Ig and complement deposits are limited to the lamina lucida. Circulating BMZ antibodies are usually present and direct IM reveals a linear deposit of IgG and complement in involved and also usually in uninvolved skin. IgA and IgM have also been demonstrated in some cases. There have been numerous reports of photoexacerbation of BP but the precise mechanism has not been documented.

In one study, two BP patients demonstrated enhanced Ig and complement deposition with evidence of a subepidermal blister at 24 hours after UV exposure of uninvolved skin. This deposition was not apparent at five hours (Cram and Fukuyama, 1972). It was impossible, however, to determine whether the deposition of immunoreactants preceded histological change. Another patient developed BP following topical treatment with fluorouracil, first at sites of application but later also on untreated normal skin (Bart and Bean, 1970). The patient denied sun exposure, systemic medications and application of other topical agents. Immunofluorescent studies of serum and blister fluid revealed basement membrane antibody titres consistent with BP.

One might perhaps conclude that an inflammatory response, of any aetiology, may precipitate clinical disease in a predisposed patient. Nevertheless, further studies of UV irradiation effects on induction or exacerbation of BP would be useful.

Of interest are recent reports of potential animal models for BP. The first of these studies used P1-2, an 18-amino acid peptide encoded for by the 230 kD BP antigen cDNA, to immunize rabbits (Hall *et al.*, 1993). All of the rabbits immunized developed antibody to P1-2, able to bind *in vitro* to the BMZ in both human and rabbit skin samples. UVB irradiation was then used to produce mild epidermal injury, inducing an enhanced inflammatory reaction in the immunized rabbits which resulted in epidermal necrosis and the sloughing of some sites at 6–9 days; histology demonstrated linear deposition of IgG and C3 at the BMZ. Control rabbits showed only mild erythema without epidermal loss and no deposition of immunoglobulin or complement. More recently, the intraperitoneal injection of sera from BP patients induced BP-like erosions and vesicles in 14–78% of neonatal mice pretreated with 600 mJ/cm² of UVB (Mitsuhashi *et al.*, 1994), a dose sufficient in controls to produce only a slight erythema and degeneration of the upper epidermal cells but not dermoepidermal separation; in addition, IMF demonstrated the linear deposition of human IgG and C3 at the dermoepidermal junctions of the affected mice, while control animals demonstrated no deposition (Mitsuhashi *et al.*, 1994). It should be noted that the above studies were primarily designed for the validation of animal models for BP and not for the study of mechanisms of photoaggravation in the disease. However, they do suggest that cutaneous UVR exposure in the condition may lead to antibody-mediated epidermal inflammation with a resulting dermoepidermal split.

ERYTHEMA MULTIFORME

Erythema multiforme (EM) is an acute, self-limiting eruption of the skin and mucous membranes, with distinctive, discrete or sometimes confluent target or iris, papular or plaque lesions in an acral distribution on the extensor surfaces, palms and soles. The pathogenesis is not fully understood but may represent an immunological hypersensitivity reaction to a normally exogenous substance, such as drug or micro-organism.

Photoaggravated EM has occasionally been reported (Anderson *et al.*, 1954; Huff and Weston, 1980; Keil, 1940), Anderson *et al.* (1954) describing an eruption following sunlight exposure that clinically resembled the disorder. It has also been reported at sites previously involved in an acute sunburn (Huff and Weston, 1980), perhaps an example of herpes simplex-induced EM, although viral changes on biopsy and viral culture were negative. Ippen (1980) also described photodermatitis multiformis acuta, in which pruritic papules, plaques, vesicles, urticaria and EM-like lesions developed after a sudden increase in light exposure, although this may conceivably have represented a form of polymorphic light eruption. Repeated exposures to UVA and UVB radiation also produced similar lesions in two of the patients. Sunlight-induced acute EM with mucous membrane lesions and the typical histological changes of the condition has also been described and this eruption closely resembled the so-called photodermatitis multiformis acuta (Helfman, 1983).

Drugs have been reported to cause photosensitive EM, a patient on phenylbutazone for acute gout developing EM three days after sun exposure (Leroy *et al.*, 1985), following which the typical erythematous target lesions on the face, neck, arms and dorsa of the hands resolved with discontinuation of treatment. EM and photosensitivity reactions to phenylbutazone have also been previously reported (Bailin and Mathaluk, 1982).

Mucosal involvement with a cutaneous photodistribution has also been noted in drug-induced EM (Leroy *et al.*, 1987), a woman using carbanilide disinfectant for daily genital cleansing along with a tetracycline-based gynaecologic tablet having developed genital haemorrhagic erosions, along with erythematous macules and papules and some target lesions. Then, 48 hours following sun exposure, cutaneous EM also developed on her face, upper chest, legs and arms; in addition, stomatitis was present but conjunctivitis was not. As a result, the medications were stopped and the lesions improved. The investigators hypothesized that the carbanilide may have been responsible for a genital form of EM and that there was then secondary solar exacerbation. Carbanilides had been reported previously to induce rare contact photosensitivity (Smith and Epstein, 1977) but EM had not been previously linked to the drug, while the tetracycline base also could have caused the photosensitivity and has, in addition, been implicated in the development of EM.

The pathogenesis of EM is unknown. However, as previously stated, it is thought that it may represent an immunological hypersensitivity reaction, as circulating immune complexes have been detected (Bushkell *et al.*, 1980), as have deposits of IgG, complement and fibrin around superficial dermal vessels (Kazmierowski and Wuepper, 1978). In addition, it has been hypothesized with respect to photoaggravated EM that sunlight may either expose inducing antigens in the skin or else attract circulating immune complexes to the sites of UVR-induced cutaneous damage.

ACTINIC LICHEN PLANUS

Actinic lichen planus (ALP) is a lichenoid eruption induced by prolonged sunlight exposure; it has also been called lichenoid melanoderma dermatitis (Verhagan and Koten, 1979), summertime actinic lichenoid eruption (Isaacson *et al.*, 1981), lichen planus tropicus (El Zawahry, 1964) and lichen planus subtropicus (Dilaimy, 1976). The condition generally develops in dark-complexioned subjects at anatomic sites undergoing prolonged UV exposure. In addition, the disease is not limited to those living in tropical or subtropical climates and although most cases have been reported in patients from the Middle East (Dilaimy, 1976), cases from Italy (Zanca and Zanca, 1978), India (Bedi, 1978), Yugoslavia (Zaharieva *et al.*, 1978), the Netherlands (Van Der Schroeff *et al.*, 1983) and the United States (Isaacson *et al.*, 1981) have also been described; disease incidence is, however, much higher in the spring and summer months. Further, ALP generally occurs in a younger age group than that described for classic lichen planus and women are affected slightly more often than men.

ALP typically presents with the insidious onset of a bluish-brown, non-scaly round or oval macule with well-defined borders, following which a slightly raised pale margin gradually develops, giving the centre of the lesion a depressed appearance. This annular configuration is characteristic for ALP. Some lesions then remain discrete, while others coalesce to form circinate plaques and all typically flatten during the winter months. The most common sites for the condition are the forehead and the dorsa of the hands. In contrast to classic lichen planus, pruritis is not a prominent feature.

Morphological variants of ALP have also been described (Isaacson *et al.*, 1981), which include in particular annular hyperpigmented plaques predominantly of the face and dorsa of the hands, chloasma-like lesions of the face and neck, dyschromic greyish-white pinhead papules with a tendency to coalesce of mostly the neck and dorsa of the hands and the lichenoid papules or plaques of classic lichen planus.

In addition, a less well-documented form of the condition has been described in India (Bhutani, 1982), being similar to lichen nitidus with pinpoint, discrete, closely aggregated, flesh-coloured or slightly hypopigmented lichenoid papules of the extensor surfaces of the arms, upper back, chest and neck, the face generally being spared. The Koebner phenomenon has also been reported in these patients and the variant is most common in young, adult females with fair skin and occurs mostly in the summer.

The diverse clinical and histological findings of ALP, which present themselves as a spectrum ranging from lichen planus to dermatitis (Verhagen and Koten, 1979), make it logical to consider ALP as not just a variant of classic lichen planus but perhaps a hybrid between lichen planus and a variety of true photosensitive disorders such as LE or polymorphic light eruption. This approach would then be consistent with Pinkus' (1973) view that not one but a spectrum of dermatoses may be associated with the lichenoid tissue reaction.

VIRAL EXANTHEMS

Herpes simplex is a viral condition commonly provoked by sun exposure or phototherapy, while vaccinia, lymphogranuloma venereum and varicella have also all been recognized as having a photosensitivity component (Blank and Rake, 1955; Pace and Owens, 1969). In particular, varicella has been known to localize in areas of cutaneous injury (Castrow and Wolf, 1973; Gilchrest and Baden, 1974), a recent series of case reports having discussed four children in whom cutaneous injury or inflammation during the period of incubation for the disorder resulted in a clinically atypical presentation (Belhorn and Lucky, 1994). Each patient had a different source of trauma, namely wasp stings on the hand, iatrogenic trauma in the neonatal period, the application of a cast after arthroscopic surgery and, in one case, extensive sun exposure but in each instance, the varicella lesions localized to the site of previous trauma. In sun-damaged areas, however, the lesions are likely to be larger, more numerous, perhaps coalescent and often apparent before those on non-exposed areas, while the classic sequential eruption is often absent. Photolocalized viral exanthems may often be misdiagnosed as drug eruptions or drug photosensitivity, thus leading to both the unnecessary discontinuation of necessary medications and the potential exposure of individuals to a contagious disease.

The exact mechanism for the photolocalization or photoexacerbation of viral exanthems is unknown, although lesions may well result from the localization and subsequent growth of viral particles in sun-damaged skin. Mims (1966) suggests several viral routes to the skin that may result in an exanthem. Small viral particles may evade the reticuloendothelial clearance system and thus localize in small blood vessels. Vessel injury may result in increased capillary permeability, allowing leakage of viral particles from vessels with a subsequent dermal inflammatory response. Other viral particles may reside intracellularly in platelets, lymphocytes, monocytes or polymorphonuclear cells. They may be transported to extravascular tissue such as the dermal and epidermal cells by diapedesis of leucocytes. UVR functions as a non-specific skin insult and may cause a localized increase in capillary permeability leading to the development of viral exanthems on sun-exposed areas. Viral particles have also been found in epidermal melanocytes in patients with recurrent herpes simplex (McNair-Scott *et al.*, 1950). One thought is that these melanocytes distribute viral particles to other epidermal cells in much the same manner as they do melanin. Exposure to sunlight could activate melanocytes and thus cause photolocalization of the viral exanthem. UVR is also known to suppress local skin immunity, thus potentially allowing for greater viral replication in sun-exposed skin. Additional UVR exposure might promote the release of various factors that may enhance viral replication. For example, prostaglandins have been shown to increase herpes simplex virus and varicella replication *in vitro*.

CUTANEOUS T-CELL LYMPHOMA

Cutaneous T-cell lymphoma (CTCL) is a neoplasm of helper T lymphocytes that initially appears in skin and eventually involves lymph nodes, internal organs and the peripheral blood. Although the aetiology is unknown, genetic factors, infection and environmental stimuli have been suggested to play a role. It is thought that the human T-cell leukaemia/lymphoma virus (HTVL), isolated from T lymphocytes of CTCL (Poiesz *et al.*, 1980), may induce transformation of skin-associated normal T lymphocytes with resultant clonal expansion of malignant cells.

Photosensitivity may occur in some CTCL patients, although it generally appears to be only a clinically mild erythema. Ive reported one case in 1964, while Volden and colleagues (Volden, 1980; Volden and Thune, 1977) later described abnormal reactions in plaque and tumour stage mycosis fungoides (MF) patients phototested against UVA, UVB and visible light. Several other investigators have also described photosensitivity in potential CTCL patients, Zugerman *et al.* (1980) having described a possible such patient with UVB sensitivity who ultimately progressed to the Sézary syndrome while Frain-Bell and Magnus (1971) reported two cases of so-called cutaneous lymphocytoma associated with solar urticaria and polymorphic light eruption. However, the actinic reticuloid variant of chronic actinic dermatitis may resemble CTCL, thus often making the differential diagnosis difficult (Neill and du Vivier, 1985; Zugerman *et al.*, 1980), and those patients may not have had CTCL at all. Thus, patients may present with a photo-induced eruption that clinically and histologically resembles severe chronic actinic dermatitis but demonstrate a lymphocytic infiltrate or circulating cells, suggestive of a diagnosis of a lymphomatous malignancy such as the Sézary syndrome (Zugerman *et al.*, 1980) or MF (Neill and du Vivier, 1985). However, patients with severe chronic actinic dermatitis alone may demonstrate such abnormalities, which then settle with treatment of the disease, and it therefore seems likely that these changes are reactive, although the possibility of malignant transformation, apparently at most very rare, should be kept in mind.

PHOTOSENSITIVE PSORIASIS

Patients with psoriasis usually benefit from exposure to sunlight or artificially produced UVR. A small number, however, exhibit worsening of their disease with such exposure (Bielecky and Kvicalova, 1964; Doyle, 1984) and estimates of the prevalence of this photosensitivity in the condition vary from 5.5% to 24% (Farber *et al.*, 1968; Lane and Crawford, 1937; Lomholt, 1963; Ros and Eklund, 1987).

In 1964, Bielecky and Kvicalova reported that photosensitive psoriatic patients did not differ in age, sex or frequency of familial incidence from non-photosensitive control psoriates. However, there was a distinctive distribution of the lesions in the photosensitive patients, most occurring on the face and the dorsa of the hands, while most of the patients had fair complexions and reduced erythemal thresholds. Frain-Bell (1982) reported similar findings, all patients in his study being susceptible to sunburn and developing psoriasis on the exposed skin of the face or hands, arguably through the Koebner phenomenon.

Ros and Eklund (1986) later sent questionnaires to 2000 psoriatic patients in Stockholm, finding a photosensitivity prevalence of 5.5%, an estimate considerably lower than that of previous studies, where numbers ranged from 14% to 24% (Farber *et al.*, 1968; Lane and Crawford, 1937; Lomholt, 1963). Of these, 43% had episodes of polymorphic light eruption which apparently led to exacerbation of their psoriatic lesions as a Koebner phenomenon. Fair skin was prevalent in these subjects, as was localization of the psoriatic lesions to the dorsa of the hands, as in Frain-Bell's (1982) study, but in contrast to his findings, Ros and Eklund (1987) found that advanced age and the female sex predominated.

It is important also to consider other common causes of photosensitivity during the evaluation of cases of apparent light-sensitive psoriasis. Thus, the occurrence of psoriasis in patients with vitiligo has been recognized for many years (Karansky and Roenigk, 1982), the vitiligo usually being clearly apparent on inspection but sometimes not in patients with very fair skin. Further, it is worth noting that when psoriasis is pustular or erythrodermic, UVR exposure may directly worsen the condition (Starke and Jillson, 1961). Finally, the possible co-existence of psoriasis with LE or porphyria, while infrequent, should also be considered in cases where the reason for any photosensitivity in psoriasis is obscure.

In summary, photosensitivity in psoriasis is well recognized but has been poorly defined. However, it now appears that many patients with the condition probably suffer attacks of polymorphic light eruption, other light sensitivity or sunburning on fair skin, followed by the development of psoriatic lesions on the affected sites by Koebnerization, to explain the phenomenon.

LIGHT-EXACERBATED ECZEMA

Exposure to UVR may induce the onset of photoallergic contact and chronic actinic dermatitis and, on occasion, also exacerbate the endogenous atopic and seborrhoeic eczemas. The most common example of the latter situation is photosensitivity in association with atopy (Frain-Bell and Scatchard, 1971) (Plate 33) in which the patient, usually female, develops eczema of the exposed areas in addition to the more typical flexural sites and may sometimes demonstrate sensitivity to UVR on phototesting. On other occasions, seborrhoeic, palmar or other unclassifiable endogenous eczemas may also spread to include eczema of the light-exposed areas and may then rarely progress to a true light-induced eczema instead (Ramsay and Kobza-Black, 1973), as may also atopic eczemas which appear to represent part of the syndrome of chronic actinic dermatitis.

Many patients with endogenous eczema state that they are worse in the summer months, particularly atopic eczema sufferers, but without a clear history that the eczema also appears on the light-exposed areas. In such circumstances, summer exacerbations of eczema may instead be due to exposure to heat or humidity rather than UVR.

TREATMENT

Treatment of all these conditions is by conventional management of the underlying disorder in addition to the restriction of light exposure and use of high-protection sunscreens. In some conditions, but not those such as LE and DM where systemic exacerbation may be possible, low-dose courses of UV phototherapy may be considered despite the light sensitivity, perhaps under initial systemic steroid or immunosuppressive cover. However, caution should be used in the early stages of treatment and other modalities sought if the condition flares uncontrollably. Conditions particularly likely to respond to such therapy, given carefully, are light-exacerbated atopic eczema and psoriasis.

REFERENCES

Anderson, D., Wallace, H.J. and Howes, W.I.B. (1954) Juvenile spring eruption. *Lancet*, **1**, 755–6.

Ansel, J.A., Luger, T.A. and Green, I. (1983) The effect of *in vitro* and *in vivo* UV irradiation on the production of ETAF activity by human and murine keratinocytes. *Journal of Investigative Dermatology*, **81**, 519–23.

Ansel, J.A., Luger, T.A., Koch, A. *et al.* (1984) The effect of *in vitro* UV irradiation on the production of IL-1 by murine macrophages and P388D1 cells. *Journal of Immunology*, **133**, 1350–5.

Baer, R.L. and Harber, L.C. (1965) Photobiology of lupus erythematosus. *Archives of Dermatology* **92**, 124–8.

Bailin, P.L. and Mathaluk, R.M. (1982) Cutaneous reactions to rheumatologic drugs. *Clinics in Rheumatic Diseases*, **2**, 493–16.

Bart, B.J. and Bean, S.F. (1970) Bullous pemphigoid following the topical use of fluorouracil. *Archives of Dermatology*, **102**, 457–60.

Bedi, T.R. (1978) Summertime actinic lichenoid eruption. *Dermatologica*, **157**, 115–25.

Beighlie, D.J. and Teplitz, R.L. (1975) Repair of UV damaged DNA in systemic lupus erythematosus. *Journal of Rheumatology*, **2**, 149–60.

Bellhorn, T.H. and Lucky, A.W. (1994) Atypical varicella exanthema associated with skin injury. *Pediatric Dermatology*, **11**, 129–32.

Bhutani, L.K. (1982) The photodermatoses as seen in tropical countries. *Seminars in Dermatology*, **1**, 175–81.

Bielecky, T. and Kvicalova, E. (1964) Photosensitivity psoriasis. *Dermatologica*, **129**, 339–48.

Biesecker, G., Lavin, L., Ziskind, M. *et al.* (1972) Cutaneous localization of the membrane attack complex in discoid and systemic lupus erythematosus. *New England Journal of Medicine*, **306**, 264–70.

Blank, H. and Rake, G.W. (1955) *Viral and Rickettsial Disease of the Skin, Eye, and Mucous Membranes of Man*, Little Brown, Boston, pp. 285–90.

Bushkell, L.L., Mackel, S.E. and Jordon, R.E. (1980) Erythema multiforme: direct immunofluorescence studies and detection of circulating immune complexes. *Journal of Investigative Dermatology*, **74**, 372–4.

Castrow, F.F. and Wolf, J.E. (1973) Photolocalized varicella. *Archives of Dermatology*, **107**, 628.

Cheong, W.K., Hughes, G.R.V., Norris, P.G. *et al.* (1994) Cutaneous photosensitivity in dermatomyositis. *British Journal of Dermatology*, **131**, 205–8.

Cleaver, J.E. (1970) DNA damage and repair in light-sensitive human skin disease. *Journal of Investigative Dermatology*, **54**, 181–95.

Cram, D.L. and Fukuyama, K. (1972) Immunohistochemistry of ultraviolet-induced pemphigus and pemphigoid lesions. *Archives of Dermatology*, **106**, 819–24.

Cram, D.L. and Winkelman, R.K. (1965) Ultraviolet-induced acantholysis in pemphigus. *Archives of Dermatology*, **92**, 7–13.

Cripps, D.J. and Rankin, J. (1973) Action spectra of lupus erythematosus and experimental immunofluorescence. *Archives of Dermatology*, **107**, 563–7.

Dilaimy, M. (1976) Lichen planus subtropicus. *Archives of Dermatology*, **112**, 1251–3.

Dovgolan, T., Elkton, K., Gharavi, A. *et al.* (1992) Enhanced membrane binding of autoantibodies to cultured keratinocytes of systemic lupus erythematosus patients after ultraviolet B/ultraviolet A irradiation. *Journal of Clinical Investigation*, **90**, 1067–76.

Doyle, J.A. (1984) Photosensitive psoriasis. *Australian Journal of Dermatology*, **25**, 54–8.

El Zawahry, M. (1964) *Skin Disease in Arabian Countries*, Vol. 2, French Institute of Oriental Archaeology, Paris, pp. 45–54.

Emerit, I. and Michelson, A.M. (1981) Mechanism of photosensitivity in systemic lupus erythematosus patients. *Proceedings of the National Academy of Science of the USA*, **78**, 2537–40.

Epstein, J.H., Tuffanelli, D.L. and Dubois, E.L. (1965) Light sensitivity and lupus erythematosus. *Archives of Dermatology*, **91**, 483–5.

Everett, M.A. and Olson, R.L. (1966) Response of cutaneous lupus erythematosus to ultraviolet light. *Journal of Investigative Dermatology*, **44**, 133–4.

Farber, E.M., Bright, R.D. and Nall, M.L. (1968) Psoriasis: a questionnaire survey of 2144 patients. *Archives of Dermatology*, **98**, 248–59.

Frain-Bell, W. (1982) What is this thing called light? (Dowling oration 1978). *Clinical and Experimental Dermatology*, **4**, 1–29.

Frain-Bell, W. and Magnus, I.A. (1971) A study of the photosensitivity factor in cutaneous lymphocytoma. *British Journal of Dermatology*, **84**, 25–31.

Frain-Bell, W. and Scatchard, M. (1971) The association of photosensitivity and atopy in the child. *British Journal of Dermatology*, **105**, 105–10.

Freeman, R.G., Knox, J.M. and Owens, D.W. (1969) Cutaneous lesions of lupus erythematosus induced by monochromatic light. *Archives of Dermatology*, **100**, 677–682.

Gahring, L., Baltz, M., Pepys, M.B. *et al.* (1984) Effects of ultraviolet radiation on production of epidermal cell lymphocyte activating factor/interleukin 1 *in vivo* and *in vitro*. *Proceedings of the National Academy of Science of the USA*, **81**, 1198–202.

Gilchrest, B. and Baden, H.P. 91974) Photodistribution of viral exanthems. *Pediatrics*, **54**, 136–8.

Gschnait, F., Pehamberger, H. and Holubar, K. (1978) Pemphigus acantholysis in tissue culture: studies on photo-induction. *Acta Dermatovenereologica (Stockholm)*, **58**, 237–9.

Hall, R.P., Murray, J.C., McCord, M.M. *et al.* (1993) Rabbits immunized with a peptide encoded for by the 230-kD bullous pemphigoid antigen cDNA develop an enhanced inflammatory response to UVB irradiation: a potential animal model for bullous pemphigoid. *Journal of Investigative Dermatology*, **101**, 9–14.

Helfman, R.J. (1983) Photodermatitis multiformis acuta. *Cutis*, **31**, 660–2.

Huff, C. and Weston, W.L. (1980) The photodistribution of erythema multiforme. *Archives of Dermatology*, **116**, 477–8.

Inderbitzen, T.M. and Katz, S.I. (1971) Pemphigus as an autoaggressive phenomenon, in *Advances in Biology of Skin*, Vol. XI, (eds W. Montagna and R.E. Billingham), Appleton-Century-Crofts, Norwalk, pp. 267–82.

Ippen, H. (1980) Photodermatitis multiformis acuta. *Dermatologische Monatsschrift*, **166**, 145–50.

Isaacson, D., Turner, M.L. and Elgart, M.L. (1981) Summertime actinic lichenoid eruption (lichen planus actinicus). *Journal of the American Academy of Dermatology*, **4**, 404–11.

Ive, F.A.(1964) Mycosis fungoides presenting as light sensitivity. *British Journal of Dermatology*, **76**, 145–9.

Jacobs, S.E. (1965) Pemphigus erythematosus and ultraviolet light. *Archives of Dermatology*, **91**, 139–41.

Jarzabek-Chorzelska, M., Zarebska, Z., Wolska, H. *et al.* (1976) Immunological phenomena induced by UV rays. *Acta Dermatovenereologica (Stockholm)*, **56**, 15–18.

Jones, S. (1992) Ultraviolet radiation (UVR) induces cell-surface Ro/SSA antigen expression by human keratinocytes *in vitro*: a possible mechanism for the UVR induction of cutaneous lupus lesions. *British Journal of Dermatology*, **126**, 546–53.

Kawashima, T., Zappi, E., Lieu, T. *et al.* (1994) Impact of ultraviolet radiation on the cellular expression of Ro/SS-A-autoantigenic polypeptides. *Dermatology*, **189** (suppl 1), 6–10.

Kazmierowski, J.A. and Wuepper, K.D. (1978) Erythema multiforme: immune complex vasculitis of the superficial cutaneous microvasculature. *Journal of Investigative Dermatology*, **71**, 366–9.

Keil, H. (1940) Erythema multiforme exudativum (Hebra): a clinical entity associated with systemic features. *Annals of Internal Medicine*, **14**, 449–94.

Kind, P., Hölzle, E., Lehmann, P. *et al.* (1987) *Histopathologic Studies of Lupus Erythematosus Experimentally Induced by UVA and UVB*. 17th World Congress of Dermatology, Berlin, p. 441.

Klein, L., Elmets, C. and Callen, J. (1995) Photoexacerbation of cutaneous lupus erythematosus due to ultraviolet A emissions from a photocopier. *Arthritis and Rheumatism*, **38**, 1152–6.

Koransky, J.S. and Roenigk, H.H. (1982) Vitiligo and psoriasis. *Journal of the American Academy of Dermatology*, **7**, 183–90.

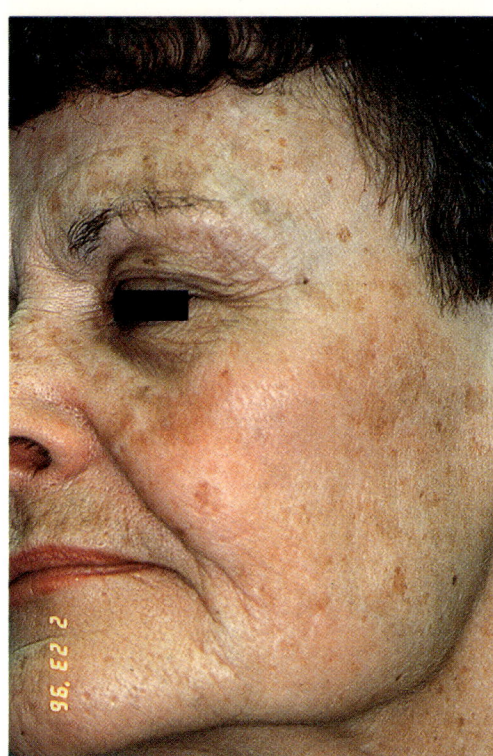

Plate 1 Mottled pigmentation, numerous lentigines and wrinkling, most pronounced around eyes and mouth, due to photoageing.

Plate 2 Coarse wrinkles around eyes, chin and mouth, as well as erythema and telangiectases on cheeks, in a middle-aged woman.

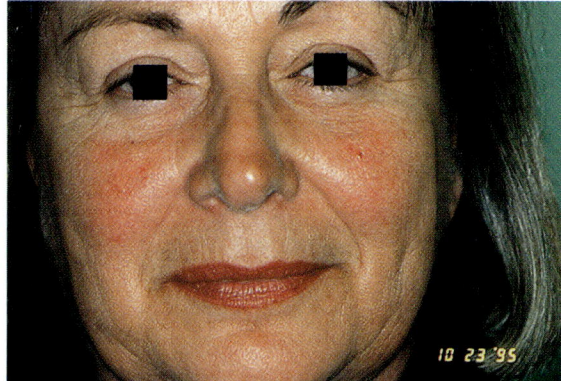

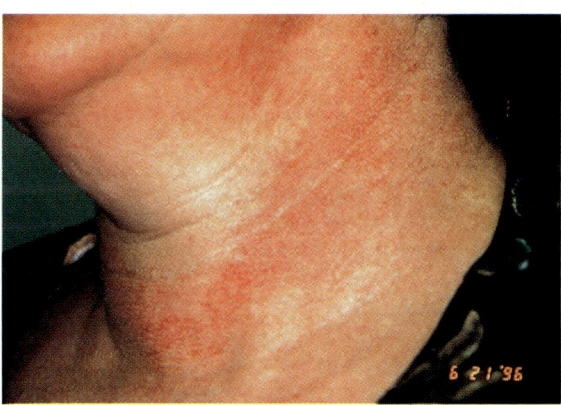

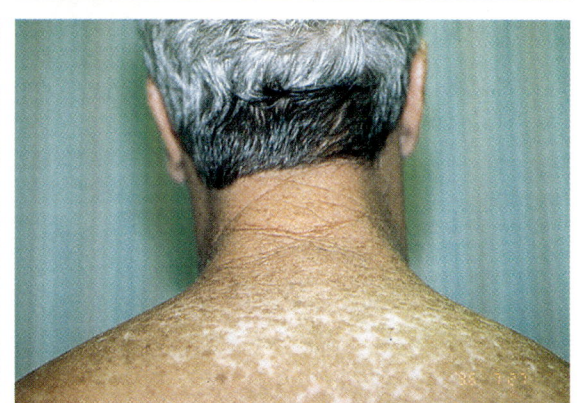

Plate 3 (above left)   Pronounced erythema and telangiectases on neck of a woman, clearly sparing relatively non-sun exposed submental region.

Plate 4 (above)   Deep criss-crossing furrows on back of outdoor labourer's neck, characteristic of cutis rhomboidalis nuchae. Also note mottled hyper- and hypopigmentation on back.

Plate 5 Solar elastosis. Amorphous basophilic masses of elastotic material are separated from epidermis by thin Grenz zone.

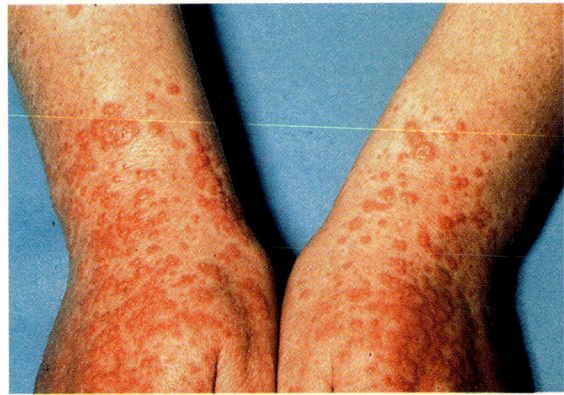

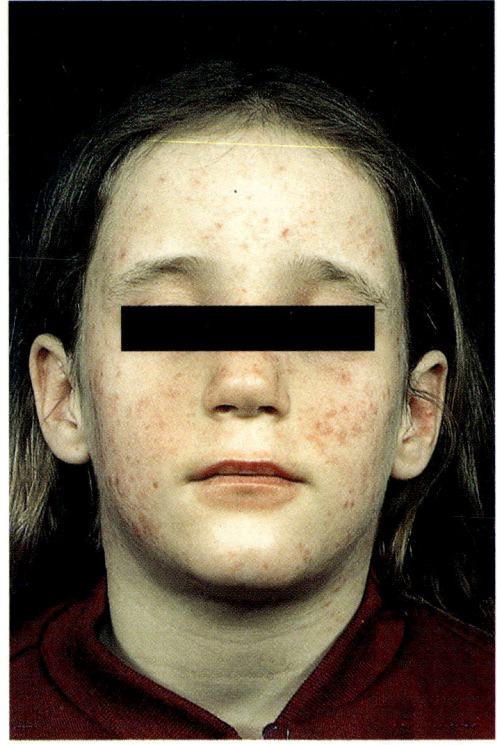

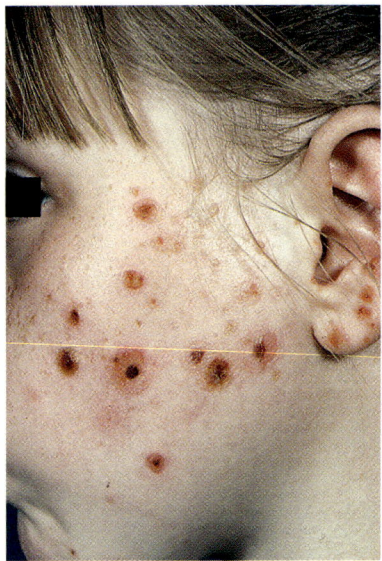

Plate 6 (top left)   Polymorphic light eruption.

Plate 7 (above)   Actinic prurigo.

Plate 8 (left)   Hydroa vacciniforme (courtesy of Addenbrooke's Hospital).

Plate 9 (left)   Eczematous changes of chronic actinic dermatitis on face and upper chest of dark-skinned patient, with sparing of protected skin of hairline, eyelids and anterior chest.

Plate 10 (below)   Eczematous changes of chronic actinic dermatitis on dorsa of hands of patient in Plate 9, with sparing of protected forearms; postinflammatory hyper- and hypopigmentation of affected skin is also present.

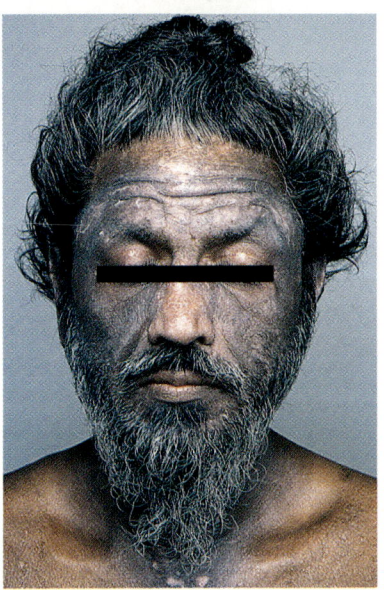

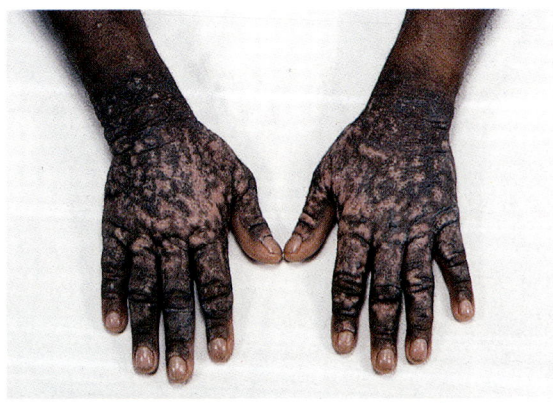

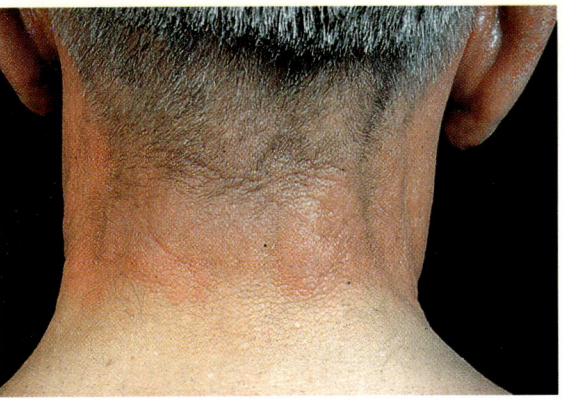

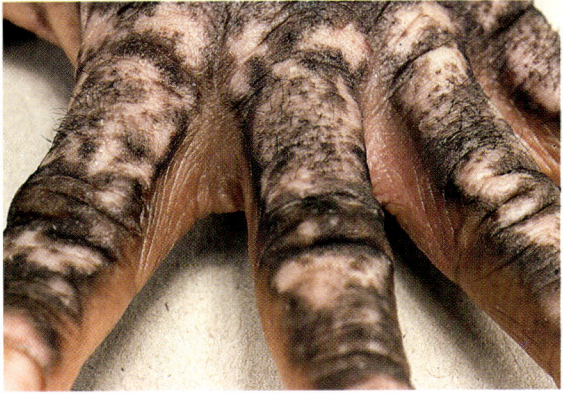

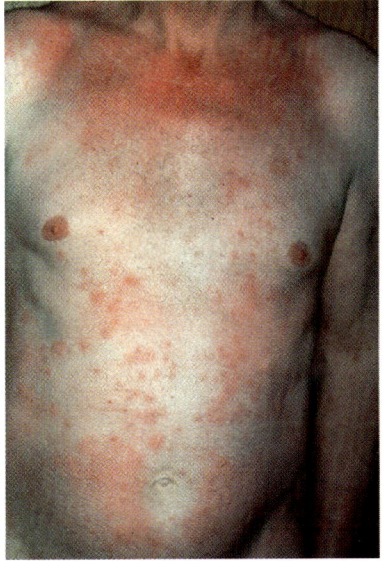

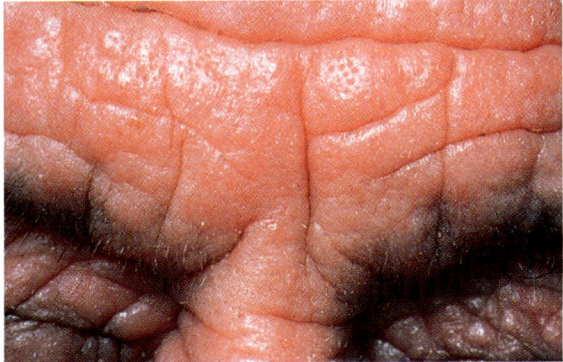

Plate 11 (top left)   Sparing of protected areas of back of neck in chronic actinic dermatitis patient (from Hawk, J.L.M. and Cheong, W.K. (1991) Eczematous photodermatoses, in *Eczema*, (ed. R. Marks), Martin Dunitz, London).

Plate 12 (top right)   Sparing of finger webs of chronic actinic dermatitis patient in Plate 9.

Plate 13 (left)   Spread of eczema in chronic actinic dermatitis patient to protected area of trunk (from Hawk, J.L.M. and Cheong, W.K. (1991) Eczematous photodermatoses, in *Eczema*, (ed. R. Marks), Martin Dunitz, London).

Plate 14 (above right)   Infiltrated skin in actinic reticuloid variant of severe chronic actinic dermatitis (from Hawk, J.L.M. and Cheong, W.K. (1991) Eczematous photodermatoses, in *Eczema*, (ed. R. Marks), Martin Dunitz, London).

Plate 15 (below left)   Histology of lesional skin of upper back of severely affected chronic actinic dermatitis patient showing florid mononuclear cell infiltrate and epidermotropism, somewhat resembling changes of cutaneous T-cell lymphoma (haematoxylin and eosin).

Plate 16 (below right)   Monochromatic and solar-simulated irradiation phototest responses of severely affected patient 24 hours after irradiation, showing abnormal monochromatic responses from 300 to 600 nm. Note the presence of patch tests.

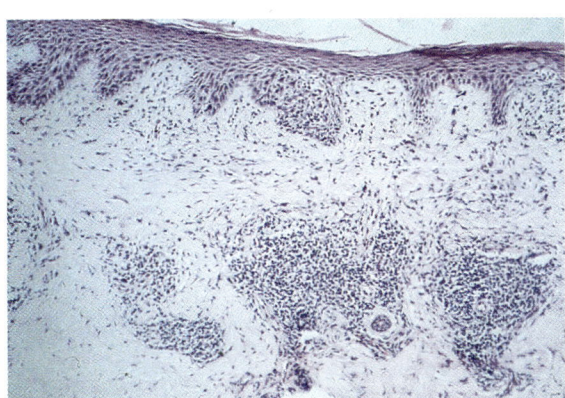

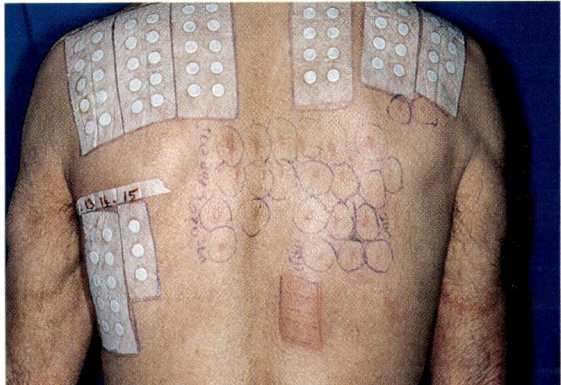

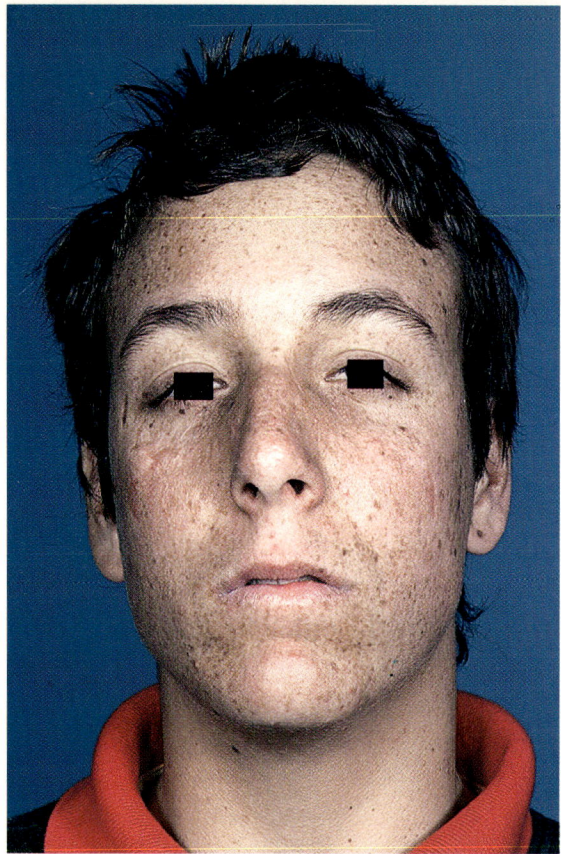

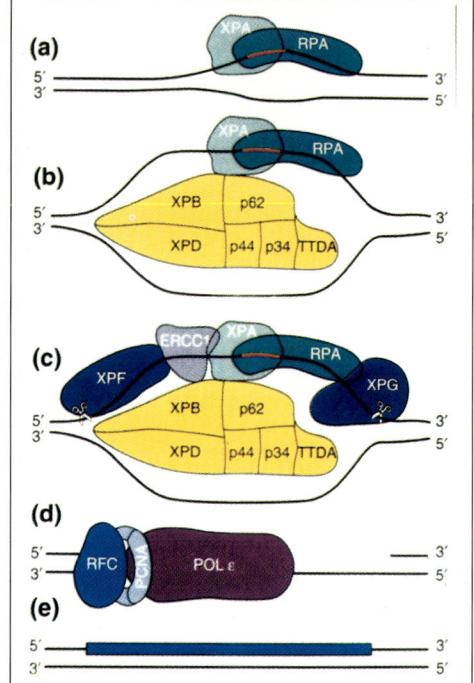

Plate 17 (above)   Dryness, telangiectasia, atrophy and scarring in a xeroderma pigmentosum patient aged 12 years.

Plate 18 (top right)   The normal DNA repair process.

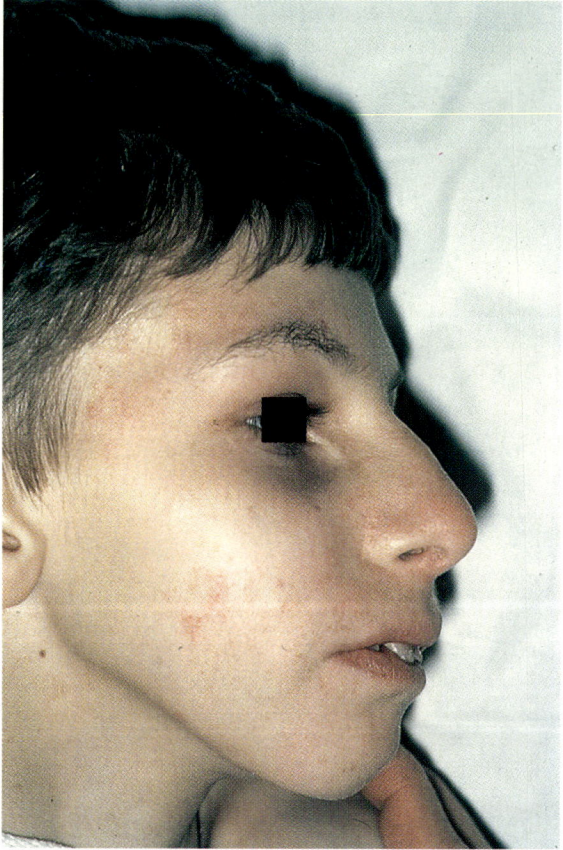

Plate 19 Prognathism, sunken eyes, thin prominent nose and lack of subcutaneous fat, producing bird-headed facies in Cockayne's syndrome (Courtesy of Dr D.J. Atherton).

Plate 20 (right)   Drug radiation interactions and possible consequences.

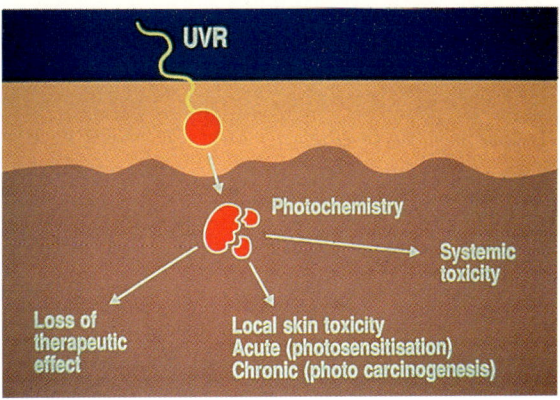

Plate 21 (below)   Severe phototoxic blistering response due to fluoroquinolone.

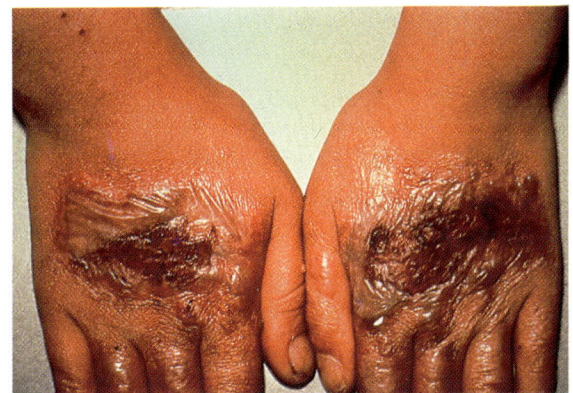

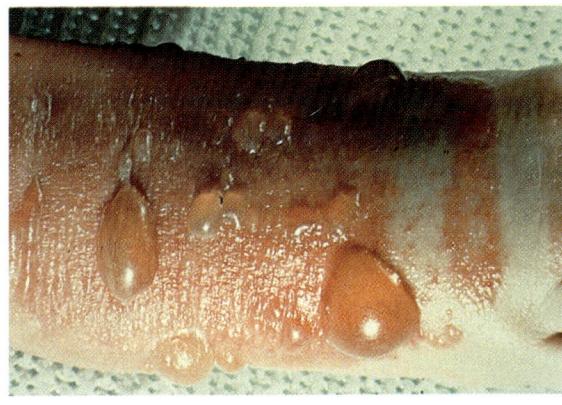

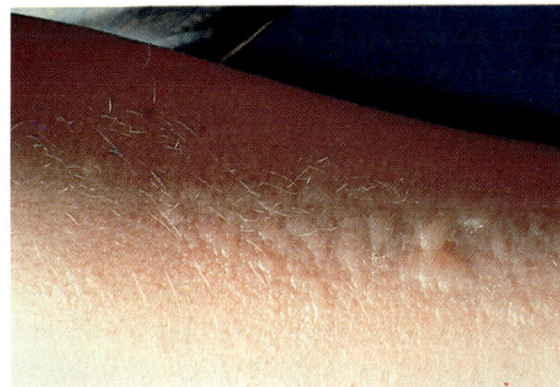

Plate 22 (above)   Phototoxic blistering following window glass-transmitted sunlight exposure in a patient on oral piroxicam.

Plate 23 (left)   Blister formation following high-dose chlorpromazine ingestion and sunlight exposure.

Plate 24 (below left)   Blistering response in a patient taking acitretin following short period of sunlight exposure.

Plate 25 (below)   Oxybenzone-induced photoallergic photopatch test response.

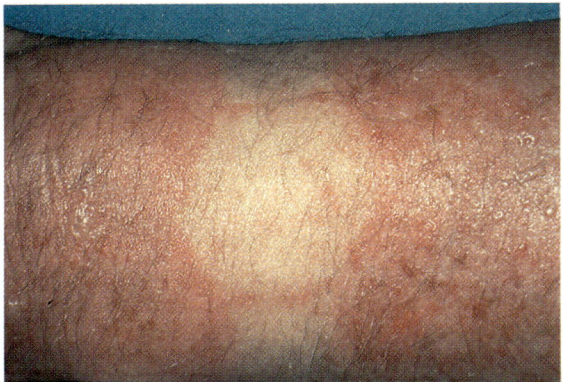

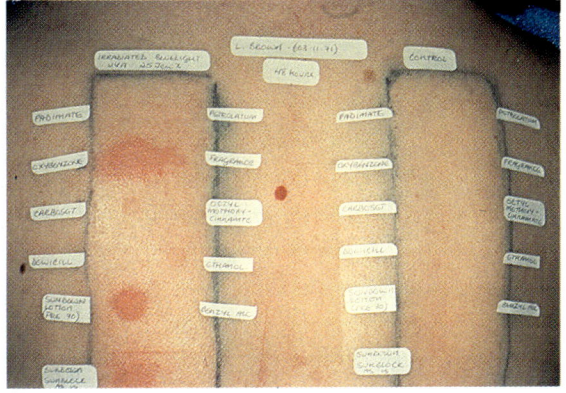

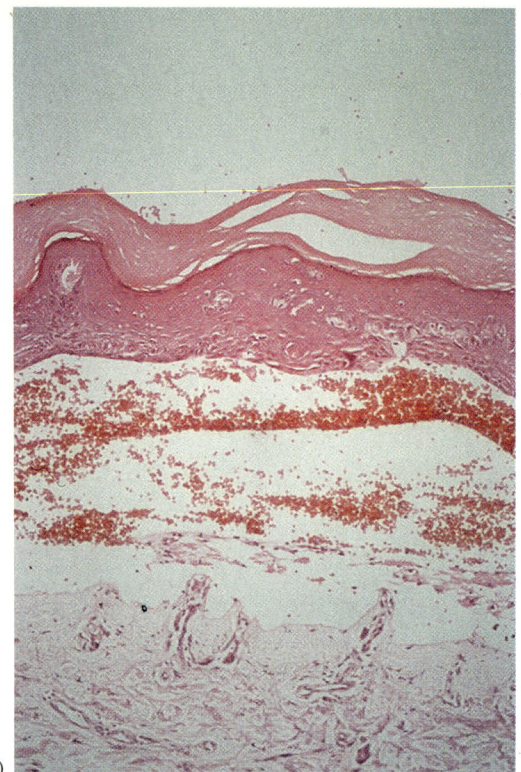

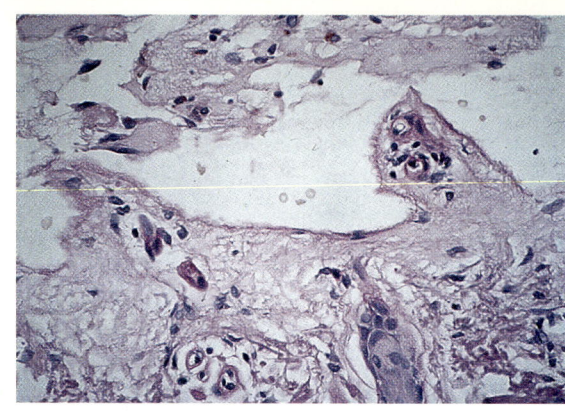

(b)

Plate 26 Porphyria cutanea tarda. (a) Subepidermal bulla (haematoxylin and eosin). (b) Hyaline material in capillary walls stained positively with periodic acid Schiff.

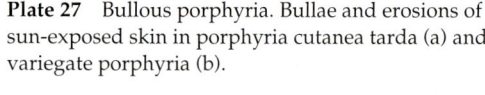

Plate 27 Bullous porphyria. Bullae and erosions of sun-exposed skin in porphyria cutanea tarda (a) and variegate porphyria (b).

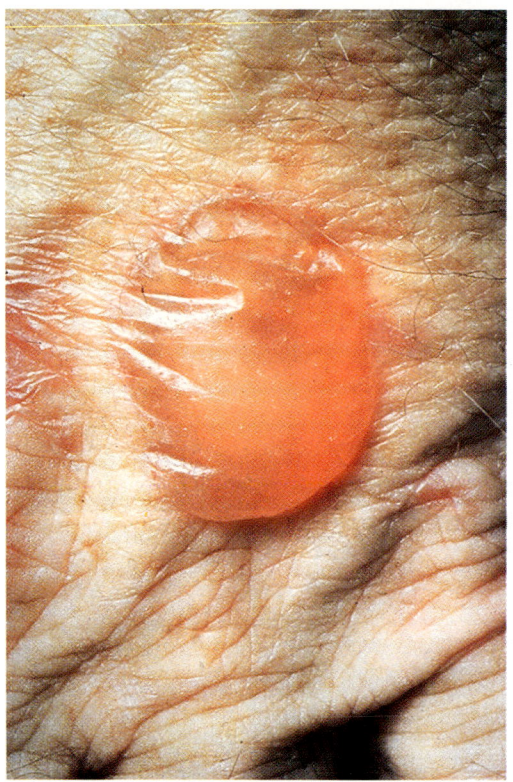

(a)

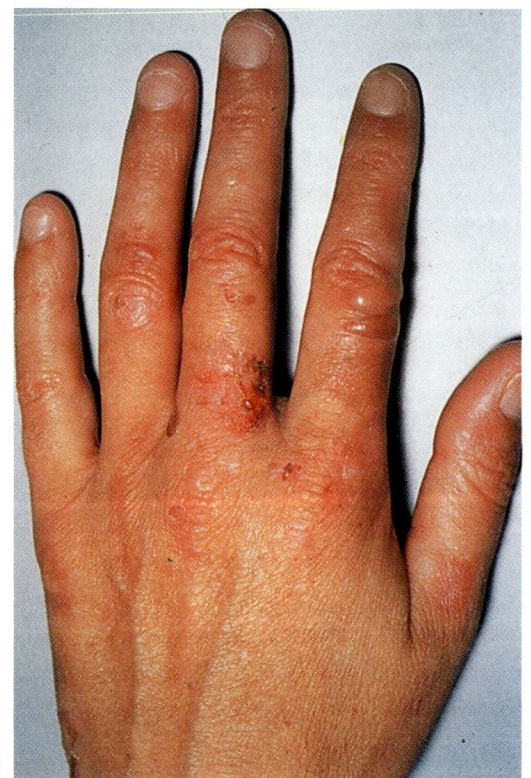

(b)

(a)

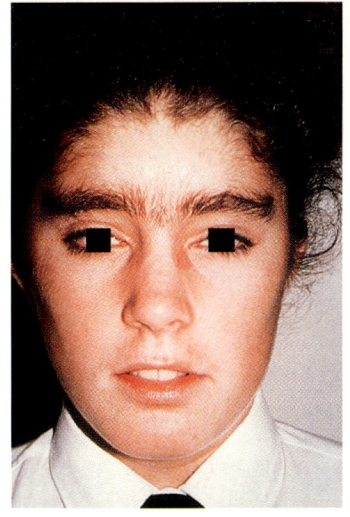

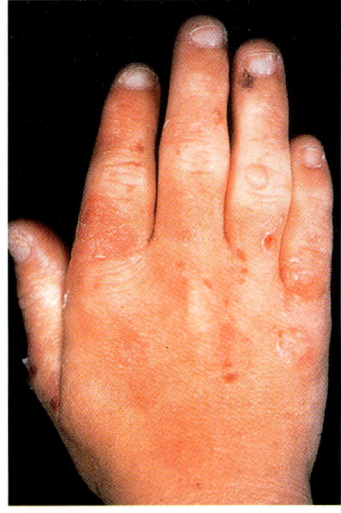

Plate 28 (left)   Hypertrichosis of porphyria cutanea tarda.

Plate 29 (right)   Homozygous variegate porphyria.

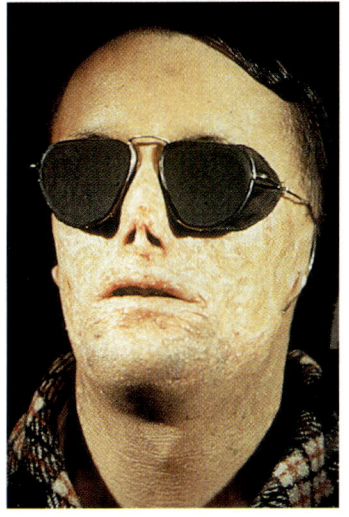

(a)

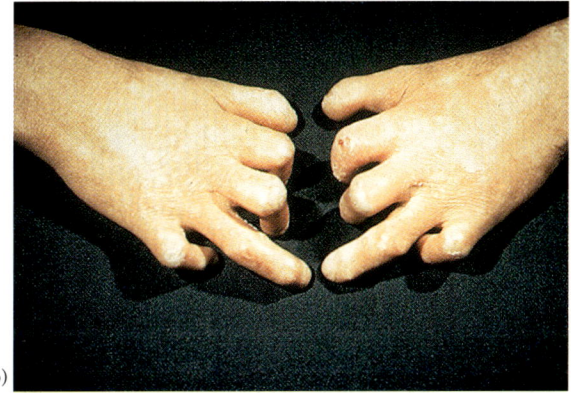

(b)

Plate 30   Congenital erythropoietic porphyria. Photomutilation of the face (a) and hands (b) in an adult with disease since infancy.

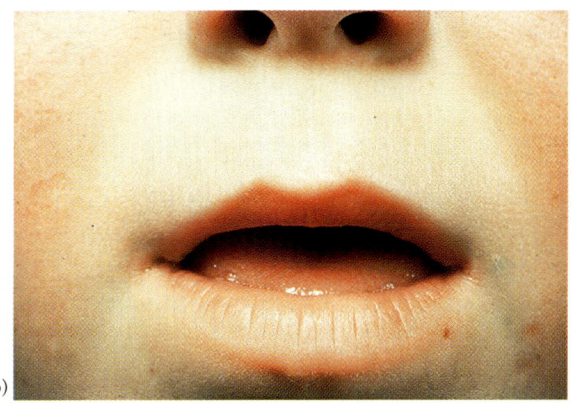

Plate 31   Erythropoietic protoporphyria. Acute purpuric (a) and chronic scarring skin lesions (b).

(a)

(b)

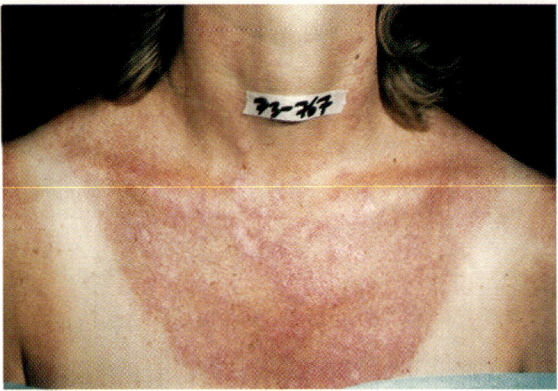
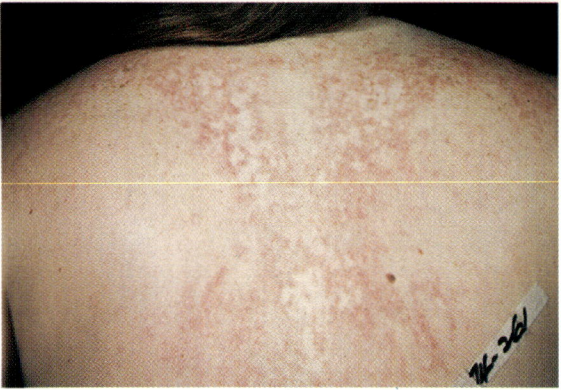

Plate 32 (above left and right)   Photoexacerbated lupus erythematosus.

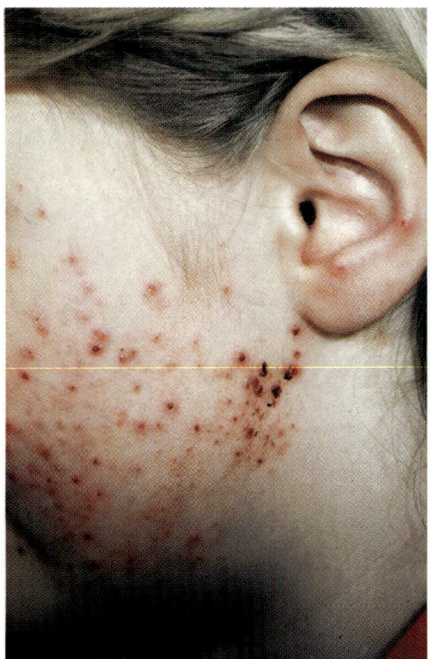
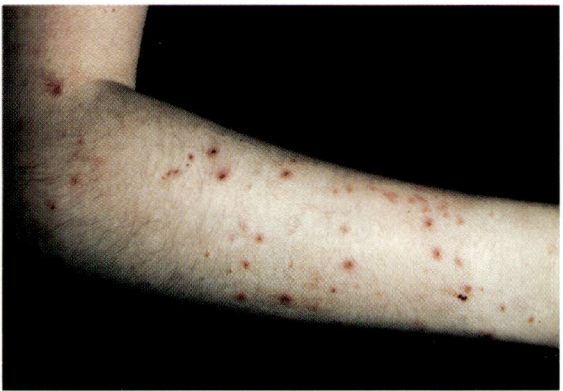

Plate 33 (left and above)   Photoexacerbated atopic eczema, somewhat resembling actinic prurigo.

Plate 34 (below left)   Diagram of a top-hat laser beam.
Plate 35 (below)   Diagram of a Gaussian laser beam.

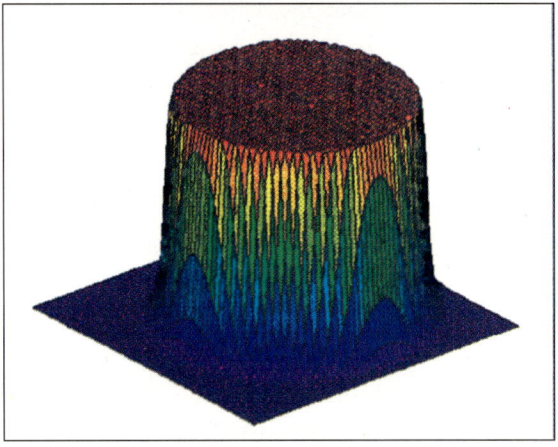
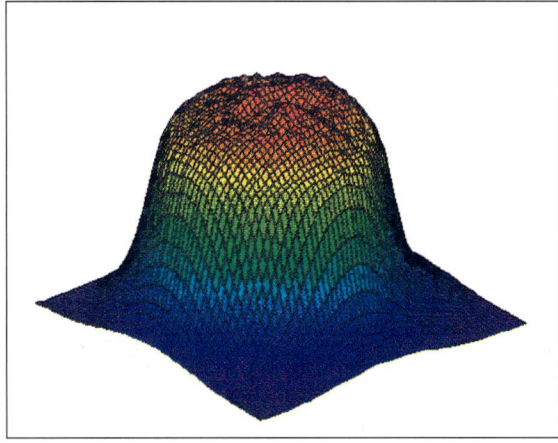

Kripke, M.L. and Morison, W.L. (1985) Modulation of immune function by UV radiation. *Journal of Investigative Dermatology*, **85**, 625–65.

Lane, C.G. and Crawford, G.M. (1937) Psoriasis. A statistical study of 231 cases. *Archives of Dermatology*, **35**, 1051–61.

LeFeber, W.P., Norris, D.A., Ryan, S.S. *et al.* (1984) Ultraviolet light induces binding of antibodies to selected nuclear antigens on cultured human keratinocytes. *Journal of Clinical Investigation*, **74**, 1545–51.

Leroy, D., DeRancourt, S. and Deschamps, P. (1987) Drug-induced EM with photodistribution and genital lesions. *Photodermatology*, **4**, 52–4.

Leroy, D., LeMaitre, M. and Deschamps, P. (1985) Photosensitive erythema multiforme apparently induced by phenylbutazone. *Photodermatology*, **2**, 176–7.

Levine, L. Seaman, E., Hammerschlag, E. *et al.* (1966) Antibodies to photoproducts of deoxyribonucleic acids irradiated with ultraviolet light. *Science*, **153**, 1666–7.

Lomholt, G. (1963) Influence of sun and sea bathing, in *Psoriasis: Prevalence, Spontaneous Course and Genetics. A Census Study on the Prevalence of Skin Diseases on the Faroe Island*, GECGAD, Copenhagen, pp. 113–14.

McNair-Scott, T.F., Blank, H., Coriell, L.L. *et al.* (1950) Pathology and pathogenesis of the cutaneous lesions of variola, vaccinia, herpes simplex, herpes zoster and varicella, in *Pathogenesis and Pathology of Viral Diseases*, (ed. J.G. Kidd), Columbia University Press, New York, pp. 74–98.

Mims, C.A. (1966) Pathogenesis of rashes in viral diseases. *Bact Rev*, **30**, 739–59.

Mitsuhashi, Y., Nakano, H., Murai, T. *et al.* (1994) Bullous pemphigoid sera induce bullous-pemphigoid-like lesions in neonatal mice pretreated with a limited dose of ultraviolet B irradiation. *Dermatology*, **189**, 76–81.

Mond, C.B., Peterson, M.G.E. and Rothfield, N.F. (1989) Correlation of anti-Ro antibody with photosensitivity rash in systemic lupus erythematosus patients. *Arthritis and Rheumatism*, **32**, 202–4.

Morison, W.L. (1983) Autoimmune disease in *Photoimmunology* (eds J.A. Parrish, W.L. Morison and M. Kripke), New York, Plenum, pp. 255–66.

Natakum, P.G. and Tan, E.M. (1973) Experimental skin lesions in mice resembling systemic lupus erythematosus. *Arthritis and Rheumatism*, **16**, 579–89.

Natali, P.G. and Tan, E.M. (1971) Immunological detection of thymidine photoproduct formation in vivo. *Radiation Research*, **46**, 506–18.

Natali, P.G. and Tan, E.M. (1972) Experimental renal disease induced by DNA-ant DNA immune complexes. *Journal of Clinical Investigation*, **51**, 345–55.

Neill, S.M. and du Vivier, A. (1985) A case of mycosis fungoides mimicking actinic reticuloid. *British Journal of Dermatology*, **113**, 497–500.

Pace, B.F. and Owens, D.W. (1969) Photosensitivity eruption following smallpox vaccination. *Cutis*, **5**, 850–3.

Pinkus, H. (1973) Lichenoid tissue reactions: a speculative review of the clinical spectrum of epidermal basal cell damage with special reference to erythema dyschromicum perstans. *Archives of Dermatology*, **107**, 840–6.

Poiesz, B.J., Ruscetti, F.W., Gazdar, A.F. *et al.* (1980) Detection and isolation of type C retrovirus particles from fresh and cultured lymphocytes of a patient with cutaneous T-cell lymphoma. *Proceedings of the National Academy of Science of the USA*, **77**, 7415–19.

Provost, T.T. and Reichlin, M. (1981) Antinuclear antibody-negative systemic lupus erythematosus. *Journal of the American Academy of Dermatology*, **4**, 84–9.

Ramsay, C.A. and Kobza Black, A. (1973) Photosensitive eczema. *Transactions of St Johns Hospital Dermatological Society*, **59**, 152–8.

Rihner, M. and McGrath, J. (1992) Fluorescent light photosensitivity in patients with systemic lupus erythematosus. *Arthritis and Rheumatism*, **35**, 949–52.

Ros, A.M. and Eklund, G. (1987) Photosensitive psoriasis: an epidemiologic study. *Journal of the American Academy of Dermatology*, **17**, 752–8.

Sinoway, P.A., Davison, C.L. and Callen, J.A. (1994) Dermatomyositis occurring during psoralen A (PUVA) therapy. *Journal of Rheumatology*, **21**, 353–6.

Smith, S.Z. and Epstein, J.H. (1977) Photocontact dermatitis to halogenated salicylanilides and related compounds. Our experience between 1967 and 1975. *Archives of Dermatology*, **113**, 1372–4.

Starke, J.C. and Jillson, O.F. (1961) Photosensitization to coal tar: a cause of psoriatic erythroderma. *Archives of Dermatology*, **84**, 935–40.

Synkowski, D.R., Reichlin, M. and Provost, T.T. (1982) Serum antibodies in systemic lupus erythematosus and correlation with cutaneous features. *Journal of Rheumatology*, **9**, 380–5.

Tan, E.M. (1968) Antibodies to deoxyribonucleic acid irradiated with ultraviolet light: detection by precipitins and immunofluorescence. *Science*, **161**, 1353–4.

Tan, E.M. (1971) Production of potentially antigenic DNA in cells, in *Immunopathology*. Sixth International Symposium, (ed. P.A. Miescher), Grune & Stratton, New York, pp. 346–9.

Tan, E.M. and Stoughton, R.B. (1969a) Ultraviolet light alteration of cellular deoxyribonucleic acid *in vivo*. *Proceedings of the National Academy of Science of the USA*, **62**, 708–14.

Tan, E.M. and Stoughton, R.B. (1969b) Ultraviolet light induced damage to deoxyribonucleic acid in human skin. *Journal of Investigative Dermatology*, **52**, 537–42.

Van Der Schroeff, J.G., Schothost, A.A. and Kanaar, P. (1983) Induction of actinic lichen planus with artificial UV sources. *Archives of Dermatology*, **119**, 498–500.

Verhagen, A.R.H.B. and Koten, J.W. (1979) Lichenoid melanodermatitis. A clinicopathologic study of 51 Kenya patients with so-called tropical lichen planus. *British Journal of Dermatology*, **101**, 651–8.

Volden, G. (1980) A study of the photosensitive factor in relation to skin lesion of mycosis fungoides patients. *Dermatologica*, **161**, 89–92.

Volden, G. and Thune, P.O. (1977) Light sensitivity in mycosis fungoides. *British Journal of Dermatology*, **97**, 279–84.

Wakizaka, A. and Okuhara, E. (1979) Immunologically active lesions induced on double-stranded DNA with ultraviolet. *Photochemistry and Photobiology*, **30**, 573–9.

Zaharieva, L., Stanoeva, L. and Konstantinov, D. (1978) Lichen planus actinicus. *Acta Dermato-Venereologica Ingosl*, **5**, 253–257.

Zamansky, G.B., Minka, D.G., Deal, C.L. *et al.* (1985) The *in vitro* photosensitivity of systemic lupus erythematosus skin fibroblasts. *Journal of Immunology*, **134**, 1571–6.

Zanca, A. and Zanca, A. (1978) Lichen planus actinicus. *International Journal of Dermatology*, **17**, 506–8.

Zugerman, C., Beaff, D. and Roenigk, H.H. Jr. (1980) Photosensitivity and Sezary syndrome. *Cutis*, **25**, 495–9.

PHOTOPROTECTION

15

Nicholas J. Lowe

Numerous investigations have documented that skin exposure to ultraviolet (UV) B and A radiation is the most important cause of cutaneous photodamage and, in particular, photocarcinogenesis and photoageing.

Most modern sunscreening agents effectively filter the UVB and to some extent UVA wavelengths, while in addition, some now contain micronized titanium or zinc oxide and are thus also capable of reflecting much of the UV and some of the infrared radiation.

There is direct evidence from animal studies that skin photoageing is reduced by sunscreen application, while there is also recent evidence in human investigations that sunscreens reduce sun-induced cutaneous premalignancies (actinic keratoses).

The regular use of effective sunscreens is therefore recommended as a logical method of reducing the incidence of cutaneous photodamage.

INTRODUCTION

The incidence of sunlight-induced skin ageing and skin cancers has been steadily increasing in many parts of the world. In particular, the incidence of both melanoma and non-melanoma skin cancer has shown a well-documented increase in several continents over the last several years (Scotto *et al.*, 1983). Many authorities are therefore recommending primary prevention programmes to reduce

Photodermatology. Edited by J.L.M. Hawk. Published in 1998 by Chapman & Hall, London. ISBN 0 412 72460 X.

this incidence of cutaneous photodamage and skin carcinogenesis and an integral component of these programmes is the use of protective clothing (Sayre and Lowe, 1982), as well as hats and effective sunscreens (Stern, 1990; Thompson *et al.*, 1993).

Most modern sunscreens have highly efficient absorptive or reflecting capabilities throughout the UVB, part of the UVA and in some instances the infrared wavelengths, while even more efficient sunscreening ingredients are steadily being developed to improve protection of the population still further (Kaidbey, 1990; Lowe *et al.*, 1988; Luftman *et al.*, 1991; Roelandts, 1991). As a result, direct evidence has at last been derived from a large population study in Australia of the effectiveness of sunscreens, demonstrating their ability to reduce the incidence of solar keratoses. Such an observation is of great importance, in that solar keratoses have been established as risk factors for basal cell carcinoma and melanoma and are known precursors of squamous cell carcinoma (Thompson *et al.*, 1993).

SUNSCREENS

In 1928, the world's first commercial sunscreen, an emulsion of benzyl salicylate and benzyl cinnamate, was developed in the United States, while in the 1930s, a 10% solution of phenyl salicylate appeared on the Australian market. In 1935, lotions of quinine oleate and quinine bisulphate then became available in the US, while in 1943, para-aminobenzoic acid (PABA) was patented, introducing this formerly popular agent followed by its derivatives. The US military also utilized red petrolatum, a physical blocking agent, as a sunblock during the Second World War, these efforts also leading to the popularization of other UV-filtering agents such as glycerol-PABA, 2-ethylhexyl salicylate, digalloyl trioleate, homomenthyl salicylate and dipropylene glycol salicylate (Shaath, 1990). Most of these early agents were directed against UVB, the portion of the sun's spectrum recognized early as being responsible for the most palpable and distressing ultraviolet (UV) effect, the familiar sunburn. Much more recently, however, Parsol 1789 (avobenzone or 4-t-butyl-4'-methoxydibenzoylmethane), an agent broadly effective against the UVA spectrum, has been marketed in combination with UVB-blocking agents, and these formulations now provide broad-spectrum chemical sun protection for the US consumer (Lowe, 1991; Lowe *et al.*, 1987). In addition, a new subclass of physical blockers, the micronized reflecting powders, has recently been made available by a variety of manufacturers which, unlike traditional physical blockers, are less visible, yet still provide broad-spectrum protection against UVR.

Future possible developments in sunscreen technology may very possibly lead to products with efficacy against UVC (which may conceivably become more important with further erosion of the ozone layer) and agents directed against infrared (Ir), which also appears to have some moderate cutaneous damage potential.

SUNSCREEN GUIDELINES IN THE UNITED STATES

The Federal Register, which was published in 1978, established guidelines for the formulation and evaluation of sunscreens marketed in the United States. These guidelines were then re-evaluated in 1988 and further revised in 1993.

The 1978 publication suggested that sun protection factors (SPF) be categorized according to the level of protection afforded, ranging from minimal sun protection for an SPF of 2–4 up to an ultrasun protection maximum for an SPF of 15. Thus, these guidelines suggested that no product exceed a maximum SPF level of 15 but in the 1993 publication, the ultrasun protection maximum was increased to 30, such SPF numbers having been achieved mainly by an increase in the concentration of the sunscreening chemicals to the maximum allowed under the monograph guidelines, although other products have achieved it by modification of their vehicle. Continuing advances have now led to SPF numbers as high as 40 or 50.

SUN PROTECTION FACTOR (SPF) DETERMINATION IN THE UNITED STATES

The Federal Register gives precise instructions on the methodology of SPF evaluation, the sun protection factor being defined as:

$$SPF = \frac{\text{Minimal erythema dose in sunscreen-protected skin}}{\text{Minimal erythema dose in non-sunscreen protected skin}}$$

Selection of subjects is of great importance in the precise determination of an SPF. Thus, in general, skin types 1–3 are ideal for these investigations (Table 15.1) and it is also suggested that such subjects avoid sun exposure or exposure to tanning beds for at least 90 days prior to study enrolment. On the other hand, darker skin types require much longer irradiation times and, in general, the longer the test irradiations, the greater the variability in minimal erythema dose (MED) determinations.

Many investigators prefer to utilize the previously non-sun exposed skin of the lower back for static SPF investigations. A MED is first determined, namely the minimum dose of UV radiation expressed as Joules per cm^2

Table 15.1 Sunscreens allowed in the USA under FDA-OTC Panel with concentration range

	Approved concentration %
Chemical	
UVA absorbers	
Oxybenzone	2–6
Sulisobenzone	5–10
Dioxybenzone	3
Methyl anthranilate	3.5–5
Azobenzone	
UVB absorbers	
Aminobenzoic acid	5–15
Amyldimethyl para-amino benzoic acid	1–5
2-Ethoxyethyl p-methoxycinnamate	1–3
Diethanolamine p-methoxycinnamate 8–10	
Digalloyl trioleate	2–5
Ethyl 4-bis (hydroxypropyl) aminobenzoate	1–5
2-Ethylhexyl-2-cyano-3,3-diphenyl-acrylate	7–10
Ethyl p-methoxycinnamate	2–7.5
Ethylhexyl salicylate	3–5
Glycerol aminobenzoate	2–3
Homomenthyl salicylate	4–25
Lawsone with dihydroxyacetone	0.25 with 3
Octyldimethyl para-amino benzoic acid	1.4–8
2-Phenylbenzimidazole-5-sulphonic acid	1–4
Triethanolamine salicylate	5–12
Physical	
Red petrolatum	30–100
Titanium dioxide	2–25

required to produce a minimal uniform skin erythema with clear margins at the borders of the exposure site. Such an exposure site is outlined by opaque adhesive metal foil fashioned to produce a template enclosing a 1 cm^2 area, which is then placed on the lower back skin and the areas of skin for testing uncovered at precisely predetermined times to ensure that the correct dose is administered. In this way an accurate MED is determined for each subject in the first 24 hours of the study.

The response to the UV exposure is determined around 24 hours following the irradiation. From previous experience, the approximate MED of each skin type with the solar simulator used is generally known and

appropriate amounts of UV radiation are then delivered to approximate that anticipated MED time.

The following day the sunscreens to be tested are applied at a concentration of 2 mg/cm^2, carefully measured with a pipette. The areas for application are marked beforehand with the help of the template noted above. Since most sunscreen products have a specific gravity of almost unity, the amount of 2 mg/cm^2 is usually conveniently measured out as 2 μl/cm^2. It is most important that the sunscreen application be absolutely uniform and the test technician must therefore be carefully trained in this technique; otherwise very large variations in SPF estimation will be obtained.

Recent studies have strongly suggested that the average individual applies far less than $2\,mg/cm^2$ of sunscreen in regular use (Gotlieb *et al.*, 1991; Stern, 1990; Thompson *et al.*, 1993), but in spite of claims that the standard should therefore be changed to a lesser density, the 1993 Federal Register continued to maintain that $2\,mg/cm^2$ was reliable, having been in use for ten years. Indeed, a change in the standard would certainly make past scientific studies difficult to interpret because precise comparisons with the new data could not be made and such a change would therefore negate ten years of data based on the $2\,mg/cm^2$ density. In addition, consumers have adjusted their method of sunscreen use to today's SPF determinations and any change in this system would thus also lead to consumer confusion.

After application, the sunscreens are allowed to dry on the skin for 15 minutes prior to irradiation. However, some sunscreens are highly protective as soon as they are applied and further investigation is required to determine just how rapidly sunscreens acquire and for how long they retain their SPF numbers.

After sunscreen application, the volunteer is again irradiated at the sunscreen-protected sites with incremental amounts of radiation based on the preliminary estimation of SPF number for that sunscreen and on a geometric formula recommended by the Federal Drugs Administration (FDA). Thus, either a very rough spectrophotometric absorption estimate of the expected SPF is obtained beforehand or else the SPF is estimated with carefully measured incremental radiation doses in a small number of volunteer patients. In this way excessive sunburning of volunteer skin is generally avoided.

The volunteers are again examined 24 hours after the second irradiation and the MEDs determined for both the sunscreen-protected and non-protected skin; the SPF is then the ratio of these results.

EUROPEAN TESTING

There are several key differences in detail between the methods for SPF determination in the United States and Europe.

Differences exist in the amounts of sunscreen application allowed. Thus, the US monograph recommends $2\,mg/cm^2$ and Australia, Japan and Britain also follow these FDA guidelines. However, the German Deutsche Institut für Normung (DIN) has recommended a concentration of $1.5\,mg/cm^2$ in the belief that this is a much closer estimate of actual sunscreen concentration during general population usage. It is the belief of the US FDA, however, that $2\,mg/cm^2$ is more easily applied in a uniform density.

Precise European methods for SPF testing have now been published under the COLIPA guidelines and the FDA and new COLIPA guidelines are now very similar with regard to the quantities of applied sunscreen, the logarithmic increase in UV doses and the spectral characteristics of the UV source.

TYPES OF ULTRAVIOLET APPARATUS AVAILABLE FOR SUNSCREEN TESTING

A wide variety of UV sources have been used worldwide for sunscreen evaluation. Thus, in the United States, the FDA monograph recommends the use of an appropriately filtered xenon arc solar simulator for the routine evaluation of sunscreens. However, the monograph also allows the use of alternative UV sources, providing satisfactory results have been obtained first for a variety of sunscreens in comparison with those of an appropriately filtered xenon arc source. The FDA has also set forth guidelines for the appropriate characteristics of solar simulators, which should provide continuous emission from 290 to 400 nm and have less than 1% of the total energy output below 290 and not more than 5% above 400 nm. In addition, there should also be satisfactory beam uniformity and no tendency to fluctuation in radiation intensity over time.

Table 15.2   Sunscreen chemicals used in Europe

European Community chemical name	Maximum concentration %
4-Aminobenzoic acid	5
N,N,N-trimethyl-4-(2-oxoborn-3-ylidene)-methyl anilinium methyl sulphate	6
Homosalate	10
Oxybenzone	10
3-Imidazole-4-glycolic acid and ethyl ester	2
2-Phenylbenzimidazole-5-sulphonic acid and salts	8
Ethyl-4-bis (hydroxypropyl) aminobenzoate	5
Ethoxylated 4-aminobenzoic acid	10
Amyl 4-dimethylaminobenzoate	5
Glycerol 1-(4-aminobenzoate)	5
2-Ethylhexyl 4-dimethylaminobenzoate	8
2-Ethylhexyl salicylate	5
3,3,5-Trimethylcyclohexyl-2-acetaminidobenzoate	2
Potassium cinnamate	2
4-Methoxycinnamic acid salts	8
Propyl 4-methoxycinnamate	3
Salicylic acid salts	2
Amyl 4-methoxycinnamate	10
2-Ethylhexyl 4-methoxycinnamate	10
Cinnoxate	5
Digalloyl trioleate	4
Mexenone	4
Sulisobenzone	5
2-Ethylhexyl 2-(4-phenylbenzoyl)-benzoate	10
5-Methyl-2-phenylbenzoxazone	4
Sodium 3,4-dimethoxyphenylglyoxylate	5
1,3-bis (4-Methoxyphenyl)propane-1,3-dione	6
5-(3,3-Dimethyl-2-norbonylidene)-3-penten-2-one	3
a'-(2-Oxoborn-3-ylidene)-p-xylene-2-sulphonic acid	6
a'-(2-Oxoborn-3-ylidene)-toluene-4-sulphonic acid and salts	6
3-(4-Methylbenzylidene)bornan-2-one	6
3-Benzylidenebornan-2-one	6
a-Cyano-4-methoxycinnamic acid and hexyl ester	5
1-p-Cumenyl-3-phenylpropane-1,3-dione	5
4-Isopropylbenzyl salicylate	4
Cyclohexyl 4-methoxycinnamate	1
1-(4-tert-Butylphenyl-3-(4-methoxyphenyl)propane-1,3-dione	5

XENON ARC SOLAR SIMULATORS

These sources are available for SPF testing with different lamp outputs, generally ranging between 150 and 5000 watts; with the 5000 watt sources, water cooling is usually required to reduce thermal damage to the reflecting mirrors within the lamp housing, as well as to reduce the amount of heat energy delivered to the subject. Suitable 1000–2500 watt sources with appropriate filtration are available from several suppliers, currently including Oriel and Kratos (USA) and a variety of UV filters are available to provide the exact UV spectrum required.

Table 15.3 Comparison with two different solar simulators of mean SPF ± SD

Sunscreen	SPF	SPF
Homosalate	3.8 ± 0.5	4.3 ± 0.5
A	15.0 ± 2.1	16.2 ± 1.6
B	9.4 ± 2.0	9.6 ± 1.6
C	15.6 ± 2.5	16.5 ± 1.5
D	16.2 ± 1.6	16.8 ± 1.6

One example of a 150 watt source is the Berger solar simulator, of which the main advantage is its portability and main disadvantage the small skin irradiation sites possible, making it suitable only for pilot or smaller sunscreen studies. In comparison with the small units, however, the 1000–2500 watt machines can fairly uniformly irradiate an area of approximately 10 × 15 cm. It is important to note that with all xenon arc sources, the careful handling of replacement lamps is absolutely essential since they may explode and cause severe injury; thus, the housing of such lamps must also be of sufficient strength to protect against such problems.

HIGH-PRESSURE METAL HALIDE SOURCES

Mercury vapour lamps have also been used for some years as UV sources for SPF testing, but the resemblance of their output to the solar spectrum has been considered poor because there are wide gaps between their individual spectral output lines in the UV range. However, this deficiency can now be improved by the use of metal iodides within the lamp envelope, which leads to a much more satisfactory emission.

We have now investigated the efficacy of the high-pressure metal halide lamp as an appropriate source for sunscreen evaluation, comparing in a series of investigations the SPF numbers obtained for a series of sunscreens with both this source and the filtered xenon arc lamp, and very similar numbers were obtained (Table 15.3). It would therefore seem reasonable to use halide sources for the evaluation of sunscreen products of SPF less than 15, major advantages being that the machine is very portable but has a higher energy output and can irradiate larger skin areas than the 150 watt xenon arc simulator.

INTERMEDIATE-PRESSURE MERCURY VAPOUR SOURCES

Previously the West German DIN system recommended by convention the use of an Osram Vitalux intermediate-pressure mercury vapour source for sunscreen SPF testing. However, although this is not a solar simulator having a mercury vapour line spectrum, comparison studies with predicted human SPF values from an *in vitro* mouse epidermal assay showed it to give similar

Table 15.4 Comparison between the properties of xenon arc, metal halide and intermediate-pressure mercury vapour sources

	Electrical power output (w)	UVR per watt	Simulation of solar spectrum	Lamp life (h)	Ease of operation	Cost of unit	Running costs	Portability
Xenon arc	150–5000	Low	Excellent	1500	Complex	High	High	Yes
								No
Metal halide	400–1000	High	Adequate	2000	Easy	Low	Low	Excellent
Intermediate-pressure mercury vapour	300	Low	Poor	2000	Easy	Low	Low	Possible

results to a xenon arc source for most sunscreens. Thus, these studies again suggest that if necessary, there are realistic alternatives to the filtered xenon arc solar simulator for sunscreen SPF testing.

OTHER SOURCES USED FOR SPF TESTING

Other UV sources previously used for SPF testing have included fluorescent sunlamp tubes, but while these have the advantages of ease of use and a consistent UV output, their major disadvantage is that they are not solar simulating, having output peaks at 313 nm and 365 nm, relatively little UVA and some UVC.

Table 15.4 summarizes differences between these various UV sources.

SUMMARY

Ideally, a test source with an output closely resembling that of the solar spectrum should be used for human SPF testing. This is clearly most closely achieved by the use of filtered xenon arc sources. However, other units, in particular the high-pressure metal halide sources, can be filtered to produce relatively acceptable spectra as confirmed by comparison studies between these sources and the filtered xenon arc, particularly for SPF values below about 15.

OUTDOOR TESTING OF SUNSCREENS

The importance of outdoor testing of sunscreens has been stressed by some authorities because of the obvious appropriateness of their evaluation in a setting relevant to regular usage. In addition, the test subjects are free to move around such that wear and tear removal of their sunscreen is much more likely than in the static laboratory solar simulator environment. There is also the important additional factor that sunlight contains larger amounts of infrared radiation than does solar-simulated radiation, but it is also clear that it

is difficult to standardize such variables, as well as the ambient humidity and degree of volunteer perspiration, for example, during such testing.

A more practical solution may therefore be intentionally to vary indoor laboratory factors such as the ambient humidity, the amount of infrared output from the source and the laboratory room temperature. In this way a sunscreen evaluation more closely allied to the usual outdoor situation may be possible in a controlled indoor environment.

WATER-RESISTANT AND VERY WATER-RESISTANT CLAIMS OF SUNSCREEN PROTECTIVENESS

The FDA monograph (1993) outlines procedures required to evaluate the resistance to water wash-off of sunscreens in rigorous conditions where the test subjects are exposed to water for different lengths of time following sunscreen application. The degrees of resistance to such wash-off are now divided into two broad groups, namely water-resistant and very water-resistant (previously waterproof) types.

A water resistance capability for a sunscreen may be claimed following the successful SPF evaluation of a test subject after two 20-minute immersions with moderate activity in water, while the very water-resistant claim requires four such immersions; Table 15.5 shows details of the protocols to be followed. For example, a portable whirlpool jacuzzi bath may be used, with steady water movement being provided by a water agitator. The sunscreens may then be applied to the lower backs of the test subjects and immersed for the appropriate amounts of time in the whirlpool bath, the water jets being directed away from the sunscreen-treated skin to avoid direct wash-off. In addition, the water temperature, pH, salinity and movement can easily be standardized in this situation, allowing simulation of different amounts of subject exercise and different

Table 15.5 Water resistance claims protocol

Action	Time (minutes)
Water resistant	
Apply sunscreen	0
In water	20
Out of water	40
In water	60
Out of water (air dry)	80
Irradiate	100
Very water resistant	
Apply sunscreen	0
In water	20
Out of water	40
In water	60
Out of water	80
In water	100
Out of water	120
In water	140
Out of water (air dry)	160
Irradiate	180

All erythema readings 24 hours after irradiation

types of water conditions, but few of these variables have been studied as yet.

RECENT TRENDS IN SUNSCREEN DEVELOPMENT

There are several important recent trends in sunscreen development. These include the increasing sun protection factor numbers, which have mainly been achieved by the use of increasing amounts of sunscreen chemical. One concern as a result of this has been a potential increased risk of irritancy and contact allergic sensitization reactions, particularly as some sunscreens are now claiming SPF numbers of 50 or so. However, it remains to be seen whether there will be an increase in topical toxicity from these.

Further areas of advancement have included the development of micronized powders for use as physical reflecting sunscreens. This has been of great importance for patients with severely photosensitive skin who are often irritated or sensitized by chemical screens, as well as being a means of reducing instantaneous infrared radiation damage, particularly as there have been suggestions that solar infrared intensity may be important as an additional cause of sun-induced skin ageing. Current sunscreens absorb infrared very poorly, but some of the newer reflectant micronized powder sunscreens appear likely to afford some protection in this area of the solar spectrum.

The future potential risks of UVC exposure, should sufficient ozone layer depletion occur in the atmosphere, may conceivably lead to a requirement to shift the absorption spectrum of sunscreens down to the UVC region. This may well be possible with many sunscreens, particularly those containing PABA esters, particularly as it has been shown that modification of the sunscreen vehicle, for example to include more polar solvents, may shift the absorption spectrum of a number of sunscreens to shorter wavelengths. Therefore, if more UVC should penetrate the earth's atmosphere in future years, it should certainly be possible to modify sunscreens to absorb at shorter UV wavelengths, although clearly if such a change in the terrestrial solar spectrum should occur, modification of the UV sources used for sunscreen protection factor testing would also be required.

In summary, significant advances in sunscreen technology and testing have been achieved in recent years. In the future, however, developments should be directed in particular to the production of more efficient and cosmetically acceptable reflecting sunscreens with enhanced photoprotection against UVA and perhaps also UVC and infrared radiation.

ACKNOWLEDGEMENT

Part of this chapter has been reprinted with permission from Lowe, N.J., Pathak, M. and Shaath, N.A. (1996) *Sunscreens: Development, Evaluation and Regulatory Aspects*, 2nd edn, Marcel Dekker, New York.

REFERENCES

Gotlieb, A., Bourget, T. and Lowe N.J. (1991) Sunscreens: effects of amounts of application of sun protection factors, in *Sunscreens: Development, Evaluation and Regulatory Aspects*, (eds N.J. Lowe and N. Shaath), Marcel Dekker, New York, pp. 441–6.

Kaidbey, K.H. (1990) The photoprotective potential of the new superpotent sunscreens. *Journal of the American Academy of Dermatology*, **22**, 449–52.

Lowe, N.J. (1991) UVA photoprotection, sunscreens – effects of amounts of application of sun protection factors, in *Sunscreens: Development, Evaluation and Regulatory Aspects*, (eds N.J. Lowe and N. Shaath), Marcel Dekker, New York, pp. 441–6.

Lowe, N.J., Dromgoole, S.H., Sefton, J. *et al.* (1987) Indoor and outdoor efficiency testing of broad spectrum sunscreen against ultraviolet A radiation in psoralen-sensitized subjects. *Journal of the American Academy of Dermatology*, **17**, 224–30.

Lowe, N.J., Weingarten, D. and Wortzman, M. (1988) Sunscreens and phototesting. *Clinics in Dermatology*, **6**(3), 40–9.

Luftman, D.B., Lowe, N.J. and Moy, R.L. (1991) Sunscreens: update and review. *Journal of Dermatologic Surgery and Oncology*, **17**, 744–6.

Roelandts, R. (1991) Which components in broad spectrum sunscreens are most necessary for adequate UVA protection? *Journal of the American Academy of Dermatology*, **25**, 999–1004.

Sayre, R.M. and Lowe, N.J. (1992) Scientific poster presentation at the American Academy of Dermatology Meeting, December.

Scotto, J., Fear, R.R. and Fraumeni, J.F. (1983) *Incidence of Non-melanoma Skin Cancer in the United States*. US Dept of Health and Human Services, Washington DC.

Shaath, N.A. (1990) Evolution of modern sunscreen chemicals, in *Sunscreens: Development, Evaluation and Regulatory Aspects*, (eds N.J. Lowe and N. Shaath), Marcel Dekker, New York, pp. 3–36.

Stern, R.S. (1990) Sunscreen use and non-melanoma skin cancer, in *Sunscreens: Development, Evaluation and Regulatory Aspects*, (eds N.J. Lowe and N. Shaath), Marcel Dekker, New York, pp. 85–92.

Thompson, S.C., Jolley, D. and Marks, R. (1993) Reduction of solar keratoses by regular sunscreen use. *New England Journal of Medicine*, **329**, 1147–51.

PHOTOTHERAPY AND PHOTOCHEMOTHERAPY

16

Bernhard Ortel and Herbert Hönigsmann

INTRODUCTION

This is an overview of the current practice of phototherapy by means of ultraviolet (UV) radiation alone and of psoralen photochemotherapy (PUVA) in the treatment of skin diseases. Both treatment modalities have well-established places in today's armamentarium of dermatologic therapy, continued clinical research having steadily helped to improve treatment protocols. Simultaneously, the understanding of mechanisms underlying the biological responses to UV exposure and psoralen photosensitization has increased and we are therefore now well prepared to minimize potential long-term side effects such as skin carcinogenesis by optimizing therapeutic strategies. Phototherapeutic regimens use repeated controlled UV exposures to alter cutaneous biology, which in this context aim at inducing the remission of skin disease, and in this chapter we will discuss the use of both unsensitized UV radiation (phototherapy in the stricter sense) and psoralen photosensitization (PUVA). The relevant treatment regimens, action spectra and other details will be described primarily with regard to psoriasis, which is the most common indication for both UVB phototherapy and PUVA, and other indications will then be discussed more briefly with reference to this background. Although UVB has been used for a longer

Photodermatology. Edited by J.L.M. Hawk. Published in 1998 by Chapman & Hall, London. ISBN 0 412 72460 X.

time than PUVA, the latter has been evaluated and validated in a more detailed and co-ordinated fashion and will thus also be discussed in more detail.

PHOTOTHERAPY

In dermatology, phototherapy traditionally means the use of artificial UVB irradiation delivered by fluorescent lamps (Farr, 1996; Van Der Leun and Van Weelden, 1986), although more recently both broad-band UVA alone and combinations of UVA with UVB have also been used (Berg *et al.*, 1994; Jekler and Laiko, 1991; Midelfart *et al.*, 1986). More recently, again, however, the use of UVAI (340–400 nm) has been advocated in addition for the treatment of a few specific inflammatory skin diseases (Kerscher *et al.*, 1995; Kowalzick *et al.*, 1995; Krutmann *et al.*, 1992; Morison, 1994).

Finally, natural sunlight may be used as a broad-band therapeutic source, but restrictions to largely mid-day outdoor exposure and the variability of climatic conditions in many locations severely limit the usefulness of this form of phototherapy; however, one major exception is phototherapy at the Dead Sea (Abels and Kattan-Byron, 1985).

PRINCIPLES AND MECHANISMS

Phototherapy is the use of ultraviolet irradiation for therapeutic purposes without the addition of an exogenous photosensitizer, the radiation being absorbed by endogenous chromophores. Photochemical reactions associated with these absorbing biomolecules then result in alterations of skin biology leading to the treatment effect; such acute effects of UV radiation are discussed in detail earlier in this volume.

The best-characterized chromophore for UVB is nuclear DNA, absorption of UV by its nucleotides leading to DNA photoproduct formation, mainly pyrimidine dimers (Cadet *et al.*, 1992). Despite the quantitative predominance of these dimers, however, the pyrimidine (6-4) pyrimidone photoproduct also formed may be biologically more significant (Petit Frere *et al.*, 1996). Many biological consequences of UV radiation have been linked to specific DNA photoproducts (Moan and Peak, 1989; Ronai *et al.*, 1992) and we have acquired a good understanding of how such products interfere with cell cycle progression and induce growth arrest for cell fate decision (Liu and Pellingo, 1995). Besides the effects on cell cycle, UV also induces prostaglandin release and alters cytokine expression and secretion (Greaves, 1986; Hruza and Pentland, 1993), while interleukins 6 and 10 seem to play important roles in inducing the systemic symptoms of UV phototoxicity and immunosuppression (Beissert *et al.*, 1995; Schwarz and Luger, 1989; Ullrich, 1995; Urbanski *et al.*, 1996). Such mechanisms may be equally important for therapeutic effectiveness and side effects, while recently, UV-induced cellular molecular effects have also been demonstrated which are independent of nuclear DNA damage. Such events involve membrane receptors and molecular signalling pathways which regulate transcriptional activity (Devary *et al.*, 1993; Warmuth *et al.*, 1994), gene expression thus potentially being altered independently of DNA damage. Such molecular regulatory mechanisms therefore indicate additional or parallel molecular pathways but do not in fact help to identify actual cellular targets and effector mechanisms in

phototherapy, during which it must be assumed generally that different pathways are modified to variable extents depending on which disease is targeted. In addition, the primary cellular target may well differ depending on the disease and the interplay of the various photobiological pathways is thus far from being completely understood. In psoriasis, for example, both epidermal keratinocytes and cutaneous lymphocytes may be targeted by UVB while alteration of cytokine expression and cell cycle arrest may also contribute to the suppression of disease activity.

ACTION SPECTRUM

An action spectrum describes the relative efficacy of a radiation-induced process as a function of wavelength. In terms of phototherapy for psoriasis, its efficacy was first evaluated and compared with its erythemogenicity in the respective UV radiation bands; Fisher (1976) noted an improved efficacy at wavelengths around 313 nm. Parrish and Jaenicke (1981) then reported a broader action spectrum, demonstrating that wavelengths shorter than 296 nm were almost ineffective against psoriasis even when several multiples of a minimal erythema dose (MED) were used for the individual exposures. In contrast, the 304 and 313 nm bands were optimally effective even with suberythemogenic doses, an action spectrum well matched by standard therapeutic UVB fluorescent lamps, which emit between 295 and 350 nm with a peak at 305. In the UVA range, erythemogenic doses are also therapeutically relevant, but require irradiation doses more than 1000 times higher than for UVB phototherapy and for those reasons are therefore not practical, particularly since the addition of UVA does not enhance the therapeutic efficacy of UVB (Diette *et al.*, 1984).

New lamps have now been designed to fit this therapeutic action spectrum better than conventional broad-band sources. A regimen with metal halide lamps giving increased output between 295 and 330 nm has been described as selective ultraviolet photo-therapy (SUP) (Schröpl, 1977), more efficient than broad-band phototherapy but less so than PUVA (Hönigsmann *et al.*, 1977), while the more recently developed 312 nm narrow-band UVB (a narrow fluorescent band at 311/312 nm emitted by the so-called Philips TL01 lamp) was introduced to meet the optimal requirements for antipsoriatic activity (Van Weelden *et al.*, 1988).

PHOTOTHERAPY REGIMENS

Before the initiation of phototherapy, it is advisable to evaluate the individual UV sensi-tivity of the patient, which is undertaken by exposing small areas (e.g. 1 cm diameter circles) of lower back skin to an incremental series of UVB irradiations, the increases being fixed amounts (e.g. 10 mJ cm^2) or fractions of the previous lower doses (e.g. 40%). The smallest dose which leads to well-circum-scribed pink erythema at 24 hours is then called the MED. Use of the visually assessed MED as the optimal reference value for dosimetry, however, is somewhat open to controversy, but its evaluation is relatively accurate and easily performed, not requiring any apparatus in addition to the phototherapy equipment. Nevertheless, use of the lower, minimal detectable erythema dose has been proposed instead as a more reliable threshold value (Van Weelden *et al.*, 1988).

The initial therapeutic UVB dose should be between 70% and 80% of the MED, treatments then being given 2–5 times weekly; as peak UVB erythema appears before 24 hours after exposure, increments may be done with each successive treatment, the rate of increase depending on the treatment frequency and effect of the preceding therapeutic exposure. The objective of such increments is generally to maintain a minimally perceptible erythema as a clinical indicator of optimal dosime-try and, for example, with thrice-weekly

treatments, increases of 40% are given if no erythema is induced and 20% for slight erythema, while if the erythema is mild but persistent, no increment at all is made. On the other hand, with daily exposures, these rates are no more than 30%, 15% and again 0%, respectively, while with more intense or painful erythema, irradiations are withheld until symptoms subside. Treatments are given until total remission is reached or no further improvement is being obtained.

PHOTOTHERAPY OF PSORIASIS

Primarily, those psoriatics with widespread, eruptive and seborrhoeic but relatively super-ficial forms of psoriasis are treated with UVB because they respond rapidly, while patients with plaque-type psoriasis may also be treated in this way if they are resistant to topical therapy or have lesions covering more than 20% of the body surface area. Although such phototherapy can be very effective, it is less efficient than PUVA in terms of both remission times and clearing of the eruption (Hönigsmann *et al.*, 1994). Besides the regi-mens outlined above, others may also be used, some based, for example, on skin type-dependent starting doses and fixed incre-ments regardless of skin reaction. In addition, the patient's head, if free of psoriasis, may be covered with UV-opaque material during exposures in order to prevent unnecessary aggravation of environmental photodamage, while in some centres, the patient's extremi-ties are given higher doses than the trunk and are exposed to as much as 150% of the dose delivered to the rest of the body. Adjunctive agents and combination therapies are also used in an attempt to improve efficacy and reduce the cumulative UVB burden so as to minimize long-term side effects.

The efficacy of phototherapy may also be enhanced by the application of hydrophobic vehicles before exposure, the altered optical properties of the psoriatic scales thereby increasing the effective UV dose to the psoriatic lesion (Lebwohl *et al.*, 1995). Thus combinations with topical tars (Tanenbaum *et al.*, 1975) (Goeckerman regimen) or anthralin (dithranol) applications (Storbeck *et al.*, 1993) (Ingram regimen) are still regularly used, but the adjunctive use of topical steroids is discouraged because it may perhaps result in reduced remission times. Systemic drugs such as retinoids increase UVB efficacy, however, particularly in patients with chronic and hyperkeratotic plaque-type psoriasis (Iest and Boer, 1989; Steigleder *et al.*, 1979), while perhaps also reducing the carcinogenic potential of the phototherapy.

The recently developed narrow-band (312 nm) phototherapy lamp has proved superior to conventional broad-band UVB with respect to both clearing efficacy and remission times (Green *et al.*, 1988; Picot *et al.*, 1992; Van Weelden *et al.*, 1988), presumably because of an improved spectral emission with respect to the therapeutic requirements. In Europe, such lamps have replaced conventional phototherapy in many areas, although in the US, they have only recently come into usage, partly due to minor technical incompatibilities. Some phototherapists consider narrow-band phototherapy to be as effective as PUVA (Tanew *et al.*, 1996; Van Weelden *et al.*, 1990), but this claim needs to be substantiated on larger patient populations. Narrow-band UVB has also been used successfully in a variety of combination therapies, such as with retinoids (Green *et al.*, 1992), anthralin (dithranol) (Karronen *et al.*, 1989; Storbeck *et al.*, 1993) and calcipotriol (Kerscher *et al.*, 1993), while the already proven antipsoriatic efficacy of sub-erythemogenic narrow-band UVB irradiation (see 'Action spectrum' above) suggests the possibility of further developments and improvements.

UVB PHOTOTHERAPY FOR OTHER INDICATIONS

UVB phototherapy has numerous other dermatological applications besides psoriasis,

the treatment schedules following the same general guidelines for psoriasis therapy but perhaps not requiring such aggressive dose adjustments. Thus, UVB is useful for the induction of tolerance in the idiopathic photodermatoses such as polymorphic light eruption (PLE) (Addo and Sharma, 1987) but has also been applied to the prevention of actinic prurigo, hydroa vacciniforme, chronic actinic dermatitis (Collins and Ferguson, 1995) and solar urticaria (Addo and Sharma, 1987). It has also been used successfully for atopic dermatitis and generalized eczema (Jekler and Larko; 1988), the pruritus associated with internal diseases such as diabetes mellitus, uraemia and primary biliary cirrhosis (Gilchrest *et al.*, 1979) and for eosinophilic pustular folliculitis (Porneuf *et al.*, 1993), pityriasis rosea (Arndt *et al.*, 1983), parapsoriasis and human immunodeficiency virus (HIV)-associated pruritic papular eruption (Pardo *et al.*, 1992). In addition, for some of these indications, reports on the use of narrow-band UVB have also been published, the therapeutic results generally being encouraging, while for PLE and atopic dermatitis, relatively large studies have demonstrated high efficacy and it can therefore be definitely recommended (Bilsland *et al.*, 1993; George *et al.*, 1993); for most of the other indications, however, narrow-band phototherapy has been explored only in relatively small groups of patients and its efficacy therefore now needs to be confirmed on a larger scale.

PHOTOTHERAPY WITH UVA

Broad-band UVA, alone and in combination with UVB, has been used for the treatment of atopic eczema (Jekler, 1992) as the addition of UVA to the therapeutic emission spectrum seems to be beneficial in this disorder. A novel approach evolving from this, which was primarily directed at the treatment of acutely exacerbated atopic dermatitis (Krutmann *et al.*, 1992), used radiation from high-output metal halide lamps filtered below 340 nm, therefore emitting UVAI (340–400 nm) but not UVAII (320–340 nm); its efficacy, however, has not been systematically compared to that of other phototherapeutic modalities effective in the disorder. Initially, doses of 100 J/cm² and more were used but more recently, medium- and low-dose regimens have also been explored (Kawalzick *et al.*, 1995). Other indications for UVAI phototherapy have also been reported, such as lupus erythematosus treated with a low-dose UVAI regimen (McGrath, 1994) and localized morphoea, which has improved with both medium- and high-dose treatments (Kerscher *et al.*, 1995). This area of phototherapy is still developing and further indications may evolve. Presumably, any improved efficacy of UVAI over other phototherapeutic modalities is related to its depth of penetration into the skin and its mode of action by both direct absorption and photosensitization mechanisms.

PHOTOCHEMOTHERAPY WITH PSORALENS

Psoralen photochemotherapy (PUVA) is the combined use of the drug psoralen (P) and long-wave UV radiation (UVA), a combination resulting in a therapeutic effect not achieved by the single components alone. Its use leads to the remission of skin disease by repeated controlled phototoxic reactions.

PRINCIPLES AND MECHANISMS

PUVA is performed by the administration of a fixed dose of psoralen at a constant interval before UVA exposure, parameters kept unaltered to make psoralen plasma levels as reproducible as possible. Initial radiation dose finding (phototoxicity testing) and dose adjustments are then undertaken by the varying UVA dose. Therefore, effective UVA dosimetry is critical for safe and efficient PUVA therapy (Parrish *et al.*, 1974; Wolff *et al.*, 1975).

Psoralens are linear furocoumarins originally derived from plants and known to be active in repigmenting vitiligo when combined with sun exposure (Pathak and Fitzpatrick, 1992). In current clinical use, 8-methoxypsoralen (8-MOP, methoxsalen) is the most commonly prescribed but 5-methoxypsoralen (5-MOP, bergapten) and the synthetic linear furocoumarin 4,5′,8-trimethylpsoralen (TMP) are also commonly utilized. These compounds are all described as bifunctional, in that they have two photoactivatable double bonds (Fig. 16.1). Currently, they are available in three oral forms, which contain crystals, micronized crystals or solubilized psoralen in a gel matrix, the liquid preparation (available for 8-MOP and 5-MOP) inducing not only earlier and higher but also more reproducible peak plasma levels than the crystalline form. Oral psoralen is metabolized by the liver and excreted in the urine within 12–24 hours, but because of a considerable hepatic first-pass effect, small alterations in dose may alter plasma levels considerably, this perhaps being a major source of the high intra- and interindividual variability of plasma levels (Brickl *et al.*,

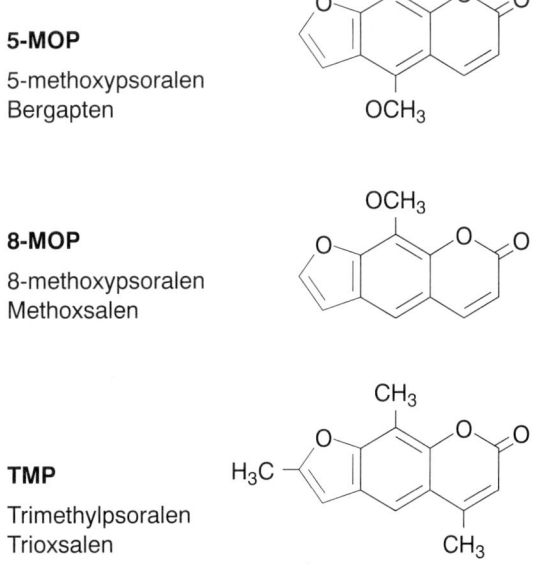

5-MOP
5-methoxypsoralen
Bergapten

8-MOP
8-methoxypsoralen
Methoxsalen

TMP
Trimethylpsoralen
Trioxsalen

Figure 16.1 Psoralens in clinical use.

1984; Herfst and De Wolff, 1983; Hönigsmann *et al.*, 1982). It is thus important for best possible reproducibility that as many parameters as possible are kept constant, such as, for example, the type and quantity of food eaten before or with the drug and time of the day the drug is taken.

Psoralen is only biologically reactive when activated by UV radiation and only in those layers of skin reached by UVA, namely the epidermis, papillary dermis and the superficial vascular plexus. Electronically excited psoralen may then undergo photochemical reactions which modify cutaneous biomolecule and skin function.

Psoralen photoreactivity with nuclear DNA seems biologically highly relevant and has been investigated thoroughly (Dall'Acqua, 1986), bifunctional psoralens reacting with DNA in three steps. First, the psoralen intercalates with the DNA double strand, a process which occurs in the absence of radiation, following which irradiation may induce a reactive double bond to form a cyclobutane adduct with an adjacent pyrimidine base; these are called 3,4 monoadducts (MA) or 4',5' MA according to the psoralen double bond involved, only the 4',5' MA being able finally to form a complete psoralen-DNA crosslink after absorbing a second photon. Under clinical conditions, MA are the more prominent adducts but the exact frequences of the psoralen-DNA photoproducts depend on both psoralen type and irradiation wavelengths (Tessman *et al.*, 1985). Although most is known about these psoralen-DNA photoproducts, other 8-MOP photochemical reactions may also contribute to the therapeutic effect (Schmitt *et al.*, 1985), excited psoralen, for example, reacting with molecular oxygen to form reactive oxygen species such as singlet oxygen, which in turn may cause cell membrane damage by lipid peroxidation or activate the cyclo-oxygenase and arachidonic acid metabolic pathways (Averbeck, 1989).

DNA-psoralen crosslinking inhibits DNA replication and causes cell cycle arrest by cellular molecular pathways which have recently been elucidated to improve our understanding of the responsible mechanisms. Thus, psoralen photosensitization leads to altered cytokine and cytokine receptor expression as well as cytokine secretion (Averbeck, 1989), thereby normalizing the pathologically altered keratinocyte differentiation and reducing proliferating epidermal cell numbers. As a result, infiltrating lymphocytes are strongly suppressed by PUVA, with variable effects on the different T-cell subsets (Vallat *et al.*, 1994), while PUVA is also far more potent at inducing lymphocyte rather than keratinocyte apoptosis at a similar level of antiproliferative activity for both cell types (Johnson *et al.*, 1996). Thus, PUVA readily induces apoptotic cell death in lymphocytes, a specific response pattern which may explain its high efficacy in both cutaneous T-cell lymphoma (CTCL) and lymphocyte-associated inflammatory skin disease.

However, although these recent findings have improved our knowledge of the pathways and mechanisms of psoralen photosensitization, the exact interactions and relative contributions of these processes to the clearing of specific diseases are not yet fully understood.

ACTION SPECTRUM

The action spectrum for 8-MOP-induced delayed erythema was originally believed to peak at 365 nm, but more recent studies have instead shown maximal activity at around 330 nm (Cripps *et al.*, 1982; Kaidsbey, 1985) while, as for phototherapy, the therapeutic efficacy of the erythema action spectrum has been evaluated only in psoriasis. Thus, while the data are harder to collect for PUVA because of the relatively high intraindividual variability of psoralen levels in plasma and skin, it currently seems that PUVA antipsoriatic activity parallels its erythema action spectrum (Brücke *et al.*, 1991; Farr *et al.*, 1991). In addition, a similar spectrum has been obtained for

8-MOP-DNA crosslinking in human skin *in vivo* (Ortel and Gange, 1990), apparently supporting the therapeutic relevance of psoralen-DNA crosslinks in the treatment of psoriasis.

The psoralen action spectrum is well covered by the broad emission of conventional therapeutic UVA fluorescent tubes, while metal halide lamps used for pure UVA phototherapy also emit a broad spectrum although with filtering in the UVB and UVC range; these are, however, also suitable for photochemotherapy and their high UVA output greatly reduces treatment times. In addition, the efficacy of broad-band as well as narrow-band (312 nm) UVB phototherapy has been shown to be enhanced in the presence of 8-MOP (Ortel *et al.*, 1993), again as might be expected in accordance with the PUVA erythema action spectrum (Sakuntabhai *et al.*, 1993).

PUVA REGIMENS

Our general recommendations are in accordance with the so-called European PUVA Study (EPS) protocol (Henseler *et al.*, 1981), the regimen requiring initial determination of the minimal phototoxic dose (MPD), in analogous fashion to MED determination, by exposure of the psoralen-sensitized lower back skin to a series of graded UVA exposures. The delayed phototoxic erythema is then visually assessed 72–96 hours later,

the smallest dose resulting in a well-circumscribed, mild erythema being the MPD. The initial therapeutic dose may then be chosen at 60–80% of the MPD and is most reliably safe if liquid psoralen preparations are used. Irradiations may be given 2–4 times weekly but dose increments not more frequently than twice, at least 72 hours apart, in order to avoid cumulative delayed cutaneous phototoxicity. During therapy, as for UVB treatment, a minimally perceptible erythema throughout may be considered a clinical indicator of good dosimetry and optimal therapeutic effect.

PUVA FOR PSORIASIS

Practically all forms of psoriasis respond to PUVA, although erythrodermic and generalized pustular psoriasis are less responsive than the more common varieties (Hönigsmann *et al.*, 1993). There are two therapeutic approaches to such treatment, however, both originally developed simultaneously and both highly efficient and thus still in use; according to their origins they are usually referred to as the American and the European regimens. Table 16.1 outlines these two methods for crystalline oral 8-MOP (Henseler *et al.*, 1981; Melski *et al.*, 1977). Our current routine treatment consists of the oral administration of 0.6–0.8 mg/kg 8-MOP liquid or 1.2–1.8 mg/kg 5-MOP liquid one or two hours before UVA exposure. For plaque-type psoriasis, treatments four times a week

Table 16.1 Protocols and therapeutic results of the European PUVA Study (EPS) and the US Co-operative Clinical Trial (USCCT)

	EPS	*USCCT*
Starting dose	1 MPD	Skin type dependent
Treatments per week	4	2–3
UVA dose increments	Individualized	Fixed
Clearing rate	88.8%	88%
Exposures	20	25
Time to clearing	5.7 weeks	12.7 weeks
Cumulative UVA dose	96 J/cm^2	245 J/cm^2

with an intermission on Wednesdays are then performed until clearing is achieved, maintenance therapy as recommended for the European regimen then being given twice weekly for four weeks at the last UVA dose used for clearing, followed finally by exposures once a week for four weeks. According to the recommendations of the British Photodermatology Group (1994), however, maintenance treatment should be considered only if relapse rapidly follows clearance and to clarify the efficacy of maintenance therapy, further studies are required.

New regimens or modifications of existing protocols have gradually been introduced to increase PUVA efficacy and reduce its side effects, one major advance being the widespread introduction of 5-MOP, leading to a much lower incidence of gastrointestinal side effects even at dosages of up to 1.8 mg/kg. In addition, after oral administration, 5-MOP is clinically less phototoxic than 8-MOP and therefore safer with regard to burning risk (Tanew *et al.*, 1988).

Another modification is an aggressive PUVA schedule which optimizes UVA irradiations by repeated phototoxic threshold determinations during the course of the therapy, treatments being given twice weekly, 72 hours apart. This procedure aims at optimized dosimetry to increase efficacy and reduce cumulative UVA doses (Carabott and Hawk, 1989), while more recently, a combination of dihydroxyacetone-induced UVA protection of uninvolved skin during PUVA has again resulted in improved psoriasis clearing (Taylor *et al.*, 1996).

PUVA for limited skin areas may be performed by topical psoralen administration, 8-MOP, for example, being used as a 0.15% solution painted on to lesions 20 minutes before exposure, while topical TMP application in bath water has been popular in Scandinavia for many years (Fischer and Alsins, 1976), but has only recently become of worldwide interest. 8-MOP may also be administered in bath water, thus avoiding

gastrointestinal side effects and apparently protecting the eyes from phototoxic insult because there is minimal systemic photosensitization. In addition, skin psoralen levels are highly reproducible and photosensitivity is less persistent than with oral administration. However, there is a higher tendency to unwanted phototoxicity, but this can be easily prevented by the use of a lower UVA starting dose at 50% of the MPD and more cautious dosimetry during the initial phases of treatment (Calzavara-Pinton *et al.*, 1993). Concentrations of 8-MOP between 0.0001 and 0.001% are used, baths being taken for 15–20 minutes and the skin carefully patted dry; UVA exposure should then take place immediately, before photosensitivity rapidly declines. TMP may also be used but is more phototoxic than 8-MOP after topical application and must therefore be used at even lower concentrations.

In a continuing quest for new psoralens with reduced side effects, the angular furocoumarin 4,6,4′-trimethylangelicin and the monofunctional 7-methylpyridopsoralen have been synthesized along with many other similar trial products. Of all the compounds tested, these two in particular have demonstrated the most promising photobiological parameters and useful antipsoriatic activity after topical application (Cristofolini *et al.*, 1990; Dubertret *et al.*, 1985) but for commercial reasons they still await further development.

As for UVB phototherapy, PUVA may be combined with a variety of adjunctive therapies. However, the efficacy of PUVA is such that these are needed only for the most severe psoriatics or the reduction of cumulative UVA doses. Nevertheless, the use of systemic retinoids with PUVA (chemophotochemotherapy or RePUVA) is one of the most potent therapeutic regimens for psoriasis (Fritsch *et al.*, 1978; Lauharanta *et al.*, 1981), the retinoid treatment perhaps being optimally initiated where possible five days before the first therapeutic irradiation, thus ridding the psoriatic lesions of their hyperkeratotic scale, helping to allow a rapid cutaneous response and reducing cumulative UVA dose by a third or more. Other combinations with, for example, cyclosporin A, methotrexate, interferon, UVB and calci-potriol have also been reported, methotrexate and calcipotriol in particular having useful effects in appropriate circumstances, but they are not yet part of standard protocols. In addition, potential synergism with regard to long-term hazards, particularly, for example, with cyclosporin A, caution against their more generalized introduction (Fitzsimons *et al.*, 1983).

PUVA FOR OTHER INDICATIONS

Vitiligo was the original indication for PUVA (Pathak and Fitzpatrick, 1992), as photoactivated psoralens not only stimulate pigment formation in normal skin but also induce the repopulation of leucoderma by surrounding melanocytes. Psoralen, 8-MOP, 5-MOP and TMP have all been used successfully in this way (Hann *et al.*, 1991; Pathak *et al.*, 1980), as have the non-psoralen compounds khellin and phenylalanine (Cormane *et al.*, 1985; Ortel *et al.*, 1988). Treatments are given 2–3 times per week, TMP being used orally at 0.6 mg/kg, which is sufficient to be therapeutically active but not to cause clinical photosensitivity, while 8- and 5-MOP dosages may be lower, at 0.3–0.6 mg/kg and 0.6–1.2 mg/kg respectively, than for psoriasis treatment in order to avoid excess phototoxicity. Phototoxic erythema of the vitiliginous skin is still the usual limiting factor for UVA dose increments and the use of topical psoralens for vitiligo treatment is therefore discouraged because of the higher risk of this. However, if there is no alternative to such therapy and the affected skin area is limited, the lower psoralen concentration range (0.1% and below) should be chosen, a 0.1% 8-MOP solution having the same efficacy as a 1% solution but leading to far fewer side effects (Grimes *et al.*, 1982).

CTCL in its early stages is another disorder optimally treated by PUVA, given its limited side effects and high efficacy (Herrmann *et al.*, 1985). The addition of systemic retinoids or interferons may also be beneficial, but more controlled investigations are required to determine precise efficacies. However, several studies in reasonably sized patient cohorts have provided data on initial CTCL response to PUVA alone, although it should be noted that varying treatment protocols, psoralen preparations and light sources were used, perhaps contributing to the heterogeneity of the published results. Nevertheless, the percentage of patients achieving complete remission during a first course of PUVA treatment was 75–100% for stage Ia, 47–100% for stage Ib, 67–83% for stage IIa, 40–100% for stage IIb and 33–100% for stage III; only a very few stage IV patients were treated with PUVA alone, the therapy being generally considered of only palliative or adjunctive value at this stage. Herrmann *et al.* (1995) have further summarized the results from five of these studies on a total of 244 patients, calculating average complete initial response rates of 90% for stage Ia, 76% for stage IIa, 59% for stage IIb and 61% for stage III.

Also of major relevance, however, are the data on long-term relapse rates and durations of disease-free intervals and according to the Swedish National Central Bureau of Statistics, it seems likely that PUVA is the reason for the significant 50% decrease in the CTCL death rate since the treatment was introduced (Swanbeck *et al.*, 1994).

Whether CTCL may be cured by PUVA remains controversial, but no other therapy seems to have a better risk:benefit ratio, particularly for early disease, while delaying more aggressive therapies by the institution of PUVA does not seem to reduce long-term survival rates. Treatment regimens follow the general recommendations for psoriasis with, for example, four exposures weekly and at least two months of maintenance therapy; in addition, individual adjustments to take account of disease variation may be required.

PLE, along with the other idiopathic photodermatoses discussed in detail earlier in this volume, is a further disorder effectively treatable by PUVA, this time as a preventive therapy (Ortel *et al.*, 1986). Regimens for PLE vary but include, for example, twice weekly gradually incrementing exposures for 3–4 weeks, which is then generally sufficient to prevent later development of the rash. Regular sun exposure may also perhaps be required to maintain protection for the summer season, although this has not been firmly established. PUVA for the treatment of other photodermatoses requires similar regimens but with low UVA dose thresholds for disease precipitation, as for example in some patients with solar urticaria, extremely careful dosimetry may be necessary, while for similar reasons, patients with chronic actinic dermatitis may often require hospitalization and concurrent systemic corticosteroid therapy in the initial PUVA phase.

A large number of additional dermatoses have also been treated on occasion with PUVA with greater or less degrees of success, these including a whole spectrum of diseases from granuloma annulare to acute graft-versus-host disease, as shown in Table 16.2.

PHOTOTHERAPY AND PUVA IN HIV-INFECTED PATIENTS

Skin disease is common in HIV-infected individuals (Stern, 1994), psoriasis and other phototherapy-sensitive dermatoses such as CTCL and vitiligo being regularly encountered (Crane *et al.*, 1991; Duvic *et al.*, 1987), while such patients also develop specific dermatoses such as pruritic papular eruption (PPE) and eosinophilic pustular folliculitis (EPF) (Bason *et al.*, 1993; Rosenthal *et al.*, 1991). However, the use of phototherapy and photochemotherapy in HIV-infected individuals has always been controversial.

First, UVB and PUVA, both able to induce systemic immune suppression, may theoretically modify patient immune status so as to lead to worsening of the HIV disease (Ullrich, 1996). Second, UV radiation, as well as psoralen photosensitization, may activate HIV promoter, which might boost viral gene transcription and eventually virus production (Morrey *et al.*, 1991). Finally, virus-induced immune suppression may promote accelerated skin carcinoma development in UVB- and PUVA-treated patients (Wang *et al.*, 1995). However, in pilot studies, UVB proved efficient and safe in the short-term for PPE, EPF and also psoriasis, the therapies not worsening the HIV disease or increasing complication rates (Meola *et al.*, 1993; Pardo *et al.*, 1992). Further, oral PUVA for psoriasis was also safe, not leading to any progression of the HIV or an increased rate of side effects (Horn *et al.*, 1994; Ranki *et al.*, 1991). It was thus concluded that UVB phototherapy and PUVA are apparently safe in HIV-positive psoriatics, while theoretical modelling of the

Table 16.2 PUVA-responsive diseases (in some diseases experience is limited to a small number of patients)

Atopic dermatitis
Chronic actinic dermatitis
Chronic hand dermatitis
Eosinophilic pustular folliculitis
Erythropoietic protoporphyria
Graft-versus-host disease (acute and chronic)
Granuloma annulare
Lichen planus
Lymphomatoid papulosis
Mycosis fungoides (cutaneous T-cell lymphoma)
Palmoplantar pustulosis
Pityriasis lichenoides
Pityriasis rubra pilaris
Polymorphic light eruption
Pruritic papular eruption of human immunodeficiency virus infection
Psoriasis
Solar urticaria
Urticaria pigmentosa
Vitiligo

putative UV-induced HIV promoter activation in human skin suggested that UVB is more likely than PUVA to activate viral transcription *in vivo* and PUVA may thus be the initial treatment of choice (Zmudzka *et al.*, 1996). Such studies are clearly encouraging, but until data from long-term observations are available, it remains ill advised to advocate the widespread use of PUVA or UVB in HIV-immunosuppressed individuals, although major hazards seem unlikely. If treatment is necessary, however, the available data and theoretical considerations suggest that UVB is more likely to be a hazard than PUVA (Morison, 1996; Zmudzka *et al.*, 1996).

SHORT- AND LONG-TERM ADVERSE EFFECTS OF UVB PHOTOTHERAPY AND PUVA

The acute adverse side effects of UVB and PUVA overdose are apparently similar, namely redness, swelling, blister formation and skin necrosis, as also seen in sunburn. However, there is a major difference in the two time courses, UVB-induced erythema peaking within 24 hours but the maximal PUVA reaction not being reached for at least 72 hours. Generalized pruritus or tingling may herald the onset of phototoxic side effects and should thus be taken as a warning sign, particularly since if large skin areas are affected, severe systemic symptoms such as fever and malaise may occur because of massive cytokine release. In such circumstances, additional measures for the alleviation of distress determined by the extent and degree of the phototoxicity may be necessary, in particular cool compresses, non-steroidal anti-inflammatory drugs and topical or even systemic corticosteroids, while future UVA dosimetry may also need adjustment. PUVA-induced pain unrelated to phototoxic burning is also rarely possible and may sometimes necessitate discontinuation of treatment. In addition, during the initial phase of PUVA with 5-MOP, an asymptomatic, transient,

maculopapular eruption not related to phototoxicity occasionally occurs, requiring symptomatic treatment only (Tanew *et al.*, 1988). Finally, photo-onycholysis and subungual haemorrhages are occasional, somewhat delayed signs of recurrent, acute, nail bed phototoxicity.

In addition to phototoxic episodes, psoralens can induce acute systemic side effects in the absence of irradiation, the most notorious being the nausea and vomiting induced by oral 8-MOP. This effect is blood level dependent, more common with 8-MOP liquid and grossly reduced by oral 5-MOP, a major reason for increased usage of this compound.

Further, accidental ocular UVB overexposure may induce photokeratitis as a result of its absorption in the conjunctiva and cornea, while UVA also penetrates the ocular lens and is itself cataractogenic at high doses. With systemic psoralen sensitization, however, psoralen-protein lens photoproducts may also be formed and the higher permeability of the juvenile ocular lens means that oral PUVA is relatively contraindicated for children younger than 12 years. However, despite the experimental animal data supporting this risk of premature cataract formation, clinical studies show no such increase in lens opacities, even in patients who have neglected careful eye protection (Calzavara-Pinton *et al.*, 1994; Cox *et al.*, 1987); on the other hand, they may sometimes suffer other ocular side effects such as conjunctival alteration instead (Calzavara-Pinton *et al.*, 1994). Notwithstanding the foregoing, eye protection is by convention mandatory during UVA exposure and also for ambient UV exposure until the evening of the treatment day.

In the long term, the cumulative adverse effects of UVB and PUVA generally resemble those associated with photoageing, or dermatoheliosis, which is the overall damage induced in skin by prolonged solar exposure. Such changes are usually confined to the permanently sun-exposed areas such as the face, neck and forearms in normal subjects, but high cumulative doses of whole-body UVB or PUVA also result in similar changes elsewhere, characterized in particular by skin pigmentary changes, xerosis, loss of elasticity, wrinkle formation and actinic keratoses. Additionally, PUVA may induce hypertrichosis, the profuse formation of dark lentigines, termed PUVA lentiginosis, and characteristic PUVA keratoses (Hönigsmann *et al.*, 1993). However, the major concern with prolonged and repeated phototherapeutic regimens is the possible induction or promotion of skin cancer (for review, see Young, 1996) and as solar radiation plays a major role in this process, PUVA patients were carefully monitored from the very beginning for the development of premalignant and malignant lesions. Such data, however, are almost all from psoriatics, as they form the largest group of patients receiving PUVA, but provide very useful information.

The cancer risk in PUVA patients is presumably related to DNA damage, but PUVA-induced downregulation of cutaneous immune responses may certainly play an additional role. In such patients, the risk of squamous cell carcinoma, but not basal cell, is significantly increased in comparison with that of matched controls, the magnitude of the increase appearing to be dose-dependent (Maier *et al.*, 1996; Stern and Laird, 1994). However, there is continuing uncertainty about the exact contribution of PUVA to these observations, many reported patients having had previous exposure to excessive sunlight and other treatments of known carcinogenicity such as for example, arsenic, UVB and immunosuppressive therapies such as methotrexate (Henseler *et al.*, 1987; Maier *et al.*, 1986). However, some authors are convinced that PUVA alone may be carcinogenic (Stern and Laird, 1994) and the male genitalia appear to be particularly susceptible, particularly in patients previously treated with tar and UVB (Stern, 1990), although it is claimed that such risk is not increased at all if only PUVA is used (Wolff and Hönigsmann, 1991).

The carcinogenicity of 5-MOP UVA therapy is unknown, but 5-MOP has shown similar activity to that of 8-MOP in *in vitro* photomutagenicity and photocarcinogenicity studies in mice (Young *et al.*, 1983).

After over 20 years of use, no substantial increase in melanoma risk has been found, even after prolonged treatment periods and high cumulative exposures (Gupta *et al.*, 1988). However, a recent study has suggested a slight increase in risk many years after the initiation of long-term therapy (Stern, 1997).

In any case, it is certainly advisable to keep cumulative UVA dosages low by utilizing UVA-sparing aggressive, therapeutic regimens without prolonged maintenance courses, which appear likely to be safer than continuous non-aggressive regimens (Gibbs *et al.*, 1986) and may perhaps slow the possible onset of PUVA carcinogenesis (Young, 1996).

Based on the results of a single Swedish study (Lindelöf *et al.*, 1982), bath PUVA seems to carry no relevant risk of carcinogenesis but since this form of therapy results in much higher epidermal psoralen concentrations than oral PUVA, the lower therapeutic UVA doses needed may conceivably induce similar numbers of mutagenic DNA lesions; on the other hand, it is just possible with bath PUVA that such lesions are concentrated at less strategically important sites. Thus, the data on long-term bath PUVA safety should be considered as encouraging in the meantime but not definitive until further information becomes available.

It is important also to compare the risks of PUVA with those of UVB phototherapy in the treatment of psoriasis. Thus, animal studies show that broad-band UVB is certainly carcinogenic but model studies indicate that the observed risk for PUVA is much higher than the calculated risk for UVB (Slaper *et al.*, 1986). As a result, there has been a marked recent trend in Europe towards use of the narrow-band 312 nm UVB lamp (Philips TL-01), although its carcinogenic risk in comparison with that of PUVA is not known.

However, it is definitely more carcinogenic than conventional broad-band UVB (for review, see Young, 1995) and it is now crucial to monitor its long-term effects.

From the information provided in this chapter and elsewhere, it is clear that the management of severe psoriatics requires long-term planning. Informed and competent physicians with appropriate experience may reach this goal by careful patient and treatment selection. Thus, for disabling psoriasis, treatment choice lies not just between high risk and complete safety but is rather a judgement among alternative options such as methotrexate, cyclosporin A, oral retinoids, PUVA and UVB, no one of which is either fully safe or fully effective. Any of this series of individual treatments and combinations may suit a given patient, but of these PUVA still has a very favourable risk:benefit ratio and so far no other single therapy (narrow-band UVB requires further confirmation) has been accepted as equally useful.

REFERENCES

Abels, D.J. and Kattan-Byron, J. (1985) Psoriasis treatment at the Dead Sea: a natural selective ultraviolet phototherapy. *Journal of the American Academy of Dermatology*, **12**, 639–43.

Addo, H.A. and Sharma, S.C. (1987) UVB phototherapy and photochemotherapy (PUVA) in the treatment of polymorphic light eruption and solar urticaria. *British Journal of Dermatology*, **116**, 539–47.

Arndt, K.A., Paul, B.S., Stern, R.S. and Parrish, J.A. (1983) Treatment of pityriasis rosea with UV radiation. *Archives of Dermatology*, **119**, 381–2.

Averbeck, D. (1989) Recent advances in psoralen phototoxicity mechanism. *Photochemistry and Photobiology*, **50**, 859–82.

Bason, M.M., Berger, T.G. and Nesbitt, L.T. Jr (1993) Pruritic papular eruption of HIV-disease. *International Journal of Dermatology*, **32**, 784–9.

Beissert, S., Hosoi, J., Grabbe, S., Asahina, A. and Granstein, R.D. (1995) IL-10 inhibits tumor antigen presentation by epidermal antigen-presenting cells. *Journal of Immunology*, **154**, 1280–6.

Berg, M., Ros, A.M. and Berne, B. (1994) Ultraviolet A phototherapy and trimethylpsoralen UVA photochemotherapy in polymorphous light eruption – a controlled study. *Photodermatology, Photoimmunology and Photomedicine*, **10**, 139–43.

Bilsland, D., George, S.A., Gibbs, N.K. and Aitchinson, T. (1993) A comparison of narrow-band phototherapy (TL-01) and photochemotherapy (PUVA) in the management of polymorphic light eruption. *British Journal of Dermatology*, **129**, 708–12.

Brickl, R., Schmid, J. and Koss, F.W. (1984) Pharmacokinetics and pharmacodynamics of psoralens after oral administration: considerations and conclusions. *National Cancer Institute Monograph*, **66**, 63–7.

British Photodermatology Group (1994) British Photodermatology Group guidelines for PUVA. *British Journal of Dermatology*, **130**, 246–55.

Brücke, J., Tanew, A., Ortel, B. and Hönigsmann, H. (1991) Relative efficacy of 335 and 365 nm radiation in photochemotherapy of psoriasis. *British Journal of Dermatology*, **124**, 372–4.

Cadet, J., Anselmino, C., Douki, T. and Voituriez, L. (1992) Photochemistry of nucleic acids in cells. *Journal of Photochemistry and Photobiology (B Biology)*, **15**, 277–98.

Calzavara-Pinton, P.G., Carlino, A., Manfredi, E. *et al.* (1994) Ocular side effects of PUVA-treated patients refusing eye sun protection. *Acta Dermatovenereologica*, **186**, 164–5.

Calzavara-Pinton, P.G., Ortel, B., Carlino, A.M., Hönigsmann, H. and De Panfilis, G. (1993) Phototesting and phototoxic side effects in bath-PUVA. *Journal of the American Academy of Dermatology*, **28**, 657–9.

Carabott, F.M. and Hawk, J.L.M. (1989) A modified dosage schedule for increased efficiency in PUVA treatment of psoriasis. *Clinical and Experimental Dermatology*, **14**, 337–40.

Collins, P. and Ferguson, J. (1995) Narrow-band UVB (TL-01) phototherapy: an effective preventative treatment for the photodermatoses. *British Journal of Dermatology*, **132**, 956–63.

Cormane, R.H., Siddiqui, A.H., Westerhof, W. and Schutgens, R.B. (1985) Phenylalanine and UVA light for the treatment of vitiligo. *Archives of Dermatological Research*, **277**, 126–30.

Cox, N.H., Jones, S.K., Downey, D.J. *et al.* (1987) Cutaneous and ocular side-effects of oral photochemotherapy: results of an 8-year follow-up study. *British Journal of Dermatology*, **116**, 145–52.

Crane, G.A., Variakojis, D., Rosen, S.T., Sands, A.M. and Roenigk, H.H. Jr (1991) Cutaneous T-cell lymphoma in patients with human immune deficiency virus infection. *Archives of Dermatology*, **127**, 989–94.

Cripps, D.J., Lowe, N.J. and Lerner, A.B. (1982) Action spectra of topical psoralens: a re-evaluation. *British Journal of Dermatology*, **107**, 77–82.

Cristofolini, M., Recchia, G., Boi, S. *et al.* (1990) 6-Methylangelicins: new monofunctional photochemotherapeutic agents for psoriasis. *British Journal of Dermatology*, **122**, 513–24.

Dall'Acqua, F. (1986) Furocoumarin photochemistry and its main biological implications, in *Current Problems in Dermatology, Vol 15. Therapeutic Photomedicine*, (eds H. Hönigsmann and G. Stingl), Karger, Basel, pp. 137–63.

Devary, Y., Rosette, C., DiDonato, J.A. and Karin, M. (1993) NF-kB activation by ultraviolet light not dependent on a nuclear signal. *Science*, **261**, 1442–5.

Diette, K.M., Momtaz, K., Stern, R.S., Arndt, K.A. and Parrish, J.A. (1984) Role of ultraviolet A in phototherapy for psoriasis. *Journal of the American Academy of Dermatology*, **11**, 441–7.

Dubertret, L., Averbeck, D., Bisagni, E. *et al.* (1985) Photochemotherapy using pyridopsoralens. *Biochimie*, **67**, 417–22.

Duvic, M., Rapini, R., Hoots, W.K. and Mansell, P.W. (1987) Human immunodeficiency virus-associated vitiligo: expression of autoimmunity with immunodeficiency? *Journal of the American Academy of Dermatology*, **17**, 656–62.

Farr, P.M. (1996) Ultraviolet phototherapy: principles and action spectra, in *The Fundamental Bases of Phototherapy*, (eds H. Hönigsmann, G. Jori and A. Young), OEMF, Milan, pp. 89–98.

Farr, P.M., Diffey, B.L., Higgins, E.M. and Matthews, J.S.N. (1991) The action spectrum between 320 and 400 nm for clearance of psoriasis by psoralen photochemotherapy. *British Journal of Dermatology*, **124**, 443–8.

Fischer, T. and Alsins, J. (1976) Treatment of psoriasis with trioxsalen baths and dysprosium lamps. *Acta Dermato-Venereologica*, **56**, 383–90.

Fisher, T. (1976) UV-light treatment of psoriasis. *Acta Dermato-Venereologica*, **56**, 473–9.

FitzSimons, C.P., Long, J. and MacKie, R.M. (1983) Synergistic carcinogenic potential of methotrexate and PUVA in psoriasis. *Lancet*, **1**, 235–6.

Fritsch, P.O., Hönigsmann, H., Jaschke, E. and Wolff, K. (1978) Augmentation of oral methoxsalen-photochemotherapy with an oral retinoic acid derivative. *Journal of Investigative Dermatology*, **70**, 178–82.

George, S.A., Bilsland, D.J., Johnson, B.E. and Ferguson, J. (1993) Narrow-band (TL-01) UVB air-conditioned phototherapy for chronic severe adult atopic dermatitis. *British Journal of Dermatology*, **128**, 49–56.

Gibbs, N.K., Hönigsmann, H. and Young, A.R. (1986) PUVA treatment strategies and cancer risk. *Lancet*, **1**, 150–1.

Gilchrest, B.A., Rowe, J.W., Brown, R.S., Steinman, T.I. and Arndt, K.A. (1979) Ultraviolet phototherapy of uremic pruritus: long-term results and possible mechanisms of action. *Annals of Internal Medicine*, **91**, 17–21.

Greaves, M.W. (1986) Ultraviolet erythema: causes and consequences, in *Current Problems in Dermatology, Vol. 15. Therapeutic Photomedicine*, (eds H. Hönigsmann and G. Stingl), Karger, Basel, pp. 18–24.

Green, C., Ferguson, J., Lakshmipathi, T. and Johnson, B.E. (1988) 311 nm UVB phototherapy – an effective treatment for psoriasis. *British Journal of Dermatology*, **119**, 691–6.

Green, C., Lakshmipathi, T., Johnson, B.E. and Ferguson, J. (1992) A comparison of the efficacy and relapse rates of narrowband UVB (TL-01) monotherapy vs. etretinate (re-TL.01) vs. etretinate-PUVA (re-PUVA) in the treatment of psoriasis patients. *British Journal of Dermatology*. **127**, 5–9.

Grimes, P.E., Minus, H.R., Chakrabarti, S.G. *et al.* (1982) Determination of optimal topical photochemotherapy for vitiligo. *Journal of the American Academy of Dermatology*, **7**, 771–8.

Gupta, A.K., Stern, R.S., Swanson, N.A., Anderson, T.F. and the PUVA Follow-up Study (1988) Cutaneous melanomas in patients treated with psoralen plus ultraviolet. *Journal of the American Academy of Dermatology*, **19**, 67–76.

Hann, S.K., Cho, M.Y., Im, S. and Park, Y.K. (1991) Treatment of vitiligo with oral 5-methoxypsoralen. *Journal of Dermatology*, **18**, 324–9.

Henseler, T., Christophers, E., Hönigsmann, H. and Wolff, K. (1987) Skin tumors in the European PUVA study: eight year follow-up of 1643 patients treated with PUVA for psoriasis. *Journal of the American Academy of Dermatology*, **16**, 108–16.

Henseler, T., Wolff, K., Hönigsmann, H. and Christophers, E. (1981) The European PUVA study (EPS): oral 8-methoxypsoralen photochemotherapy of psoriasis. A cooperative study among 18 European centres. *Lancet*, **1**, 853–7.

Herfst, M.J. and De Wolff, F.A. (1983) Intra-individual and interindividual variability in 8-methoxypsoralen kinetics and effect in psoriatic patients. *Clinical Pharmacology and Therapeutics* **34**, 117–25.

Herrmann, J.J., Roenigk, H.H. Jr and Hönigsmann, H. (1995) Ultraviolet radiation for treatment of cutaneous T-cell lymphoma. *Hematology and Oncology Clinics of North America*, **9**, 1077–88.

Hönigsmann, H., Calzavara-Pinton, P.G. and Ortel, B. (1994) Phototherapy and photochemotherapy, in *Psoriasis*, (ed. L. Dubertret), ISED, Brescia, pp. 135–500.

Hönigsmann, H., Fitzpatrick, T.B., Pathak, M.A. and Wolff, K. (1993) Oral photochemotherapy with psoralens and UVA (PUVA): principles and practice, in *Dermatology in General Medicine*, 4th edn, (eds T.B. Fitzpatrick *et al.*), McGraw-Hill, New York, pp. 1728–54.

Hönigsmann, H., Fritsch, P. and Jaschke, E. (1977) UV-Therapie der Psoriasis. Halbseitenvergleich zwischen oraler Photochemotherapie (PUVA) and selektiver UV-Phototherapie (SUP). *Zeitschrift für Hautkrankheiten*, **52**, 1078–82.

Hönigsmann, H., Jaschke, E., Nitsche, V. *et al.* (1982) Serum levels of 8-methoxypsoralen in two different drug preparations. Correlation with photosensitivity and UVA dose requirements for photochemotherapy. *Journal of Investigative Dermatology*, **79**, 233–6.

Horn, T.D., Morison, W.L., Farzadegan, H., Zmudzka, B.Z. and Beer, J.Z. (1994) Effects of psoralen plus UVA radiation (PUVA) on HIV-1 in human beings: a pilot study. *Journal of the American Academy of Dermatology*, **31**, 735–40.

Hruza, L.L. and Pentland, A.P. (1993) Mechanisms of UV-induced inflammation. *Journal of Investigative Dermatology*, **100**, 35S–41S.

Iest, J. and Boer, J. (1989) Combined treatment of psoriasis with acitretin and UVB phototherapy compared with acitretin alone and UVB alone. *British Journal of Dermatology*, **120**, 665–70.

Jekler, J. (1992) Phototherapy of atopic dermatitis with ultraviolet radiation. *Acta Dermato-Venereologica*, **171** (suppl.), 1–37.

Jekler, J. and Larkö, O. (1988) UVB phototherapy of atopic dermatitis. *British Journal of Dermatology*, **119**, 697–705.

Jekler, J. and Larkö, O. (1991) Phototherapy for atopic dermatitis with ultraviolet A (UVA), low-dose UVB and combined UVA and UVB: two paired-comparison studies. *Photodermatology, Photoimmunology and Photomedicine*, **8**, 151–6.

Johnson, R., Staiano-Coico, L., Austin, L. *et al.* (1996) PUVA treatment selectively induces a cell cycle block and subsequent apoptosis in human T-lymphocytes. *Photochemistry and Photobiology*, **63**, 566–71.

Kaidbey, K.H. (1985) An action spectrum for 8-methoxypsoralen-sensitized inhibition of DNA synthesis *in vivo*. *Journal of Investigative Dermatology*, **85**, 98–101.

Karvonen, J., Kokkonen, E.L. and Ruotsalainen, E. (1989) 311 nm UVB lamps in the treatment of psoriasis with the Ingram regimen. *Acta Dermatovenereologica*, **69**, 82–5.

Kerscher, M., Dirschka, T. and Volkenandt, M. (1995) Treatment of localised scleroderma by UVA1 phototherapy. *Lancet*, **346**, 1166.

Kerscher, M., Volkenandt, M., Plewig, G. and Lehmann, P. (1993) Combination phototherapy of psoriasis with calcipotriol and narrow-band UVB. *Lancet*, **342**, 9.

Kowalzick, L., Kleinheinz, A., Weichenthal, M. *et al.* (1995) Low dose versus medium dose UV-A1 treatment in severe atopic eczema. *Acta Dermato-Venereologica*, **75**, 43–5.

Krutmann, J., Czech, W., Diepgen, T. *et al.* (1992) High-dose UVA1 therapy in the treatment of patients with atopic dermatitis. *Journal of the American Academy of Dermatology*, **26**, 225–30.

Lauharanta, J., Juvakoski, T. and Lassus, A. (1981) A clinical evaluation of the effects of an aromatic retinoid (Tigason), combination of retinoid and PUVA, and PUVA alone in severe psoriasis. *British Journal of Dermatology*, **104**, 325–32.

Lebwohl, M., Martinez, J., Weber, P. and De Luca, R. (1995) Effects of topical preparations on the erythemogenicity of UVB: implications for psoriasis phototherapy. *Journal of the American Academy of Dermatology*, **32**, 469–71.

Lindelöf, B., Sigurgeirsson, B., Tegner, E., Larkö, O. and Berne, B. (1992) Comparison of the carcinogenic potential of trioxsalen bath PUVA and oral methoxsalen PUVA. A preliminary report. *Archives of Dermatology*, **128**, 1341–4.

Liu, M. and Pellingo, J.C. (1995) UV-B/A irradiation of mouse keratinocytes result in p53-mediated WAF-1/CIP-1 expression. *Oncogene*, **10**, 1955–60.

McGrath, H. Jr (1994) Ultraviolet-A1 irradiation decreases clinical disease activity and autoantibodies in patients with systemic lupus erythematosus. *Clinical and Experimental Rheumatology*, **12**, 129–35.

Maier, H., Schemper, M., Ortel, B. *et al.* (1996) Skin tumours in photochemotherapy for psoriasis.

A single centre follow-up of 496 patients. *Dermatology*, **193**, 185–91.

Melski, J.W., Tanenbaum, L., Fitzpatrick, T.B., Bleich, H.L. and Parrish, J.A. (1977) Oral methoxsalen photochemotherapy for the treatment of psoriasis: a cooperative clinical trial. *Journal of Investigative Dermatology*, **68**, 328–35.

Meola, T., Soter, N.A., Ostreicher, R., Sanchez, M. and Moy, J.A. (1993) The safety of UVB phototherapy in patients with HIV infection. *Journal of the American Academy of Dermatology*, **29**, 216–20.

Midelfart, K., Stenvold, S.E. and Volden, G. (1986) Combined UVB and UVA phototherapy of atopic eczema. *Dermatologica*, **171**, 95–8.

Moan, J. and Peak, M.J. (1989) Effects of UV radiation of cells. *Journal of Photochemistry and Photobiology (B Biology)*, **4**, 21–34.

Morison, W.L. (1994) UVA-1 phototherapy of lupus erythematosus. *Lupus*, **3**, 139–41.

Morison, W.L. (1996) PUVA therapy is preferable to UVB phototherapy in the management of HIV-associated dermatoses. *Photochemistry and Photobiology*, **64**, 267–8.

Morrey, J.D., Bourn, S.M., Bunch, T.D. *et al* (1991) *In vivo* activation of human immunodeficiency virus type I long terminal repeat by UV type A (UV-A) light plus psoralen and UV-B light in the skin of transgenic mice. *Journal of Virology*, **65**, 5045–51.

Ortel, B. and Gange, R.W. (1990) An action spectrum for the elicitation of erythema in skin persistently sensitized by photobound 8-methoxypsoralen. *Journal of Investigative Dermatology*, **94**, 781–5.

Ortel, B., Perl, S., Kinaciyan, T., Calzavara-Pinton, P.G. and Hönigsmann, H. (1993) Comparison of narrow-band (311 nm) UVB and broad-band UVA after oral or bath-water 8-methoxypsoralen in the treatment of psoriasis. *Journal of the American Academy of Dermatology*, **29**, 736–40.

Ortel, B., Tanew, A. and Hönigsmann, H. (1988) Treatment of vitiligo with khellin and ultraviolet A. *Journal of the American Academy of Dermatology*, **18**, 693–701.

Ortel, B., Tanew, A., Wolff, K. and Hönigsmann, H. (1986) Polymorphous light eruption: action spectrum and photoprotection. *Journal of the American Academy of Dermatology*, **14**, 748–53.

Pardo, R.J., Bogaert, M.A., Penneys, N.S., Byrne, G.E. and Ruiz, P. (1992) UVB phototherapy of the pruritic papular eruption of the acquired immunodeficiency syndrome. *Journal of the American Academy of Dermatology*, **26**, 423–8.

Parrish, J.A. and Jaenicke, K.F. (1981) Action spectrum for phototherapy of psoriasis. *Journal of Investigative Dermatology*, **76**, 359–62.

Parrish, J.A., Fitzpatrick, T.B., Tanenbaum, L. and Pathak, M.A. (1974) Photochemotherapy of psoriasis with oral methoxsalen and long wave ultraviolet light. *New England Journal of Medicine*, **291**, 1207–11.

Pathak, M.A. and Fitzpatrick, T.B. (1992) The evolution of photochemotherapy with psoralens and UVA (PUVA): 2000 BC to 1992 AD. *Journal of Photochemistry and Photobiology (B Biology)*, **14**, 3–22.

Pathak, M.A., Mosher, D.B., Parrish, J.A. and Fitzpatrick, T.B. (1980) Relative effectiveness of three psoralens and sunlight in repigmentation of 365 vitiligo patients. *Journal of Investigative Dermatology*, **74**, 252.

Petit Frere, C., Clingen, P.H., Arlett, C.F. and Green, M.H. (1996) Inhibition of RNA and DNA synthesis in UV-irradiated normal human fibroblasts is correlated with pyrimidine (6–4) pyrimidone photoproduct formation. *Mutation Research*, **354**, 87–94.

Picot, E., Meunier, L., Picot-Debeze, M.C., Peyron, J.L. and Meynadier, J. (1992) Treatment of psoriasis with a 311-nm UVB lamp. *British Journal of Dermatology*. **127**, 509–12.

Porneuf, M., Guillot, B., Barneon, G. and Guilhou, J.J. (1993) Eosinophilic pustular folliculitis responding to UVB therapy. *Journal of the American Academy of Dermatology*, **29**, 259–60.

Quinn, A.G., Diffey, B.L., Craig, P.S. and Farr, P.M. (1994) Definition of the minimal erythema dose used for diagnostic phototesting. *British Journal of Dermatology*, **131**, 56.

Ranki, A., Puska, P., Mattinen, S., Lagerstedt, A. and Krohn, K. (1991) Effect of PUVA on immunologic and virologic findings in HIV-infected patients. *Journal of the American Academy of Dermatology*, **24**, 404–10.

Ronai, Z.A., Lambert, M.E. and Weinstein, I.B. (1992) Inducible cellular responses to ultraviolet light irradiation and other mediators of DNA damage in mammalian cells. *Cell Biology and Toxicology*, **6**, 105–26.

Rosenthal, D., LeBoit, P.E., Klumpp, L. and Berger, T.G. (1991) Human immunodeficiency virus-associated eosinophilic folliculitis. A unique dermatosis associated with advanced human immunodeficiency virus infection. *Archives of Dermatology*, **127**, 206–9.

Sakuntabhai, A., Diffey, B.L. and Farr, P.M. (1993) Response of psoriasis to psoralen-UVB photochemotherapy. *British Journal of Dermatology*, **128**, 296–300.

Schmitt, I., Chimenti, S. and Gasparro, F. (1995) Psoralen-protein photochemistry – the forgotten field. *Journal of Photochemistry and Photobiology (B Biology)*, **27**, 101–5.

Schröpl, F. (1977) Zum heutigen Stand der technischen Entwicklung der selektiven Phototherapie. *Der Deutsche Dermatologe*, **25**, 499–504.

Schwarz, T. and Luger, T.A. (1989) Effect of UV irradiation on epidermal cell cytokine production. *Journal of Photochemistry and Photobiology (B Biology)*, **4**, 1–13.

Slaper, H., Schothorst, A.A. and Van Der Leun, J.C. (1986) Risk evaluation of UVB therapy for psoriasis: comparison of calculated risk for UVB therapy and observed risk in PUVA-treated patients. *Photodermatology*, **3**, 271–83.

Steigleder, G.K., Orfanos, C.E. and Pullmann, H. (1979) Retinoid-SUP-Therapie der Psoriasis. *Zeitschrift für Hautkrankheiten*, **54**, 19–23.

Stern, R.S. (1994) Epidemiology of skin disease in HIV infection: a cohort study of health maintenance organization members. *Journal of Investigative Dermatology*, **102**, 34S–37S.

Stern, R.S. and Laird, N. for the Photochemotherapy Follow-up Study (1994) The carcinogenic risks of treatments for severe psoriasis. *Cancer*, **73**, 2759–64.

Stern, R.S., Nichols, K.T. and Vakeva, L.H. (1997) Malignant melanoma in patients treated for psoriasis with methoxsalen (psoralen) and ultraviolet A radiation (PUVA). The PUVA Follow-Up Study. *New England Journal of Medicine*, **336**, 1041–5.

Stern, R.S. and members of the Photochemotherapy Follow-up Study (1990) Genital tumors among men with psoriasis exposed to psoralens and ultraviolet A (PUVA) radiation and ultraviolet B radiation. *New England Journal of Medicine*, **322**, 1093–7.

Storbeck, K., Hölzle, E., Schurer, N., Lehmann, P. and Plewig, G. (1993) Narrow-band UVB (311 nm) versus conventional broad-band UVB with and without dithranol in phototherapy for psoriasis. *Journal of the American Academy of Dermatology*, **28**, 227–31.

Swanbeck, G., Roupe, G. and Sandström, M.H. (1994) Indications of a considerable decrease in the death rate in mycosis fungoides by PUVA treatment. *Acta Dermato-Venereologica*, **74**, 465–6.

Tanenbaum, L., Parrish, J.A., Pathak, M.A., Anderson, R.R. and Fitzpatrick, T.B. (1975) Tar phototoxicity and phototherapy for psoriasis. *Archives of Dermatology*, **111**, 467–70.

Tanew, A., Fijan, S. and Hönigsmann, H. (1996) Halfside comparison study on narrow-band UV-B phototherapy versus photochemotherapy (PUVA) in the treatment of severe psoriasis. *Journal of Investigative Dermatology*, **106**, 212.

Tanew, A., Ortel, B., Rappersberger, K. and Hönigsmann, H. (1988) 5-methoxypsoralen (Bergapten) for photochemotherapy. *Journal of the American Academy of Dermatology*, **18**, 333–8.

Taylor, C.R., Kwangsustich, C., Hruza, L. *et al.* (1996) *Dihydroxyacetone-enhanced PUVA for Psoriasis: A Pilot Study. 12th International Congress of Photobiology*, Vienna, Austria, p. 262.

Tessman, J.W., Isaacs, S.T. and Hearst, J.E. (1985) Photochemistry of the furan-side 8-methoxypsoralen-thymidine monoadduct inside the DNA helix. Conversion to diadduct and to pyrone-side monoadduct. *Biochemistry*, **24**, 1669–76.

Ullrich, S.E. (1995) Modulation of immunity by ultraviolet radiation: key effects on antigen presentation. *Journal of Investigative Dermatology*, **105**, 30S–36S.

Ullrich, S.E. (1996) Does exposure to UV radiation induce a shift to a Th-2-like immune reaction? *Photochemistry and Photobiology*, **64**, 254–8.

Urbanski, A., Schwarz, T., Neuner, P. *et al.* (1990) Ultraviolet light induces increased circulating interleukin-6 in humans. *Journal of Investigative Dermatology*, **94**, 808–11.

Vallat, V., Gillaudeau, P., Battat, L. *et al.* (1994) PUVA bath therapy strongly suppresses immunological and epidermal activation in psoriasis: a possible cellular basis for remittive therapy. *Journal of Experimental Medicine*, **180**, 283–96.

Van Der Leun, J.C. and Van Weelden, H. (1986) UV-B phototherapy: principles, radiation sources, regimens, in *Current Problems in Dermatology, Vol. 15. Therapeutic Photomedicine*, (eds H. Hönigsmann and G. Stingl), Karger, Basel, pp. 39–54.

Van Weelden, H., De La Faille, H.B., Young, E. and Van Der Leun, I.C. (1988) A new development in UVB phototherapy of psoriasis. *British Journal of Dermatology*, **119**, 11–19.

Van Weelden, H., De La Faille, H.B., Young, E. and Van Der Leun, J.C. (1990) Comparison on narrow-band UV-B phototherapy and PUVA photochemotherapy in the treatment of psoriasis. *Acta Dermato-Venereologica*, **70**, 212–15.

Wang, C.Y., Brodland, D.G. and Su, W.P. (1995) Skin cancers associated with acquired immunodeficiency syndrome. *Mayo Clinic Proceedings*, **70**, 766–72.

Warmuth, I., Harth, Y., Matsui, M.S., Wang, N. and DeLeo, V.A. (1994) Ultraviolet radiation induces phosphorylation of the epidermal growth factor receptor. *Cancer Research*, **54**, 374–6.

Wolff, K. and Hönigsmann, H. (1991) Genital carcinoma in psoriasis patients treated with photochemotherapy. *Lancet*, **1**, 439.

Wolff, K., Hönigsmann, H., Gschnait, F. and Konrad, K. (1975) Photochemotherapie bei Psoriasis. Klinische Erfahrungen bei 152 Patienten. *Deutsche Medizinische Wochenschrift*, **100**, 2471–7.

Young, A.R. (1995) Carcinogenicity of UVB phototherapy assessed. *Lancet*, **345**, 1431–2.

Young, A.R. (1996) Photochemotherapy and skin carcinogenesis: a critical review, in *The Fundamental Bases of Phototherapy*, (eds H. Hönigsmann, G. Jori and A.R. Young), OEMF, Milan, pp. 77–87.

Young, A.R., Magnus, I.A., Davies, A.C. and Smith, N.P. (1983) A comparison of the phototumorigenic potential of 8-MOP and 5-MOP in hairless albino mice exposed to solar simulated irradiation. *British Journal of Dermatology*, **108**, 507–18.

Zmudzka, B.Z., Miller, S.A., Jacobs, M.E. and Beer, J.Z. (1996) Medical UV exposures and HIV activation. *Photochemistry and Photobiology*, **64**, 246–53.

THE PHOTOBIOLOGY AND THEORETICAL APPLICATIONS OF LASERS

17

Robert M. Herd, Jeffrey S. Dover and Kenneth A. Arndt

INTRODUCTION

HISTORY

In 1917, through the vision of Albert Einstein, the stimulated emission of electromagnetic (EM) radiation was first conceived (Einstein, 1917). The theory was that a photon of a certain EM energy could stimulate an already excited atom possessing the equivalent transition energy to emit another photon of that energy. The validity of this hypothesis was confirmed in a practical experiment ten years later, but the world had to wait until 1960 for the development of the first equipment to employ this technique – the laser, an acronym of light amplification by stimulated emission of radiation (Maiman, 1960). This construction of synthetic ruby surrounded by a helical flashlamp heralded the start of the laser revolution.

Some of today's most commonly used lasers, in particular including the neodymium-doped yttrium aluminium garnet (Nd:YAG), carbon dioxide (CO_2), organic dye and argon varieties, appeared in the early years. These opened up a wide range of applications, particularly in the communications, defence and music industries, which were subsequently further developed. The expansion of the

Photodermatology. Edited by J.L.M. Hawk. Published in 1998 by Chapman & Hall, London. ISBN 0 412 72460 X.

technique into medicine, however, began in the early 1960s, when the accessibility of the eye and skin made them the objects of research into the new technology. Further medical applications were then discovered when the argon and CO_2 lasers were introduced in the early 1970s. Research in the 1980s further enhanced understanding of laser–tissue interactions, following which a plethora of new devices provided many novel ways of treating a host of difficult conditions.

ELECTROMAGNETIC RADIATION AND LASERS

The majority of laser emissions fall in or close to the visible EMR wavelengths between 400 and 700 nm (Fig. 17.1), short wavelength X-rays and gamma rays merely causing a non-specific ionization of tissue molecules, far infrared energy instead heating them indiscriminately and imprecisely.

However, although visible light of low energy impacts the skin constantly with little discernible effect, large amounts of such energy directed at a localized area of skin may lead, through its absorption by appropriate chromophores, to specific changes which can be controlled precisely by adjusting the size, shape, duration and intensity of the incident beam.

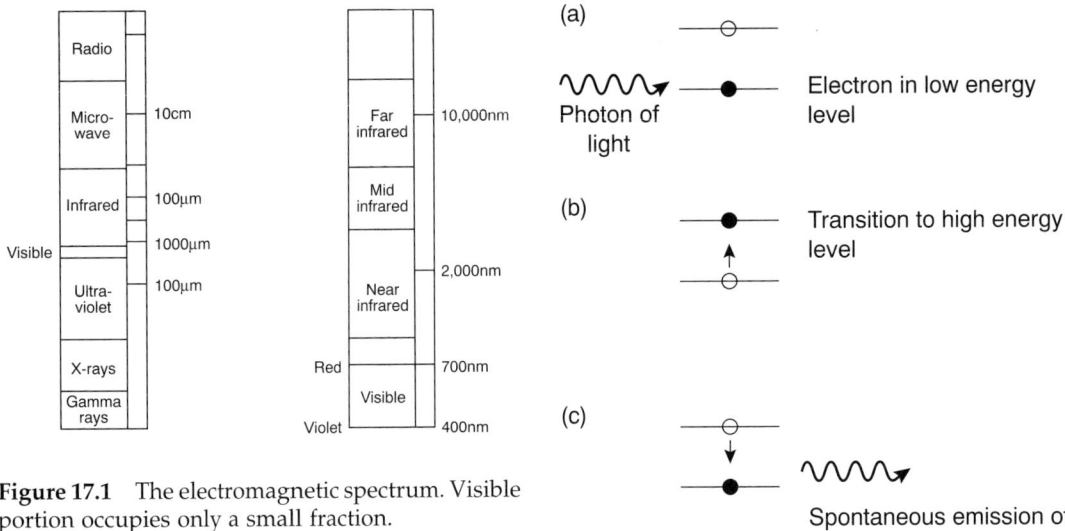

Figure 17.1 The electromagnetic spectrum. Visible portion occupies only a small fraction.

SPONTANEOUS AND STIMULATED EMISSION

Electrons surrounding an atom or molecule may exist at more than one energy level, usually the lowest or resting state, where they are stable. However, this energy may be increased or diminished in discrete steps or quanta of EMR energy known as **photons**, leading to a corresponding change in the energy level of the electron (Fig. 17.2). For example, an electron in the resting state, following the absorption of a photon of light of the correct wavelength, moves to one of its excited states. However, it is generally unstable in this new state and as a result drops back to its resting state, thus re-releasing a photon of energy. This form of generation of EMR is called **spontaneous emission**. However, such emission can also be stimulated. Thus, although during spontaneous emission there is always a drop to a lower energy state, this transition can occur earlier if the electron is first stimulated by another photon of equivalent energy, in this instance resulting in the release of two photons with identical energies, directions and phases (Fig. 17.3), a process known as **stimulated emission**.

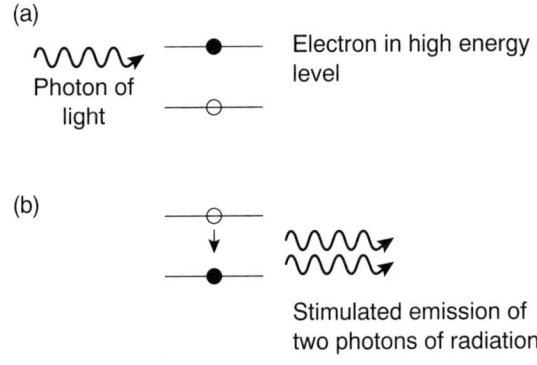

Figure 17.2 (a) Electron in the resting state. (b) Electron after absorption of energy changes to its excited state. (c) Spontaneous emission of radiation

(a)
Photon of light — Electron in high energy level

(b)
Stimulated emission of two photons of radiation

Figure 17.3 Stimulated emission. (a) Absorption of another photon of equivalent energy. (b) Stimulated emission of radiation: two photons of identical energy in the same direction and in perfect phase.

The photons released during stimulated emission are then of the correct energy to stimulate further emissions from excited atoms of the same type. However, in normal circumstances the majority of atoms are in the resting state such that stimulated emission is a rare event and only when the majority move into the excited state does such emission become likely. This increase in the proportion of excited atoms is a prerequisite for laser function and is called **population inversion**, photons then having a higher than even chance of encountering an excited electron to stimulate a further photon emission of the same energy, which may then do the same again. To induce such a population inversion with its associated high frequency of stimulated emissions, an external electrical, chemical or light source is necessary, in a process known as **pumping**.

These mechanisms are used directly in the construction of a laser (Fig. 17.4). Thus, an external source of energy is needed to create a population inversion in the laser chamber, while photons produced in the axis of the chamber during the stimulated emission process are reflected off mirrors at either end to stimulate further emissions again in the same axis. One of the mirrors, however, is only partially reflective, thus allowing some of the energy to escape to form the laser beam.

The so-called gain medium in the laser chamber where energy amplification occurs may be a solid (e.g. synthetic ruby), liquid (e.g. organic dye) or gas (e.g. CO_2), each having distinctive atomic energy transitions which determine the wavelength of the emitted light. There are various ways of pumping the system from an external power source as well and examples of these are described later.

PROPERTIES OF LASER RADIATION

MONOCHROMATICITY

Laser radiation is very different from that from an electric light or the sun and contains only a very narrow band of wavelengths as compared with the white light from other sources, which consists of a wide spectrum. Laser radiation is thus essentially **monochromatic**.

COHERENCE

Laser radiation beams from any given source travel virtually parallel to one another, their divergence being measured in fractions of a degree, in contrast to those of an electric light which diverge quite markedly (Fig. 17.5). This minimal divergence is called **spatial coherence** or **collimation** and allows a laser beam to be transmitted over long distances without loss of intensity or to be focused to a small spot with very high power density. The photons of laser radiation are also essen-

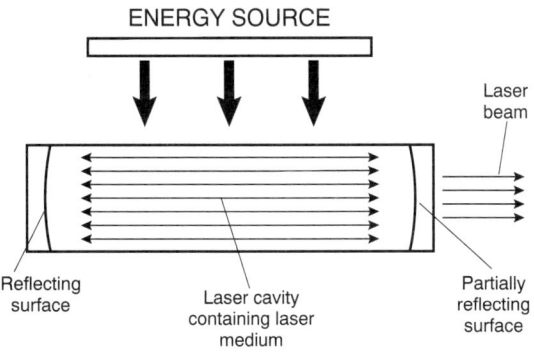

Figure 17.4   The production of laser radiation.

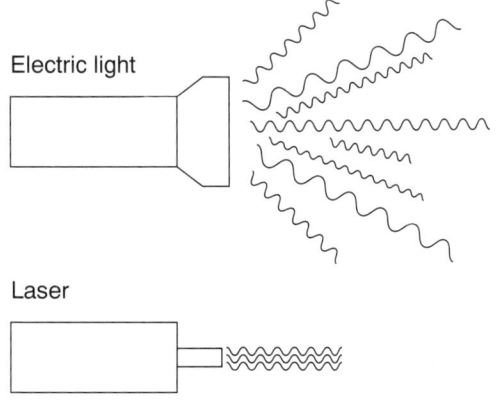

Figure 17.5   The contrast between light from an electric light and a laser.

tially in phase with each other or **temporally coherent**.

Radiation from a laser is thus analogous to a marching band of soldiers, the emitted photons marching in time with one another so as to have equal strides (monochromaticity) and aligned rows (temporal coherence) and columns with fixed spacings between them (spatial coherence). On the other hand, white light is equivalent to a crowded street of individuals walking at different paces with different stride lengths and in different directions. Many of the advantages of laser surgery are attributable to these properties.

RADIOMETRY

Laser novices may be alienated by the terminology of power and energy. However, such fundamental language is needed to describe precisely the complexities of laser radiation and its interactions with skin and four simple definitions only are required, namely of energy, power, fluence (energy density, radiation dose) and irradiance (Fisher, 1993).

Energy is work or the potential to accomplish work and is measured in joules. **Power** is the rate at which such energy is expended and is measured in watts (joules per second). Joules are thus a suitable measure of energy of a single output burst, from a pulsed laser, whereas watts should be used to denote the prolonged emission of a continuous wave device.

Energy and power thus quantify the radiation output as it leaves a laser, but also needed is a measure of the radiation reaching the skin, which in turn depends on the area of skin over which it is spread and the radiation beam profile. This incident radiation is denoted as the **energy density, radiation dose** or **fluence**. In other words:

Energy density = Joules per unit area,

Generally   = $\dfrac{\text{Joules}}{\text{cm}^2}$

Thus, if a pulsed laser with energy per pulse of 10 J is focused to a 1 cm spot size (radius 0.5 cm), then the area of the spot is $\pi r^2 = \pi \times (0.5)^2$ and the energy density is

$$\frac{10}{\pi \times (0.5)^2} = 12.7 \text{ J per cm}^2$$

If the same energy is then focused to a spot size of 0.5 cm, the area of the new spot is $\pi r^2 = \pi \times (0.25)^2$ and the energy density is now:

$$\frac{10}{\pi \times (0.25)^2} = 50.9 \text{ J per cm}^2$$

Halving the spot size therefore increases the energy density at the target by a factor of 4, and as a general rule, the energy density is thus inversely proportional to the square of the radius of the spot size. Conversely, to achieve the same energy density with a spot size of one half the previous diameter, the laser energy output would have to be reduced by a factor of 4.

Irradiance refers to the intensity, or dose rate, of a continuous wave laser beam and is measured in watts per cm². Calculations similar to those above show the same relationship between spot size and irradiance as between spot size and fluence. Thus, irradiance is inversely proportional to the square of the radius of the spot size.

LASER TIME DEPENDENCE

Lasers can be divided into two categories, namely continuous wave (CW) and pulsed (Fig. 17.6). In the CW mode, lasers work unremittingly and deliver constant power. Examples are the argon and CW dye lasers used for vascular coagulation, while a similar effect results from quasi-CW devices such as the copper vapour laser, which emits a train of pulses at a frequency of 15 000 per second, so fast that the skin responds as if to a continuous beam of light

One limitation of CW lasers is their low peak power and while they can be shuttered

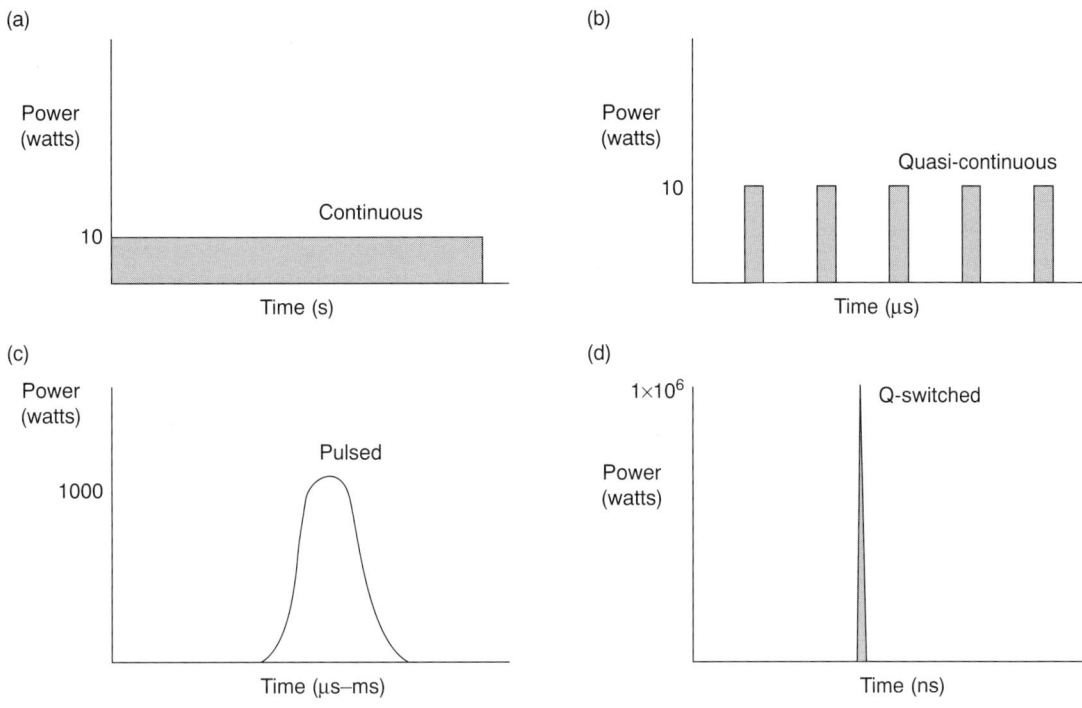

Figure 17.6 The time dependence of (a) continuous, (b) quasi-continuous, (c) pulsed-dye and (d) Q-switched lasers.

to produce short emission times, they are still not the equivalent of pulsed lasers, which produce short emissions of high peak power. True pulsed lasers for cutaneous surgery produce pulses of 1 ms or shorter, for skin resurfacing and vascular anomalies and of 1 μs to 1 ms and for pigmented disorders. In addition, these last are also usually **Q-switched** or **mode locked**, Q referring to the quality of the laser chamber which may be changed suddenly to produce a short, intense light, the value of Q being the ratio of the energy stored in the laser cavity to the energy uselessly dissipated and usually constant; thus, if the laser is run with most of the energy allowed to disperse, the Q ratio is low. A sudden change in the optical properties of the laser cavity may then be used to increase the amount of energy stored, thus creating a sudden population inversion in the lasing medium and a short burst of high energy light, an alteration known as **Q switching**.

BEAM TYPE

A change in the profile of a laser beam can also alter the tissue effect as much as a change in the fluence. Thus, some laser beams have an identical energy across their whole area, referred to as a top-hat distribution (Plate 34), while others have more energy centrally and are called Gaussian beams (Plate 35). Tissue effects vary because a Gaussian beam has a greater effect centrally and less peripherally than a top-hat beam of identical spot size and a knowledge of the beam profile is thus clearly pertinent, particularly when a laser from a different manufacturer is used (Jackson *et al.*, 1996).

SKIN OPTICS

When a laser beam strikes the skin, there are various possible outcomes: it can be reflected or transmitted and scattered and absorbed or transmitted and scattered before passing again out of the skin (Fig. 17.7). However, the Grotthus–Draper Law states that a tissue effect can only occur if the radiation is absorbed and thus neither the 4–7% of the light reflected from nor that passed through a tissue has any effect (Anderson and Parrish, 1981). On the other hand, a chromophore in the skin absorbs specific wavelengths selectively and if its absorption spectrum is known, laser light of that wavelength can then be directed at it to produce a desired tissue effect.

Tailoring the laser wavelength to a skin chromophore is not, however, easy. The principal chromophores in the skin are haemoglobin, water and melanin (Fig. 17.8) and since over the visible radiation spectrum, the depth of penetration is dependent on absorption by them and scattering, it is essentially inversely related to wavelength; thus, the longer the wavelength, the deeper the penetration (Fig 17.9) (Parrish and Deutsch, 1984). However, a relative optical window exists in the region 600–1300 nm in that at wavelengths below 300 nm, there is strong absorption by melanin and also by protein, urocanic acid and DNA, while between 300 nm and 600 nm

haemoglobin and melanin are the significant chromophores and over 1300 nm, despite the longer wavelengths, the penetration is relatively shallow because of the absorption of radiation by water, the dominant chromophore at this end of the spectrum

The difficulty in selecting a wavelength for a chromophore can be illustrated by the example of haemoglobin, which has an absorption peak at 420 nm, too short for treating cutaneous vascular lesions such as port-wine stains because penetration is only 100 μm, to the region of the dermoepidermal junction. Clearly, to have a biological effect on dermal vessels it is necessary for the radiation to penetrate more deeply with a longer wavelength such as 577 nm (Fig. 17.8), at which, although the haemoglobin absorption is now significantly less than at its 420 nm peak, it is more efficient because sufficient radiation now penetrates to the dermis.

TISSUE INTERACTIONS

THERMAL EFFECTS

Laser light can only impose a tissue effect when absorbed and converted into energy, mostly heat. The biological effect is determined by the temperature achieved. Cell injury and subsequent inflammation and repair occur after increases of only 5–10°C

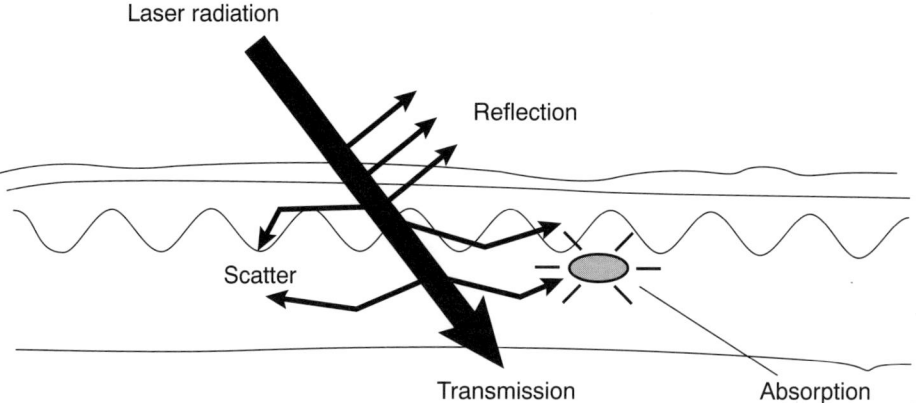

Figure 17.7 Laser radiation can be reflected, scattered, absorbed or transmitted.

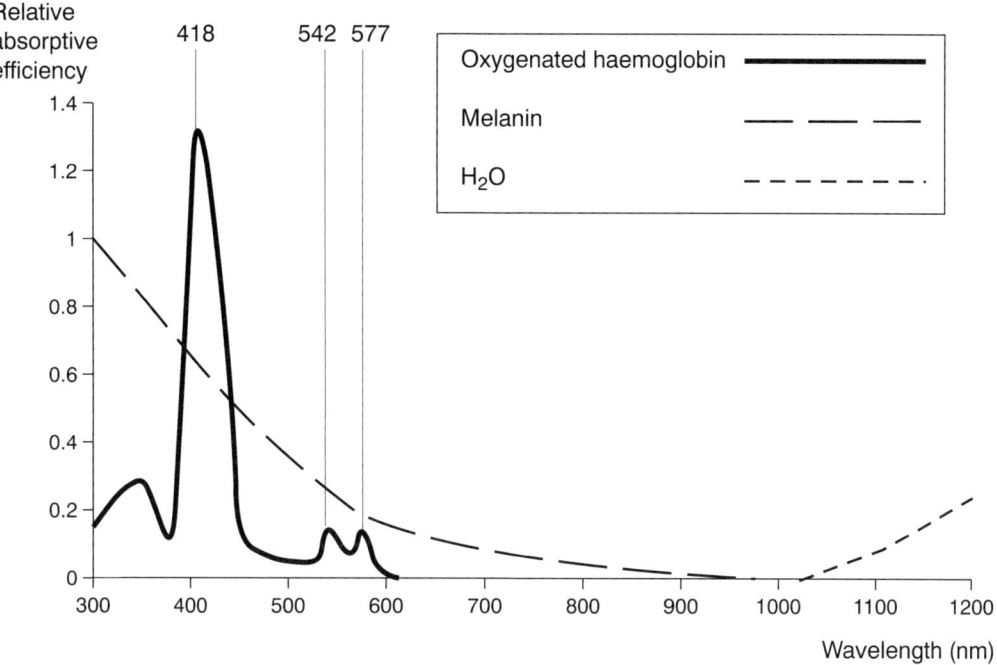

Figure 17.8   The absorption spectra of the principal skin chromophores: melanin, oxyhaemoglobin and water. Haemoglobin has absorption peaks at 418nm, 542nm and 577nm.

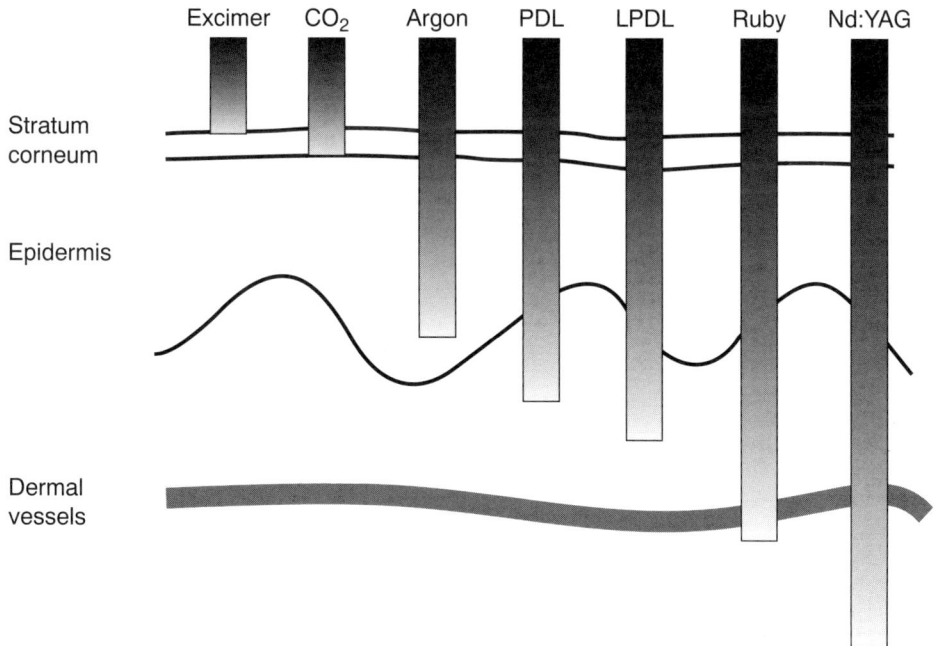

Figure 17.9   Comparative depth of penetration of some commonly used medical lasers (PDL, pulsed-dye laser; LPDL, long-pulsed-dye laser).

(Parrish and Deutsch, 1984), while higher temperatures below 100°C denature macro-molecules, for instance by breaking Van Der Waal's bonds. Most proteins are denatured above 60°C and DNA above 70°C (Anderson and Parrish, 1983). At temperatures of over 100°C, the intracellular water temperature exceeds boiling point and vaporization can occur, the steam produced causing a rapid increase in pressure that damages cells and blood vessels. Further heating at these temperatures then leads to desiccation and charring.

To achieve the desired alteration in skin structures, the temperature rise and resultant effect must be reproducible with heat conduction taken into account. When light is absorbed heat loss begins immediately by conduction to adjacent tissues in all directions, a process known as **thermal relaxation**. The speed of thermal relaxation varies according to the thermal relaxation time (TRT) of the tissue, defined as the time it takes for a structure to cool to half the temperature to which it was heated. Small objects cool faster than large ones: melanosomes of 0.5–1 μm have a shorter TRT (around 1 μs) than capillaries measuring 10–100 μm (around 1 ms). The TRTs of some important skin chromophores are shown in Table 17.1.

The tissue effect is caused by the primary influence of laser energy heating a chromophore, and from the secondary spread of heat to the adjacent tissues. The extent of the thermal damage is influenced first by the height of the temperature achieved, which

determines the damage to the target, and second by the length of time the target is at that temperature, which in turn is influenced by heat conduction, and thus the extent of overall tissue damage is governed by the fluence and pulse duration, along with the tissue heat conduction.

MECHANICAL EFFECTS

Lasers also cause photomechanical effects (Sigrist and Kneubuhl, 1978; Watanabe *et al.*, 1988). Thus, when the pulse duration is shorter than the TRT of the target, there is a sudden thermoelastic expansion within the target caused by spatially localized heating, which generates acoustic waves and damages surrounding structures.

With very short pulses, the rate of temperature rise can be remarkable, leading to a very steep temperature gradient between the target and its surroundings. Thus, when the pulsed-dye laser is used to treat blood vessels with a 1.5 μs pulse width, the estimated rate of temperature rise in the target erythrocytes is 10^7°C per second (Anderson and Parrish, 1981; Garden *et al.*, 1986), which may be responsible for initiating pressure waves to cause vessel rupture.

There is also evidence for photoacoustic damage when pigmented lesions are treated with Q-switched lasers, in that melanosomes, the target in the treatment of endogenous pigmentation, rupture to cause mechanical damage to the melanocyte (Anderson *et al.*, 1989; Ara *et al.*, 1990; Polla *et al.*, 1987). Further, the mechanical damage to tattoo pigment during laser treatment may similarly be the primary mechanism of pigment destruction and removal (Taylor *et al.*, 1991).

SELECTIVE PHOTOTHERMOLYSIS

The concept of selective photothermolysis follows directly from an understanding of laser–tissue interactions, the ultimate aim of

Table 17.1 Estimated thermal relaxation times of some important skin structures

Structure	Size	Thermal relaxation time (approx)
Melanosome	0.5-1 μm	1 μs
Cell	10 μm	300 μs
Blood vessel	50 μm	1 ms
	100 μm	5 ms
	200 μm	20 ms

laser surgery being to direct energy precisely at a specific chromophore in the skin such as blood or melanin without causing any change in the adjacent tissues.

Three variables must be taken into account to achieve such microscopic precision (Anderson and Parrish, 1983). First, the wavelength must be absorbed more avidly by the target tissue than surrounding structures, which can be achieved, for instance if blood vessels are the target, by the choice of a haemoglobin absorption peak. Second, the fluence must be sufficiently high to impart enough thermal energy to alter the target tissue. Third, the exposure duration must be less than the time necessary for cooling of the target, a pulse width exceeding the TRT instead causing non-specific thermal damage through heat diffusion to surrounding tissues. On the other hand, if the pulse width is too short, either vaporization or shockwave damage may occur or, in the case of vascular lesions, insufficient damage may be delivered to the vessel wall to destroy the target fully. Thus, the selection of these three variables forms the essence of selective photothermolysis.

By the choice of a wavelength satisfactorily absorbed by the target tissue, it should be possible to select a pulse duration and fluence that will selectively damage the target. Thus, the flashlamp-pumped pulsed-dye laser was designed to treat children with port-wine stains and the calibre of the ectatic vessels in such lesions is 10–40 μm with a calculated TRT of 0.05–1.0 ms. For these reasons, the original pulsed-dye laser was designed with a wavelength of 577 nm corresponding to one of the absorption peaks of haemoglobin, along with a 350–450 μs pulse width falling directly within the range of predicted TRTs. Pulsed dye laser treatment of port-wine stains in children has since been shown to be of proven benefit in clinical practice.

Not all port-wine stains are alike, lesions varying according to site, vessel diameter, vessel depth and vessel wall thickness. The pulsed-dye laser should be able to treat vessels of 10–40 μm diameter down to the optical penetration depth, but in practice vessels at the lower end of this range and over 100 μm in diameter are not destroyed (Fiskerstrand *et al.*, 1996; Hohenleutner *et al.*, 1995) the simple explanation being that the pulse duration is too long for small vessels and too short for large ones. More work on varying pulse width, wavelength, fluence and spot size is necessary to overcome these difficulties.

Selective photothermolysis has also been applied to the treatment of pigmented lesions, a melanosome 0.5 μm in diameter having a TRT of about 250 ns, and as theory predicts, the Q-switched ruby laser, with its wavelength of 694 nm and pulse width of 25–40 ns, slightly less than the TRT, selectively destroys these particles.

CLINICAL LASER SYSTEMS

CO$_2$ LASER

Wavelength (nm)	Type	Target	Clinical applications
10 600	CW	H$_2$O	Tissue vaporization, surgical cutting
	Pulsed	H$_2$O	Resurfacing

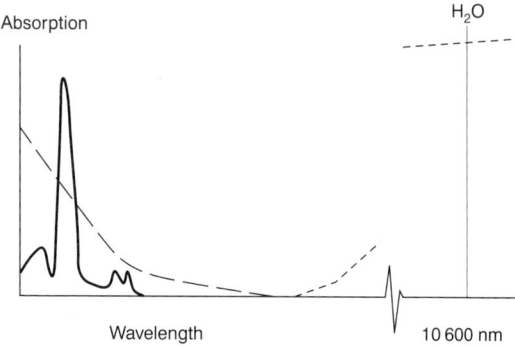

The CO$_2$ laser was first developed in 1964 and is now frequently used in modern dermatological practice (Patel *et al.*, 1964). It emits light at 10 600 nm in the infrared part of the spectrum, a wavelength strongly absorbed by intra- and extracellular water. When the CO_2 laser is defocused with an exposure time of less than 1 ms, it penetrates only to about 20–30 μm in skin (Polanyi, 1983), although the tissue effects from heat diffusion are deeper.

The CO_2 laser was first developed as a continuous beam surgical cutting tool. Focused to a spot size of 0.1–0.2 mm, it generates irradiances of 50–100 000 W/cm² and cutting with it is relatively bloodless (Slutzki *et al.*, 1977). In addition, it has been thought by some to reduce the severity of postoperative pain by destroying sensory nerve endings. However, its use as a cutting instrument is limited by unwanted damage to adjacent tissues, the zone of residual thermal damage of 200–600 μm not only interfering with the ability of the pathologist to assess surgical margins but also slowing wound healing. This limitation was therefore addressed by the development of pulsed CO_2 lasers and superpulsed lasers with a higher peak power and a rapid pulse train of 200–1000 Hz. More detailed evaluation has not, after all, shown them to produce more precise tissue cutting or a significant reduction in the zone of thermal injury.

The use of CO_2 lasers for skin resurfacing has now created a major surge of interest (Hruza and Dover, 1996) and to be effective, such lasers must produce a consistent thin zone of thermal damage at the target area. The thermal relaxation time of the 20–30 μm of water that absorbs CO_2 laser radiation is less than 1 ms (Walsh and Deutsch, 1988), while the energy required to ablate this depth of tissue is 5 J/cm². It therefore follows from selective photothermolysis theory that the ideal laser for skin resurfacing would have a pulse duration of less than 1 ms and a fluence of 5 J/cm² per pulse or an equivalent energy for the speed of beam movement for a CW laser. Two classes of CO_2 laser have now been designed to meet these requirements and have been used successfully for cosmetic resurfacing, the first being pulsed lasers with

pulse durations between 60 μs and 1 ms, the second scanned CW CO_2 lasers with dwell times of less than 1 ms and power that gives a fluence of around 5 J/cm², thus resulting in a tissue effect similar to that of the pulsed lasers.

CONTINUOUS-WAVE VISIBLE LIGHT LASERS

CW lasers deliver constant power to target tissue and have three parameters which need to be varied by the operator, namely the power, spot size and speed of movement of the beam; such operator dependence thus leads to results that vary between laser surgeons, depending on their experience. For example, too much energy applied to any one area increases the likelihood of side effects such as scarring and pigmentary change, although control can be enhanced by fixing of the pulse duration by means of an electronic or mechanical shutter.

CW visible light lasers are mainly used in the treatment of benign vascular and superficial pigmented lesions, most commonly port-wine stains, facial telangiectasia, venous lakes, cherry angiomas, angiokeratomas, lentigines and junctional naevi.

Argon laser

Wavelengths (nm)	Type	Target
488 and 514	CW	Blood vessels

Absorption

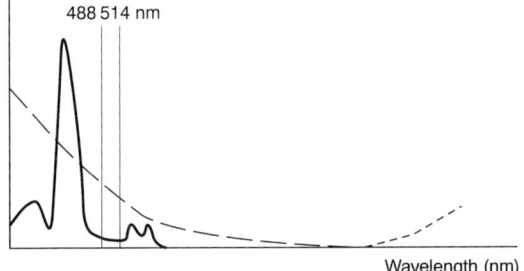

The argon laser was the first such device used to treat port-wine stains and remained the treatment of choice until the late 1980s. The principal emission peaks of 488 nm and 514 nm are fairly well absorbed by haemoglobin and should cause minimal thermal damage to surrounding tissue. However, they do not coincide precisely with the absorption peaks of the chromophore, such that non-absorbed energy is dissipated by scattering, leading to thermal damage. Further non-specific heating occurs secondary to heat conduction from the primary target. At low energies, melanin in the epidermis is in fact the principal chromophore creating heat and thermal damage (Neumann *et al.*, 1992), while at higher energies thermal damage can be detected in the dermis to a depth of 0.6 mm, partly from heat conduction from the epidermis and partly from the effects of radiation absorbed there.

The argon laser is used predominantly for port-wine stains with nodular areas and although most patients have satisfactory outcomes, total clearing of such lesions is uncommon (Cosman, 1980). Thus 75% of patients can expect good to excellent results (Apfelberg *et al.*, 1980; Cosman, 1980) but even with optimal expertise, side effects may include hypertrophic scarring in up to 4% of patients (Silver, 1986), along with textural change and permanent hypopigmentation in up to 30% (Dixon *et al.*, 1984). The tracing technique with this laser is highly effective in the thermal sealing of telangiectatic vessels and because the device causes no post-treatment purpura, as may be seen the pulsed-dye laser, it is ideal for the treatment of facial telangiectasia. Further, in an effort to limit the potential for thermal damage, computerized scanners have been developed and shown to increase the reproducibility of therapy and reduce the incidence of side effects (Dover *et al.*, 1995; Mordon *et al.*, 1989; Sheehan-Dare and Cotterill, 1994). However, scanned visible light lasers such as the argon device have never demonstrated selective vascular destruction in clinical settings but cause non-specific thermal effects instead, and are thus less effective than pulsed-dye lasers for treating vascular lesions (Achauer *et al.*, 1990).

Copper vapour laser

Wavelengths (nm)	Type	Target
511	Quasi-CW	Pigment
578	"	Blood vessels

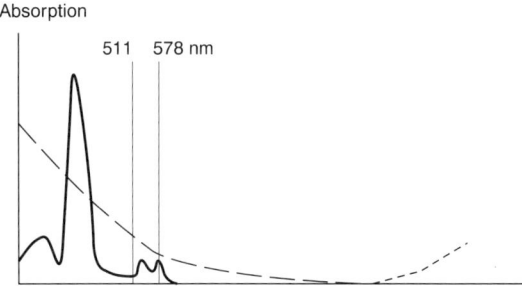

Absorption

511   578 nm

Wavelength (nm)

Copper vapour lasers incorporated elemental copper to enable the emission of either green light at 511 or yellow light at 578 nm, thus producing a train of pulses with a repetition rate of 15 000 per second and pulse duration of 20–40 ns, rapid enough to have a tissue effect similar to that of a CW laser. The 578 nm band coincides with one of the absorption peaks of oxyhaemoglobins, suitable for the treatment of vascular lesions, while the 511 nm line is used to target melanin.

The copper vapour laser used in conjunction with a computerized scanner appears histologically to have an advantage over the argon device in the treatment of port-wine stains (Neumann *et al.*, 1992). Thus, the 578 nm wavelength appears to cause less epidermal damage than the output from the argon laser, while dermal disruption is confined to the blood vessels and surrounding collagen. In practice, however, such an apparent improvement in selectivity has not yielded clinical results significantly better than those of the argon laser (Neumann *et al.*, 1993) and although some darker port-wine stains do appear to respond more favourably, the associated side effects of textural and pigmentary change are still seen as frequently (Sheehan-Dare and Cotterill, 1993).

Argon-pumped dye and krypton lasers

Argon-pumped dye

Wavelengths (nm)	Type	Target
529–640	CW	Blood vessels

Krypton

Wavelengths (nm)	Type	Target
521, 530, 568	CW	Blood vessels

Two further CW lasers are also worthy of mention. The argon-pumped dye device, basically energized by a conventional argon laser, has a fluorescent organic dye as its lasing medium, the emission wavelength being determined by the specific dye used. For instance, rhodamine dyes can emit anywhere between 529 and 640 nm, although they are most often chosen to discharge at wavelengths of 577 or 585 nm for the treatment of vascular lesions. The main theoretical advantage of this device over the basic argon is the precision afforded by the use of yellow light at 577 nm, which coincides with the absorption peak of haemoglobin, but this advantage has yet to be shown to produce superior clinical results.

The krypton laser is the newest CW device for the treatment of vascular lesions, emitting energy at 568 nm for the targeting of blood vessels, with two further bands at 521 and 530 nm for the treatment of pigmented lesions. It can be used in a similar fashion to the argon laser, but clinical experience is still limited (Wheeland, 1993). However, the initial excitement generated by the introduction of these precise instruments for the targeting of blood vessels has not been followed up by the expected clinical benefits, no clinical data having yet demonstrated results significantly better than those obtained with the argon laser.

PULSED LASERS FOR VASCULAR LESIONS

The successful treatment of benign vascular lesions has clearly presented a major challenge to laser technology. However, theory predicts that a wavelength of 577 nm, one of the absorption peaks of oxyhaemoglobin, along with a pulse duration of 1–10 ms, is optimal for the selective destruction of lesions of the dermal vasculature (Anderson and Parrish, 1983; Anderson *et al.*, 1983; Van Gemert *et al.*, 1986). Thus, the pulsed-dye laser was built to conform to these parameters, although the longest pulse width attainable was somewhat short of the theoretically optimal 1–10 ms duration.

Flashlamp-pumped pulsed-dye laser

Wavelength (nm)	Type (pulse width)	Target (diameter)	Clinical applications
585	Pulsed (450 μs)	Blood vessels (30–100 μm)	Port-wine stains Small-calibre telangiectasia

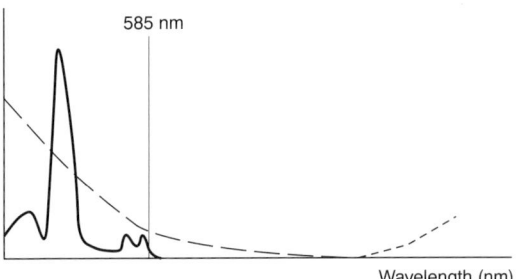

Absorption

585 nm

Wavelength (nm)

The lasing medium in the flashlamp-pumped pulsed-dye laser is a fluorescent organic dye dissolved in a liquid solvent and housed in a transparent cell. Its chemical structure and the solvent and additives used with it dictate its operating lifetime which is limited by dye decomposition as a result of intense heat and radiation exposure, particularly in the ultraviolet part of the spectrum; however, rhodamine 6G dye has a long lifetime and is often employed. The cell containing the dye is then surrounded by a flashlamp capable of producing a pulse duration of 450 μs.

The radiation penetration depth of the pulsed-dye laser is 0.2 mm below the dermo-epidermal junction (Nakagawa *et al.*, 1985) which can, however, be increased to 0.5–1.2 mm by extension of the wavelength from the original 577 to 585 nm (Tan *et al.*, 1989). In this report, 590 nm in fact penetrated less deeply than 585 nm for the same fluence, but longer wavelengths require more energy for similar efficacy, and therefore deeper penetration with 590 nm and longer wavelengths remains a possibility (Levins *et al.*, 1991). Side effects have been minimal except for purpura lasting up to 14 days, the severity depending on fluence and spot size (Lanigan, 1995).

The pulse duration of 450 μs for this laser is at the lower end of the range of TRTs for skin vasculature, namely between 200 and 3000 μs for vessels of 10–40 μm diameter. Because of increases in port-wine stain vessel calibres with age, the pulsed-dye laser treats children more efficiently than adults (Achauer *et al.*, 1990; Ashinoff and Geronemus, 1991; Reyes and Geronemus, 1990; Tan *et al.*, 1989).

Prolongation of the pulse duration to 1–10 ms may improve pulsed-dye laser results (Dierickx *et al.*, 1995) but an increase in energy density is necessary to achieve this (Garden *et al.*, 1986), proven in practice by the use of the 532 nm Nd:YAG laser. This has a pulse width adjustable between 1 and 30 ms and when tested on port-wine stains, proved to be most effective with 3 or 5 ms pulses and fluences of 15 or 20 J/cm² (Dierickx *et al.*, 1996).

Long-pulsed dye laser

Wavelengths (nm)	Type (pulse width)	Target (diameter)	Clinical applications
595, 600	Pulsed (1.5 ms)	Vessels (up to 1 mm)	Facial telangiectasia Arborizing leg veins

Absorption

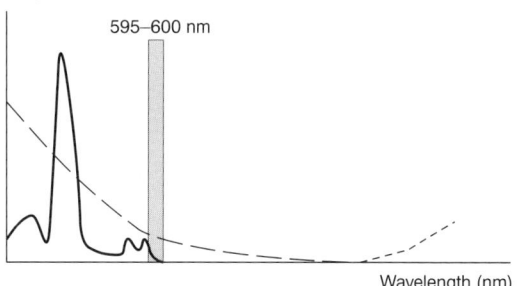

595–600 nm

Wavelength (nm)

The 585 nm, 450 μs, pulsed-dye laser has become established as the standard mode of treatment for port-wine stains and small-calibre telangiectasia but for larger vessels, a longer pulse width is required. As a result, there are now lasers capable of pulsing for 1.5 ms at 595–600 nm and in trials using an elliptical spot for the treatment of arborizing leg veins, best results were obtained at 590 nm and were better than those of alternative existing lasers (Garden and Bakus, 1996; Grossman *et al.*, 1996).

Potassium titanyl phosphate lasers

Wavelength (nm)	Type (pulse width)	Target (diameter)	Clinical applications
532	Pulsed (1–100 ms)	Vessels (up to 1 mm)	Facial telangiectasia Arborizing leg veins

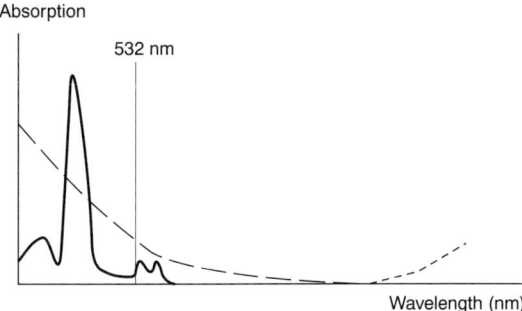

Absorption

532 nm

Wavelength (nm)

The requirement for long pulses, not easily attainable with the pulsed-dye laser, has instead been met by development of the potassium titanyl phosphate (KTP) laser. Three have been introduced with the capability of emitting pulse durations in the 1–100 ms range at 532 nm. The first is pulsed, with pulse duration of 2–10 ms (Coherent, Versapulse), the second is pumped by a diode laser to give a train of Q-switched microsecond pulses conjoined to the desired duration of 1–100 ms (Continuum Biomedical), while the third also emits a train of Q-switched pulses, this time to durations of 1–30 ms (Laserscope, Orion). Preliminary trials on port-wine stains have shown the last of these to be safe and effective (Dierickx *et al.*, 1996), while all three lasers are being studied for their efficacy in treating ectatic facial vessels and leg veins.

PULSED LASERS FOR PIGMENTED LESIONS

CW lasers have been used for the removal of unwanted cutaneous pigment since the 1960s. However, many new devices, principally short-pulsed lasers, have recently been developed for the elimination of both endogenous and exogenous pigment. Thus, the chromophore in exogenous decorative tattoos is the pigmented ink particle, while that in endogenous pigmented lesions is melanin.

CW lasers, particularly the CO_2, argon, copper vapour and krypton lasers, have all been used for the removal of cutaneous pigment, but with mixed success. For instance, the CO_2 laser, at low fluences, can successfully treat lentigines as a result of the superficial absorption of its radiation by cutaneous water, followed by conduction of the heat produced thereby through the epidermis (Dover *et al.*, 1988). However, all such lasers cause non-specific damage and the resultant thermal diffusion may lead to unwanted collateral injury with scarring and pigmentary change.

Melanin is contained in melanosomes, 0.5–1.0 µm intracellular organelles, which have been shown to be the primary target in skin during the treatment of endogenous hyperpigmentation (Dover *et al.*, 1989; Murphy *et al.*, 1983; Polla *et al.*, 1987). Its absorption spectrum ranges from below 300 to over 1000 nm and therefore it lends itself readily to treatment with a wide variety of lasers (Anderson *et al.*, 1989; Murphy *et al.*, 1983), usually selected to avoid the absorption peaks of other skin chromophores and to penetrate to the desired depth. When the efficacy of wavelengths between 504 and 750 nm was compared, the lowest caused the greatest specific injury, perhaps because absorption is highest there (Sherwood *et al.*, 1989). For deeper pigment, such as that encountered with the naevus of Ota, for example, longer wavelengths which penetrate more deeply are better. Further, by selective photothermolysis theory, the pulse duration for thermal confinement should be between 70 and 250 ns (Anderson *et al.*, 1983; Parrish and Deutsch, 1984). In fact research has shown that treatment with pulse durations below 100 ns causes melanosome rupture, as theory would predict, and that when the fluence threshold for melanosome disruption is reached, nuclear damage also occurs, possibly from a thermomechanical effect by the fast-expanding melanosome (Ara *et al.*, 1990). However, damage is also caused by pulse widths of 300 ns, above the predicted TRT of melanosomes, perhaps because heat conduction damages the melanocyte as well as the melanosome (Kurban *et al.*, 1992).

Tattoos have also been subjected to laser treatment since the 1960s, treatment with short-pulsed lasers resulting in the fragmentation of ink particles and the selective death of pigment-containing cells, with release of their pigment (Taylor *et al.*, 1991). Some ink is then lost in scale crust and some in lymphatics, while some is rephagocytosed. Damage to collagen is also apparent but is limited to the area immediately surrounding the damaged cells.

Photoacoustic effects are known to be important in tattoo removal (Ara *et al.*, 1990) and for exploitation of the concept of mechanical confinement, the use of pulse widths in the subnanosecond domain may be necessary to minimize the disruption to surrounding tissue. This is analogous to thermal confinement in the theory of selective photothermolysis, namely the limiting of mechanico-acoustic rather than heat spread, and may be an area for future development (Kilmer *et al.*, 1996; Ross *et al.*, 1996).

Q-switched ruby laser

Wavelength (nm)	Type (pulse width)	Target	Clinical applications
694	Q switched (25 ns)	Pigment	Endogenous and exogenous pigment

Absorption

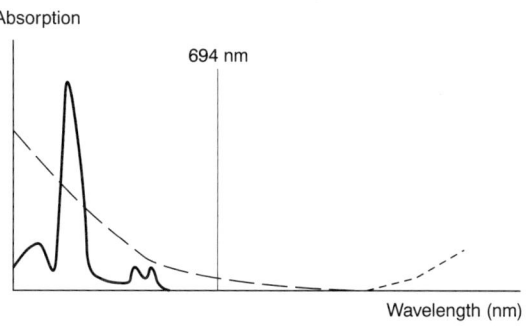

694 nm

Wavelength (nm)

The first laser to be developed was a pulsed ruby, with the Q-switched mode later offering higher fluences over a shorter duration. The active medium therein is sapphire (Al_2O_3) doped with chromium to form a red crystal and energized by a flashlamp to emit 694 nm red light. This is well absorbed by melanin and tattoo pigments and has thus been used for the treatment of a wide variety of endogenous and exogenous pigmented lesions.

Q-switched Nd:YAG laser

Wavelength (nm)	Type (pulse width)	Target	Clinical applications
1064	Q switched (5–15 ns)	Pigment	Black tattoos
532 (frequency doubled)	"	"	Red tattoos, melanin

Absorption

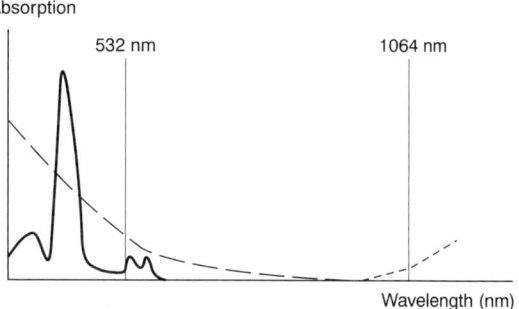

532 nm   1064 nm

Wavelength (nm)

The Nd:YAG (neodymium-doped yttrium aluminium garnet) is designed in similar fashion to the ruby, but emits in the near-infrared range at 1064 nm.

Use of the CW Nd:YAG laser has been limited by its lack of specificity and although its 1064 nm radiation penetrates to a depth of 3.7 mm, it is mostly absorbed by water, thereby causing non-specific heating and fibrosis (Apfelberg *et al.*, 1987; Landthaler *et al.*, 1986). It is thus mainly used in the Q-switched mode for the treatment of pigmented lesions. The 1064 nm energy can also be frequency doubled to produce 532 nm light by passing it through a potassium titanyl phosphate crystal (KTP), also known as the KTP laser, as described above.

The near-infrared 1064 nm radiation can treat black tattoos, and has caused leucotrichia in guinea pigs (Anderson *et al.*, 1989), while the 532 nm wavelength removes melanin and red ink (Kilmer and Anderson, 1993; Kilmer *et al.*, 1994).

Q-switched alexandrite laser

Wavelength (nm)	Type (pulse width)	Target	Clinical applications
755	Q switched (100 ns)	Pigment	Tattoos

Absorption

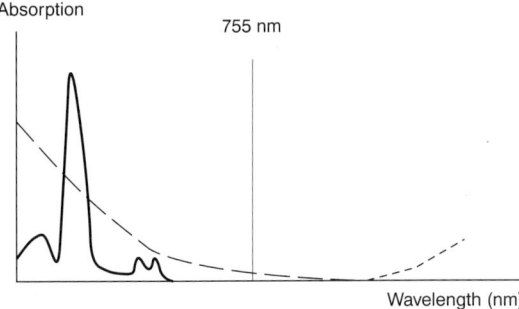

The alexandrite laser is one of a new group of solid-state lasers, containing chromium-doped $BeAl_2O_4$. It can be tuned between 701 and 826 nm but is usually operated at 755 nm, falling between the ruby and the Nd:YAG, and has a 100 ns pulse duration. Like the ruby and Nd:YAG, the active medium is the impurity in the crystal, pumped by a flash-lamp. Recently introduced, it appears to remove black, blue and green tattoos as well as the Q-switched ruby laser (Fitzpatrick and Goldman, 1994; Hodersdal *et al.*, 1996; Stafford *et al.*, 1995).

Pigmented lesion pulsed-dye laser

Wavelength (nm)	Type (pulse width)	Target	Clinical applications
510	Pulsed (300 ns)	Melanin	Epidermal pigment

Absorption

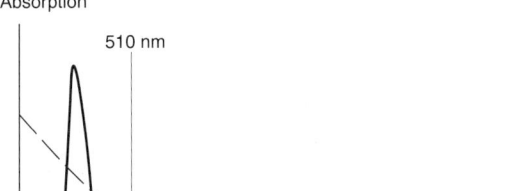

This device was designed to have a pulse width suitable for the targeting of epidermal pigment. The lasing medium is a coumarin-containing dye. It is pumped by a flashlamp and emits green light at a wavelength of 510 nm with a pulse duration of 300 ns. Animal studies revealed these parameters to be ideal for the treatment of pigment in miniature black pig skin (Sherwood *et al.*, 1989), while subsequent human trials have also yielded encouraging results with benign epidermal pigmented lesions (Fitzpatrick *et al.*, 1993).

BROAD-BAND LIGHT SOURCES

A new type of machine discharging filtered broad-band light from a flashlamp has recently been introduced. This is not a laser but works on similar principles, emitting radiation between 515 nm and the near-infrared range and incorporating filters to cut off the radiation at the lower end of this spectrum. Computer software imbues these devices with a flexibility not normally available in a laser but their uncertain internal complexities shroud them in a certain mystique. One to three pulses with adjustable pulse widths, interpulse delays and fluences are possible. Such devices have been used to treat cutaneous vascular lesions and pigmented disorders but ideal parameters for reproducible results have not yet been fully established.

REFERENCES

Achauer, B.M., Vander Kam, V.M. and Miller, S.R. (1990) Clinical experience with the pulsed-dye laser in the treatment of capillary malformations (port-wine stains): a preliminary report. *Annals of Plastic Surgery*, **25**, 344–52.

Anderson, R.R. and Parrish, J.A. (1981) The optics of human skin. *Journal of Investigative Dermatology*, **77**, 13–19.

Anderson, R.R., and Parrish J.A. (1983) Selective photothermolysis: precise microsurgery by selective absorption of pulsed radiation. *Science*, **220**, 524–7.

Anderson, R.R., Jaenicke, K.F. and Parrish, J.A. (1983) Mechanisms of selective vascular changes caused by dye lasers. *Lasers in Surgery and Medicine*, **3**, 211–15.

Anderson, R.R., Margolis, R.J., Watenabe, S. *et al.* (1989) Selective photothermolysis of cutaneous pigmentation by Q-switched Nd:YAG laser pulses at 1064, 532 and 355 nm. *Journal of Investigative Dermatology*, **93**, 28–32.

Apfelberg, D.B., Maser, M.R., Lash, H. *et al.* (1980) Progress report on extended clinical use of the argon laser for cutaneous lesions. *Lasers in Surgery and Medicine*, **1**, 71–83.

Apfelberg, D.B., Smith, T., Lash, H. *et al.* (1987) Preliminary report on use of the neodymium-YAG laser in plastic surgery. *Lasers in Surgery and Medicine*, **7**, 189–98.

Ara, G., Anderson, R.R., Mandel, K.G. *et al.* (1990) Irradiation of pigmented melanoma cells with high intensity pulsed radiation generates acoustic waves and kills cells. *Lasers in Surgery and Medicine*, **10**, 52–9.

Ashinoff, R. and Geronemus, R.G. (1981) Flashlamp-pumped pulsed dye laser for port-wine stains in infancy: earlier versus later treatment. *Journal of the American Academy of Dermatology*, **24**, 467–72.

Clayman, L., Fuller, T and Beckman. H. (1978) Healing of continuous-wave and rapid super-pulsed, carbon dioxide laser-induced bone defects. *Journal of Oral Surgery*, **36**, 932–7.

Cosman, B. (1980) Experience in the argon laser therapy of port wine stains. *Plastic and Reconstructive Surgery*, **65**, 119–29.

Dierickx, C.C., Casparian, J.M., Venugopalan, V. *et al.* (1995) Thermal relaxation of port-wine stain vessels probed *in vivo*: the need for 1-10 millisecond laser pulse treatment. *Journal of Investigative Dermatology*, **105**, 709–14.

Dierickx, C.C., Farinelli, W.A., Flotte, T. *et al.* (1996) Effect of long-pulsed 532 nm Nd:YAG laser on portwine stains (PWS). *Lasers in Surgery and Medicine*, **16** (suppl 8), 33.

Dixon, J.A., Huether, S. and Rotering, R. (1984) Hypertrophic scarring in argon laser treatment of port-wine stains. *Plastic and Reconstructive Surgery*, **73**, 771–7.

Dover, J.S., Smoller, B.R., Stern, R.S. *et al.* (1988) Low-fluence carbon dioxide laser irradiation of lentigines. *Archives of Dermatology*, **124**, 1219–24.

Dover, J.S., Margolis, R.J., Polla, L.L. *et al.* (1989) Pigmented guinea pig skin irradiated with Q-switched ruby laser pulses. *Archives of Dermatology*, **125**, 43–9.

Dover, J.S., Geronemus, R., Stern, R.S. *et al.* (1995) Dye laser treatment of port-wine stains: comparison of the continuous wave dye laser with a robotized scanning device and pulsed dye laser. *Journal of the American Academy of Dermatology*, **32**, 237–40.

Einstein, A. (1917) Zur Quantentheorie der Strahlung. *Physiologische Zeitschrift*, **18**, 121–8.

Fisher, J.C. (1983) The power density of a surgical laser beam. *Lasers in Surgery and Medicine*, **2**, 301–15.

Fiskerstrand, E.J., Svaasand, L.O., Kopstad, G. *et al.* (1996) Photothermally induced vessel-wall necrosis after pulsed dye laser treatment: lack of response in port-wine stains with small sized or deeply located vessels. *Journal of Investigative Dermatology*, **107**, 671–5.

Fitzpatrick, R.E. and Goldman, M.P. (1984) Tattoo removal using the alexandrite laser. *Archives of Dermatology*, **130**, 1508–14.

Fitzpatrick, R.E., Goldman, M.P. and Ruiz-Esparza, J. (1993) Laser treatment of benign pigmented epidermal lesions using a 300 nsecond pulse and 510 nm wavelength. *Journal of Dermatologic Surgery and Oncology*, **18**, 341–7.

Garden, J.M. and Bakus, A.D. (1996) Treatment of leg veins with high energy pulsed dye laser. *Lasers in Surgery and Medicine*, **8** (suppl), 34.

Garden, J.M., Tan, O.T., Kerschmann, R. *et al.* (1986) Effect of dye laser pulse duration on selective cutaneous vascular injury. *Journal of Investigative Dermatology*, **87**, 653–7.

Grossman, M.C., Bernstein, L.J., Kauvar, A.N.B. *et al.* (1996) Treatment of leg veins with a long pulse tunable dye laser. *Lasers in Surgery and Medicine*, **16** (suppl 8), 35.

Hodersdal, M., Bech-Thomsen, N. and Wulf, H.C. (1996) Skin reflectance-guided laser selections for treatment of decorative tattoos. *Archives of Dermatology*, **132**, 403–7.

Hohenleutner, U., Hilbert, M., Wlotzke, U. *et al.* (1995) Epidermal damage and limited coagulation depth with the flashlamp-pumped pulsed dye laser: a histochemical study. *Journal of Investigative Dermatology*, **104**, 798–802.

Hruza, G.J. and Dover, J.S. (1996) Laser skin resurfacing. *Archives of Dermatology*, **132**, 451–5.

Jackson, B.A., Arndt, K.A. and Dover, J.S. (1996) Are all 585 nm pulsed dye lasers equivalent? *Journal of the American Academy of Dermatology*, **34**, 1000–4.

Kilmer, S.L. and Anderson, R.R. (1993) Clinical use of the Q-switched ruby and the Q-switched Nd:YAG (1064 nm and 532 nm) lasers for treatment of tattoos. *Journal of Dermatologic Surgery and Oncology*, **19**, 330–8.

Kilmer, S.L., Wheeland, R.G., Goldberg, D.J. *et al.* (1994) Treatment of epidermal pigmented lesions with the frequency-doubled Q-switched NdYAG laser. *Archives of Dermatology*, **130**, 1515–19.

Kilmer, S.L., Fitzpatrick, R.E., Da Silva, L.B. *et al.* (1996) Picosecond and femtosecond laser treatment of tattoo ink. *Lasers in Surgery and Medicine*, **16** (suppl 8), 36.

Kurban, A.K., Morrison, P.R., Trainor, S.W. *et al.* (1992) Pulse duration effects on cutaneous pigment. *Lasers in Surgery and Medicine*, **12**, 282–7.

Landthaler, M., Haina, D., Brunner, R. *et al.* (1986) Neodymium-YAG laser therapy for vascular lesions. *Journal of the American Academy of Dermatology*, **14**, 107–17.

Lanigan, S.W. (1995) Patient-reported morbidity following flashlamp-pumped pulsed tunable dye laser treatment of port-wine stains. *British Journal of Dermatology*, **133**, 423–5.

Levins, P.C., Grevelink, L.M. and Anderson, R.R. (1991) Action spectrum of immediate and delayed purpura in human skin using a tunable pulsed dye laser. *Journal of Investigative Dermatology*, **96**, 588.

Maiman, T.H. (1960) Stimulated optical radiation in ruby. *Nature*, **187**, 493–4.

Mordon, S.R., Rotteleur, G., Buys, B. *et al.* (1989) Comparative study of the "point-by-point technique" and the "scanning technique" for laser treatment of port-wine stain. *Lasers in Surgery and Medicine*, **9**, 398–404.

Murphy, G.F., Shepard, R.S., Paul, B.S. *et al.* (1983) Organelle-specific injury to melanin-containing cells in human skin by pulsed laser irradiation. *Laboratory Investigation*, **49**, 680–5.

Nakagawa, H., Tan, O.T. and Parrish, J.A. (1985) Ultrastructural changes in human skin after exposure to pulsed laser. *Journal of Investigative Dermatology*, **84**, 396–400.

Neumann, R.A., Knobler, R.M., Leonhartsberger, H. *et al.* (1992) Comparative histochemistry of port-wine stains after copper vapor laser (578 nm) and argon laser treatment. *Journal of Investigative Dermatology*, **99**, 160–7.

Neumann, R.A., Leonhartsberger, H., Bohler-Sommeregger, K. *et al.* (1993) Results and tissue healing after copper-vapor laser (at 578 nm) treatment of port wine stains and facial telangiectasias. *British Journal of Dermatology*, **128**, 306–12.

Parrish, J.A. and Deutsch, T.F. (1984) Laser photomedicine. *IEEE Journal of Quantum Electronics*, **QE-20**, 1386–96.

Patel, C.K.N., McFarlane, R.A. and Faust, W.L. (1964) Selective excitation through vibrational energy and optical maser action in N_2–CO_2. *Physiological Reviews ABCD*, **13**, 617–9.

Polanyi, T.G. (1983) Laser physics: medical applications. *Otolaryngeal Clinics of North America*, **16**, 753–74.

Polla, L.L., Margolis, R.J., Dover, J.S. *et al.* (1987) Melanosomes are a primary target of Q-switched ruby laser irradiation in guinea pig skin. *Journal of Investigative Dermatology*, **89**, 281–6.

Reyes, B.A. and Geronemus, R. (1990) Treatment of port-wine stains during childhood with the flashlamp-pumped pulsed dye laser. *Journal of the American Academy of Dermatology*, **23**, 1142–8.

Ross, E.V., Naseef, G.S., Kelly, M.W., *et al.* (1996) Response of tattoos to a picosecond laser. *Lasers in Surgery and Medicine*, **16** (suppl 8), 38.

Sheehan-Dare, R.A. and Cotterill, J.A. (1993) Copper vapour laser treatment of port-wine stains: clinical evaluation and comparison with conventional argon laser therapy. *British Journal of Dermatology*, **128**, 546–9.

Sheehan-Dare, R.A. and Cotterill, J.A. (1994) Copper vapour laser (578 nm) and flashlamp-pumped tunable dye laser (585 nm) treatment of port wine stains: results of a comparative study using test sites. *British Journal of Dermatology*, **130**, 478–82.

Sherwood, K.A., Murray, S., Kurban, A.K. *et al.* (1989) Effect of wavelength on cutaneous pigment using pulsed irradiation. *Journal of Investigative Dermatology*, **92**, 717–20.

Sigrist, M.W. and Kneubuhl, F.K. (1978) Laser-generated stress waves in liquids. *Journal of the Acoustic Society of America*, **64**, 1652–63.

Silver, L. (1986) Argon laser photocoagulation of port-wine stain hemangiomas. *Lasers in Surgery and Medicine*, **6**, 24–8.

Slutzki, S., Shafir, R. and Bornstein, L.A. (1997) Use of the carbon dioxide laser for large excisions with minimal blood loss. *Plastic and Reconstructive Surgery*, **60**, 250–5.

Stafford, T.J., Lizek, R., Boll, J. *et al.* (1995) Removal of colored tattoos with the Q-switched alexandrite laser. *Plastic and Reconstructive Surgery*, **95**, 313–20.

Tan, O.T., Murray, S. and Kurban, A.K. (1989) Action spectrum of vascular specific injury using pulsed irradiation. *Journal of Investigative Dermatology*, **92**, 868–71.

Taylor, C.R., Anderson, R.R., Gange, R.W. *et al.* (1991) Light and electron microscopic analysis of tattoos treated by Q-switched ruby laser. *Journal of Investigative Dermatology*, **97**, 131–6.

Van Gemert, M.J.C., Welch, A.J. and Amin, A.P. (1986) Is there an optimal laser treatment for port wine stains? *Lasers in Surgery and Medicine*, **6**, 76–83.

Walsh, J.T. and Deutsch, T.F.(1988) Pulsed CO_2 laser tissue ablation: measurement of the ablation rate. *Lasers in Surgery and Medicine*, **8**, 264–75.

Watanabe, S., Flotte, T.J., Macauliffe, D.J. *et al.* (1988) Putative photoacoustic damage in skin induced by pulsed ArF excimer laser. *Journal of Investigative Dermatology*, **90**, 761–6.

Wheeland, R.G. (1993) Treatment of port-wine stains for the 1990s. *Journal of Dermatologic Surgery and Oncology*, **19**, 348–56.

APPENDIX A
IRRADIATION TESTING OF THE SKIN

Peter M. Farr

INTRODUCTION

Irradiation testing of the skin (phototesting) may be performed for a number of reasons, particularly:

- the diagnosis of a photosensitive disorder;
- the monitoring of disease activity in a photosensitive disorder or the assessment of its response to treatment;
- the choice of an appropriate irradiation dose for phototherapy (UVB or psoralen photochemotherapy (PUVA));
- the investigation of some aspect of the biological response to ultraviolet exposure by normal or diseased skin (for example, the assessment of erythema, histological changes or inflammatory mediator production).

In general, two techniques are most commonly used:

1. the exposure of a number of relatively small areas of skin to incremental doses of ultraviolet radiation at one or more wavelengths. The threshold response for erythema (minimal erythema dose) may then be judged visually or else measured quantitatively;
2. the exposure of a rather larger area of skin to broad-spectrum radiation from an appropriate source with the intention of provoking the lesions of a photosensitivity disorder suspected clinically.

MINIMAL ERYTHEMA DOSE TESTING

Measurement of the cutaneous minimal erythema dose (MED) is used to judge the threshold erythemal sensitivity of the skin to a particular light source or waveband of radiation. This information may then be used to diagnose or exclude a photosensitivity disorder in which abnormal erythemal responses are typically found, such as, for example, chronic actinic dermatitis, drug-induced photosensitivity or xeroderma pigmentosum. MED testing may also be used to assess skin erythemal sensitivity prior to the administration of phototherapy.

RADIATION SOURCE

The choice of light source for MED testing will be determined to a large extent by the purpose of the test. For example, if the phototesting is being undertaken to enable choice of a starting dose for PUVA or UVB phototherapy, it is clearly important that the testing lamp should have the same spectrum as that used for the therapy. For diagnostic phototesting, on the other hand, it is necessary to measure the MED to UVB, UVA and, on occasions, visible light. Thus, measurement of the UVB MED alone, although technically easy, does not provide sufficient information for accurate diagnosis. Full investigation of this type requires the use of an irradiation monochromator (a xenon arc lamp with associated diffraction grating), with which discrete wavebands may be selected. A flexible, liquid-filled light guide coupled to the irradiation monochromator is a convenient method of transmitting the radiation to the skin surface, thus allowing precise positioning of the target and a sharply defined small irradiation field of between 4 and 10 mm in diameter. The availability of this type of source is generally restricted to laboratories with a particular interest in photosensitivity disorders, the equipment being expensive and requiring careful maintenance while experience in operation technique and the interpretation of results is also essential. The emission from a xenon arc lamp such as this can also be used with suitable optical filters to provide a simulated solar spectrum or broad-band UVA for lesion provocation.

Appropriate fluorescent lamps (e.g. Philips TL-12 or TL-01) can also be used, more simply but still reliably, to measure a broad-band UVB MED. For this, small areas for irradiation on the skin surface can be delineated with ultraviolet-opaque material and different exposure times may then be used to achieve an incremental series of doses. Alternatively, a simple method for the achievement of a graded series of doses with a single exposure through a series of wire optical attenuators has been described (Diffey and Oliver, 1985). On the other hand, the irradiance from UVA fluorescent lamps is too low to allow satisfactory UVA MED testing. However, some authors have suggested a simplified test, whereby a single dose of around $10–20 \, J/cm^2$ is given from PUVA-type fluorescent lamps and any erythemal reaction present at 24 hours is taken to indicate an increased sensitivity to UVA. However, a negative reaction should not be taken necessarily to indicate a normal UVA response, since patients with mild to moderate UVA sensitivity would not be identified by such simplified testing.

Although generally designed for the irradiation of large areas of skin, optically filtered high-pressure metal halide lamps (e.g. UVASUN 3000, Mutzhas, Munich) normally have sufficient irradiance within the wavelength interval 340–400 nm to allow UVA MED testing, but are too expensive for just occasional use.

BODY SITE

The skin of the back is the most commonly used site for MED testing as it provides a relatively large area of skin with a reasonably uniform response. Testing should, however, be avoided on skin within approximately 3 cm of either side of the midline overlying the vertebral column because of decreased sensitivity at that site. In addition, there are variations in sensitivity, for example minimally on opposite sides of the back at the same vertebral level (mean coefficient of variation 6%), and much more markedly between areas on the upper, mid and lower back (mean coefficient of variation 22%) (Farr and Diffey, 1984), the skin on the lower back and buttocks being significantly less sensitive than at other dorsal sites (Farr and Diffey, 1984; Rhodes and Friedmann, 1992).

RADIATION DOSE SERIES

The dose–response relationship for ultraviolet erythema follows an S-shaped curve if the dose is plotted on a logarithmic scale (Diffey and Farr, 1991). It thus follows that a dose series intended to allow useful assessment of the MED will be most informative if a geometric series of dose increments, in which successive doses increase by a fixed ratio or percentage, rather than an arithmetic series, in which they increase by a fixed amount, is used. For example, a geometric series is given below that might be used to determine the MED at 300 nm, where the median value for normal subjects is around $28 \, mJ/cm^2$:

Dose (mJ/cm^2) 5 7 10 14 20 28 40 56 80

The successive doses in this example have been increased in each case by a factor of √2 or approximately 40%. Smaller dose increments (10% or 20%) could theoretically be used to define the MED more precisely, but the imprecision of visual assessment and the variation in sensitivity of the skin, even over the back, make this of questionable value.

DEFINITION OF THE CUTANEOUS MED

Different definitions are in common use for the intensity of erythema that should be taken as the MED. These range from the dose required to achieve a just perceptible erythema to that which just produces a uniform redness with sharp borders. Any normal range for the MED will thus clearly be influenced by the definition used and variations in this may make valid comparisons difficult between the results obtained in different photodermatology units. These problems may then be compounded by the frequent use of multiples of the MED in clinical research. For example, the intensity of a skin reaction caused by three times the dose required for a just perceptible erythema is far different from that caused by three times the dose to produce a sharp-bordered erythema. Interobserver variability may make these difficulties even worse, but there is limited evidence for less variability of this type if the just perceptible erythema definition is used (Quinn *et al.*, 1994).

TIME OF MED OBSERVATION

In diagnostic phototesting, recording of the MED at a single time point (usually 24 hours after irradiation) is usually sufficient, although additional readings may occasionally be required in the diagnosis of certain cases of drug-induced photosensitivity, solar urticaria, erythropoietic protoporphyria and xeroderma pigmentosum and in the assessment of psoralen-sensitized skin.

WAVELENGTHS USED FOR MED TESTING

As a bare minimum for diagnostic phototesting, MEDs must be measured at least at one waveband in the UVB region and one in the UVA. However, photodermatology units with an irradiation monochromator usually test more reliably but more lengthily at three or more wavebands from around 300 to 365 nm (British Photodermatology Group, 1992), while testing at visible light wavelengths may also be necessary in patients with solar urticaria and severe chronic actinic dermatitis.

NORMAL MED RANGE

Because of the differences between units in phototesting equipment, testing techniques, definitions of the MED and populations under study, it is not possible to quote precise normal MED ranges for a particular waveband and it is instead necessary for individual testing centres to establish their own, locally relevant, normal ranges.

However, the 95% confidence intervals for normal subject MEDs (skin types I–IV) on the untanned skin of the back are known to encompass a 4–6-fold range for both UVA and UVB and a strong positive correlation exists between the MEDs for UVA and those for UVB (Diffey and Farr, 1989). In addition, the MEDs in a given spectral waveband and for a normal population have a positively skewed, log-normal distribution (Mackenzie, 1983) and it is therefore preferable to quote average MED values as the median, or geometric mean, rather than the arithmetic mean.

MEASUREMENT OF CUTANEOUS ERYTHEMA

A number of instruments are available commercially for the objective measurement of cutaneous erythemal intensity (Diffey and Farr, 1991) and are used mainly to study the dose–response characteristics of the ultraviolet erythemal reaction. They have not, however, been shown to improve on visual assessment of the MED for routine diagnostic photo-testing.

CUTANEOUS LESION PROVOCATION

Lesion provocation testing is used primarily as a confirmatory diagnostic assay in patients suspected of having one of the idiopathic photosensitivity disorders, most commonly polymorphic light eruption. However, in other disorders, for example, lupus erythematosus, photoprovocation experiments have also provided information concerning the wavebands responsible for disease worsening, but such testing would not normally be regarded as diagnostically useful.

RADIATION SOURCE FOR LESION PROVOCATION

For lesion provocation, it is usually necessary to irradiate a considerably larger area than for MED testing. Fluorescent UVA lamps such as those used for PUVA are often suitable, as also are optically filtered high-pressure metal halide (e.g. UVASUN 3000, Mutzhas, Munich) and xenon arc solar-simulating sources, while UVB fluorescent lamps may also occasionally be useful. However, the irradiation monochromator is generally sufficient for such provocation only in solar urticaria, the small irradiation field rarely being suitable in the other disorders.

POLYMORPHIC LIGHT ERUPTION

As lesion provocation may be successful in around 90% of patients with polymorphic light eruption (Hölzle *et al.*, 1982) this may be a useful diagnostic test, particularly when lupus erythematosus is in the differential diagnosis. In such patients with normal MEDs, broad-band UVA exposure of a large area of skin (100 cm^2 or more) with suberythemal doses, for example 10–20 J/cm^2, from a PUVA-type fluorescent lamp frequently induces lesions between four and 12 hours after irradiation, which then persist for 24–48 hours.

The dose required for a positive result may vary between patients by a factor of 4 (McFadden and Larsen, 1986), while repeated daily exposure over 2–4 days make positive tests more likely (Neumann *et al.*, 1987). On the other hand, false-negative results may occur if the testing is performed on tanned or recently sun-exposed skin or at sites at which the rash does not normally occur after sun exposure. The UVA dose required for a positive response may be considerably reduced in the small group of patients with abnormal MEDs to UVA and if there is any clinical suggestion of such increased sensitivity, MED testing should be undertaken first. On occasions, lesions may instead be triggered by UVB, repeated exposures to 2–3 MEDs sometimes being required (Miyamoto, 1989).

SOLAR URTICARIA

The weal and flare response in patients with solar urticaria generally appears within five minutes of irradiation, becoming maximal by around 15 minutes and fading over a period of an hour or so. In most cases, the triggering waveband is wide, for example encompassing the UVA and blue light regions, but in some cases may be restricted to one narrow region. Generally, only small areas of skin around 10 mm in diameter need be exposed to produce diagnostic lesions, but the test sites should be quite widely spaced as the flare reaction can spread considerably. An irradiation monochromator is best for detailed investigation of the action spectrum in the ultraviolet and visible regions, although broad-band UVA or UVB sources are also useful, if less detailed. In addition, the filtered output from a slide projector with a quartz halogen bulb has been used for the investigation of visible light responses (Horio, 1978).

OTHER DISORDERS

Repeated daily exposure of small areas of skin to radiation between 330 and 360 nm has been shown to induce intraepidermal vesicles in patients with hydroa vacciniforme (Sunohara *et al.*, 1988), while broad-band UVA exposure has also achieved lesion provocation (Hölzle *et al.*, 1987). In addition, lesions may be provoked by UVA in some patients with actinic prurigo (British Photodermatology Group, 1992), but this aspect of that disease has been poorly studied. Finally, minimal erythema responses are usually normal in patients with lupus erythematosus, but in around 60% of patients with the subacute form of the disease 40% with the discoid form and 25% with systemic disease, lesions may be provoked by multiple daily exposures to broad-band UVA, UVB or both (Lehmann *et al.*, 1990). Such a reaction is usually more delayed in onset and persistent than that provoked by similar exposure in patients with polymorphic light eruption.

REFERENCES

British Photodermatology Group (1992) Diagnostic phototesting in the United Kingdom. *British Journal of Dermatology*, **127**, 297–9.

Diffey, B.L. and Farr, P.M. (1989) The normal range in diagnostic phototesting. *British Journal of Dermatology*, **120**, 517–24.

Diffey, B.L. and Farr, P.M. (1991) Quantitative aspects of ultraviolet erythema. *Clinical Physics and Physiological Measurement*, **12**, 311–25.

Diffey, B.L. and Oliver, R.J. (1985) An inexpensive luminaire for diagnostic phototesting to UVB radiation. *Photodermatology*, **2**, 260–2.

Farr, P.M. and Diffey, B.L. (1984) Quantitative studies on cutaneous erythema induced by ultraviolet radiation. *British Journal of Dermatology*, **111**, 673–82.

Hölzle, E., Plewig, G., Hofmann, C. and Roser-Mass, E. (1982) Polymorphous light eruption. *Journal of the American Academy of Dermatology*, **7**, 111–25.

Hölzle, E. Plewig, G. and Lehmann, P. (1987) Photodermatoses – diagnostic procedures and their interpretation. *Photodermatology*, **4**, 109–14.

Horio, T. (1978) Photoallergic urticaria induced by visible light. *Archives of Dermatology*, **114**, 1761–4.

Lehmann, P., Hölzle, E., King, P., Georz, G. and Plewig, G. (1990) Experimental reproduction of skin lesions in lupus erythematosus by UVA and UVB radiation. *Journal of the American Academy of Dermatology*, **22**, 181–7.

Mackenzie, L.A. (1983) The analysis of the ultraviolet radiation doses required to produce erythemal responses in normal skin. *British Journal of Dermatology*, **108**, 1–9.

McFadden, N. and Larsen, T.E. (1986) Polymorphous light eruption: the properties of a UVA-induced PMLE patient group. *Photodermatology*, **3**, 36-40.

Miyamoto, C. (1989) Polymorphous light eruption: successful reproduction of skin lesions, including papulovesicular light eruption, with ultraviolet B. *Photodermatology*, **6**, 69–79.

Neumann, R.A., Pohl-Markl, H. and Knobler, R.M. (1987) Polymorphous light eruption: experimental reproduction of skin lesions by whole-body UVA irradiation. *Photodermatology*, **4**, 252–6.

Quinn, A.G., Diffey, B.L., Craig, P.S. and Farr, P.M. (1994) Definition of the minimal erythema dose used for diagnostic phototesting. *British Journal of Dermatology*, **131** (Suppl 44), 56.

Rhodes, L.E. and Friedmann, P.S. (1992) A comparison of the ultraviolet B-induced erythemal response of back and buttock skin. *Photodermatology, Photoimmunology and Photomedicine*, **9**, 48–51.

Sunohara, A., Mizuno, N., Sakai, M., Kawabe, Y. and Sakakibara, S. (1988) Action spectrum for UV erythema and reproduction of the skin lesions in hydroa vacciniforme. *Photodermatology*, **5**, 139–45.

APPENDIX B
PHOTOPATCH TESTING OF THE SKIN

Ian R. White

TYPES OF REACTION

Photosensitivity reactions caused by cutaneous exposure to or the ingestion of certain substances are of four types:

- contact (topical) photoallergic;
- contact (topical) phototoxic;
- systemic photoallergic;
- systemic phototoxic.

The first two types occur when the photoreactivity is caused by topical (contact) exposure to an agent and the latter two types by systemic absorption of an agent. Systemic reactivity is most commonly attributable to drug ingestion and topical phototoxicity to plants (phytophototoxic). Photopatch testing is primarily a tool for evaluating the reactions caused by contact photoallergens.

In considering photocontact reactions, the appreciation of the condition of chronic actinic dermatitis (CAD) is important. This condition presents with chronic eczematous changes on light-exposed areas with or without spread elsewhere. There are abnormal monochromatic irradiation skin tests, with reduced minimal erythema doses (MEDs) to UVB irradiation and often to longer wavelengths. Within the spectrum of CAD are the self-perpetuating persistent, light-related eczematous disorders, including those following or associated with photoallergic contact dermatitis, contact dermatitis and photosensitivity associated with systemic medication leading to presumed persistent photosensitivity from endogenous photoallergen (Norris and Hawk, 1990). In particular, persistent light reactivity (PLR) is that subgroup of CAD in which there is evidence of hypersensitivity to an apparently relevant photoallergen but to which there is no apparent current exposure.

CONTACT PHOTOALLERGENS

Numerous contact photoallergens have been described. However, in most instances, reports that substances may be photoallergens have been poorly documented or have been only rarely and sporadically observed as such. A comprehensive list of such reported topical photoallergens has been published (De Groot *et al.*. 1994), but this is not a critical review and it is probable that many are errors.

PHOTOALLERGENS IN PERSPECTIVE

Only a small number of substances have been responsible for the majority of cases of contact photoallergy. In the decade before 1975, the halogenated salicylanilides, used as antibacterial agents in soaps for instance, caused an epidemic of photosensitivity reactions. This problem was first identified by Wilkinson (1962), who described the clinical sign of sparing of a small area of skin behind the ears in those photosensitive individuals with eczematous changes on their faces, a sign known as Wilkinson's triangle. Once halogenated salicylanilides had been removed from the domestic environment, this epidemic settled, although a very few affected individuals have remained with the PLR form of CAD.

In 1978 musk ambrette, used mainly as a fragrance fixative in toiletries, was identified as a photoallergen by Larsen. During the next few years, musk ambrette became an important and common photoallergen, with allergic contact dermatitis also occurring. Following the identification of the problem and the lowering of the quantities of musk ambrette in toiletries, the incidence of new cases of musk ambrette photosensitivity fell dramatically. Use of musk ambrette is now prohibited by law in Europe and most other major markets, although it is still widely used in some Asian countries, with large quantities continuing to be exported from China.

In more recent years there has been appreciable population exposure to ultraviolet (UV) radiation-screening agents, brought about by the greater use of such preparations as the cutaneous photocarcinogenic and photoageing potential of sunlight has been realized by the public. Contact and photocontact sensitivity to these organic UV filters became a problem as a result, but again, once those agents responsible for the majority of adverse reactions were identified, they were removed from the market.

In Europe and the USA contact photoallergy is now rare and legislation requires manufacturers to evaluate the safety of substances before marketing. The stringent guidelines for such evaluation now ensure that it is unlikely that significant photoallergens will again enter the consumer market.

MUSK AMBRETTE

Musk ambrette was used extensively as a fragrance enhancer in many perfumed toiletries and in high concentrations (up to 4%) in aftershaves. It was also present in other products such as soaps, hair sprays, furniture polish and in fruit-flavoured edibles such as

yoghurts and sweets. Under the recommendations of the International Fragrance Research Association (FRA), the concentrations used, especially in male toiletries, were reduced and it was then prohibited altogether. Paralleling the reduction in population exposure, there was a rapidly reducing incidence of musk ambrette photosensitivity and new cases should not now occur in Europe or the USA.

Other so-called nitromusks, musk tibetine, musk xylene, musk ketone and moskene are not photosensitizing in the same way as musk ambrette and crossreactions to these are not frequent (Cronin, 1984).

Musk ambrette typically caused photosensitivity in males and different clinical types occurred (Cronin, 1984), the majority of patients presenting with patches of eczema on their faces where aftershaves had been patted on to cheeks and chin; fewer presented with more widespread eczema on the light-exposed areas and the appearances of CAD.

Although the majority of the affected subjects experienced clearance of their skin condition once any obvious contact with musk ambrette had ceased, in a few cases, even after the careful removal of known sources, even connubial (LeRoy and Dompmartin, 1989), of musk ambrette from the environment, there was a persistence of the photoreactivity. Such musk ambrette-related CAD has been treated by photoprotection, PUVA (Lindberg *et al.*, 1986), azathioprine (Cirne de Castro *et al.*, 1986) and cyclosporin.

UV RADIATION-ABSORBING AGENTS

Population exposure to organic UV radiation-absorbing agents has increased considerably recently, with a consequent increase in the number of adverse reactions (Thune, 1984). In addition, the incorporation of UV radiation absorbers into toiletries, to increase their shelf life by protecting against photodegradation (English *et al.*, 1987), has magnified the problem.

The main groups of UV absorbers are para-aminobenzoic acid (PABA) and its derivatives, cinnamates, benzophenones and dibenzoylmethanes, the last of these, with excellent long-wave UV radiation-absorbing properties, being particularly popular in Europe (English and White, 1986; Schauder and Ippen, 1986, 1988).

UV radiation-absorbing agents can cause an allergic or photoallergic contact dermatitis presenting acutely and having the features of allergic contact dermatitis associated with the more common allergens. However, because UV radiation-screening cosmetics are generally applied liberally to the skin before exposure to sunlight, such photoallergic contact reactions to the UV radiation-absorbing substance may be misinterpreted as an idiopathic light sensitivity response. Additionally, other individuals using sunscreens to treat an idiopathic photodermatosis may secondarily acquire allergy or photoallergy to the UV radiation-absorbing substance, which may then exacerbate the pre-existing condition. Such an example has been demonstrated in a case of photoallergy to 2-ethoxy-p-methoxycinnamate in an Asian who regularly used the screen but who had CAD as well and previously documented negative photopatch tests (Murphy and White, 1987). In such cases, the sunscreen may appear to cause an undue persistence of the light-related dermatosis.

In the past, care was also necessary in the evaluation of contact and photocontact reactions to some UV radiation-absorbing substances and especially to PABA and its derivatives, some of these reactions being caused by contaminants in the product (Bruze *et al.*, 1988).

DIAGNOSTIC DIFFICULTIES

Chronic eczema of the light-exposed areas may be due to true, so-called idiopathic CAD or to other factors. Musk ambrette reactions, for example, can present with a pattern of photosensitivity identical to such idiopathic

light sensitivity. More commonly, however, a chronic eczema of the exposed area is not due to photosensitivity but to airborne contact allergy. This may be seen, for instance, with phosphorus sesquisulphide present in some matches but more globally with Compositae (Asteraceae) dermatitis. Airborne allergic contact dermatitis characteristically involves the eyelids and extends to involve the skin under the chin and behind the ears, but this is not always so; conversely, in CAD there may be involvement of these shaded areas, although they are typically spared in these light-related conditions.

COMPOSITAE

Allergic contact dermatitis to Compositae can mimic CAD morphologically (English *et al.*, 1989; Hjorth *et al.*, 1976) while in addition, both these conditions are worse in the summer months when there is increased exposure to both sunlight and Compositae allergens. Further, it is accepted that Compositae sensitivity predisposes to the development of photosensitivity (Frain-Bell and Johnson, 1979) and the clinical evolution of this process has been described (Murphy *et al.*, 1990a).

Patch testing with the leaves or flowers of a Compositae plant will not always detect Compositae dermatitis because of variations of content of the allergens between species and seasonal differences. On the other hand, occlusive patch tests performed with some commercially available oleoresin extracts have caused false-positive irritant reactions, while open tests with these allergens have given false-negative results.

However, the development of a sesquiterpene lactone mix by Ducombs and Benezra (Ducombs *et al.*, 1990) has now given reliability in the detection of Compositae sensitivity. This preparation consists of a 0.1% dilution of an equal mixture of alantolactone, costunolide and dehydrocostuslactone, the latter two substances appearing to be most important, and is not irritant nor likely to produce active sensitization at this concentration. As an alternative, 1% costus oil may also detect the majority of Compositae-sensitive individuals, but contains a variable amount of allergen and may be sensitizing. A Compositae mix has also been developed by Hausen (Wrangsjö *et al.*, 1990) and contains the oleoresins of five species of Compositae.

PHOTOPATCH TESTING

There can be diagnostic difficulties between allergic contact dermatitis, photoallergic contact dermatitis and photodermatoses of the CAD type. The purpose of this protocol for photopatch testing is therefore to provide an adequate screen for those allergens which can mimic photoallergic reactions, as well as to detect true photoallergens.

CHANGES IN IMPORTANCE OF PHOTOALLERGENS

There are both temporal and geographic variations in those photoallergens to which an individual is likely to be exposed. For example, new cases of halogenated salicyl-anilide photosensitivity amongst the UK general population should not occur, as this agent has not been available for over two decades. However, such compounds may still be in use in some developing countries and the possibility remains of contact with them in imported goods. There has also been a dramatic fall in the number of new cases of photoallergy to musk ambrette, while banning of 6-methylcoumarin from fragrances has in addition removed exposure to this photoallergen. In the UK, photocontact dermatitis to the antimicrobial agent Fentichlor has not been reported as a result of domestic exposure for over a decade (Norris *et al.*, 1988), but current domestic use in Scandinavia has led to recent photoallergy to it in these countries. Further, adverse reactions to organic UV radiation-absorbing

compounds have steadily increased as population exposure has increased, varying with changes in popularity from country to country and season to season. However, selection of less sensitizing agents has led to a decrease in the frequency of reactions.

Because of these temporal and geographical factors, there can be no single, simple series of allergens which is a comprehensive screen for photoallergy in all countries, while on the other hand an excessively extensive series may be appropriate for use in specialized centres only.

STANDARD LIGHT ('PHOTOPATCH' TEST) SERIES

In Scandinavia, a series of allergens for use in photopatch testing has been agreed which suited their circumstances (Jansén *et al.*, 1982) and results from this series have been published (Thune *et al.*, 1988). In Germany, on the other hand, a different series of allergens was developed (Hölzle *et al.*, 1987) and in the USA a further series again (DeLeo and Harber, 1986). Finally, at the St John's Institute of Dermatology in the United Kingdom, the photopatch test series is regularly reviewed and changed at intervals as appropriate. The current series now appears to suit the United Kingdom domestic exposure to photoallergens, as well as detecting those allergens which may mimic photosensitivity or should be considered in the evaluation of an eczema of the light-exposed areas (Table B.1).

A working party of the British Photodermatology Group has also established an appropriate core list of photoallergens for routine testing (Table B.2) (Ibbotson *et al.*, 1997).

UVA DOSE

As a rule, photoallergens are active in the UVA region (310–400 nm), but there are rare exceptions in this and sulphanilamide and diphenhydramine are examples of compounds with action spectra involving the

Table B.1 St John's Institute of Dermatology scheme of allergens for photopatch testing

Not for irradiation
Extended European standard series of contact allergens
A series of facial and cosmetic contact allergens
Light series
Drugs, as appropriate: suitable dilution
Other contact substances, as appropriate: suitable dilution
Patient's own products, as appropriate: suitable dilution

For irradiation (light series)

Musk ambrette	5% pet.
Para-aminobenzoic acid (PABA)	10% pet.
Butylmethoxydibenzoylmethane (Parsol 1789)	10% pet.
Isoamyl-4-methoxycinnamate	10% pet.
2-Ethyl-4-dimethyl-aminobenzoate	10% pet.
Octylmethoxycinnamate (Parsol MCX)	10% pet.
2-Phenyl-5-benzimidazole sulphonic acid	10% pet.
Benzophenone-3 (oxybenzone)	10% pet.
3-(4-Methylbenzylidene)-camphor	10% pet.
Drugs, as appropriate: suitable dilution	
Other contact substances, as appropriate: suitable dilution	
Patient's own products, as appropriate: suitable dilution	

Table B.2 British Photodermatology Group core list of photocontact allergens

PABA (para-aminobenzoic acid)	5 or 10% pet.
Octyldimethyl PABA	2 or 10% pet.
Octylmethoxycinnamate (Parsol MCX)	2 or 10% pet.
Benzophenone-3 (oxybenzone)	2 or 10% pet.
Butylmethoxydibenzoylmethane (Parsol 1789)	2 or 10% pet.
Musk ambrette	1 or 5% pet.
Patient's own products (dilute as appropriate)	

UVB. For normal investigations, however, UVA is used for photopatch testing.

There are significant differences in opinion as to the amount (dose, measured in J/cm^2) of UVA radiation considered appropriate for use during photopatch testing for the successful elicitation of allergic photocontact reactions.

In Scandinavia, a $5 J/cm^2$ dose of UVA has been recommended, or one half a minimal erythema dose (MED) of UVA, whichever is the smaller. In Düsseldorf, Germany, $10 J/cm^2$ has been used while in the USA, a range of $5-15 J/cm^2$ has been suggested but $10 J/cm^2$ has been usual. At St John's Institute of Dermatology, $5 J/cm^2$ is now used for routine photopatch testing but this may be reduced for individuals with a known or presumed low MED or increased for dark-skinned subjects; $5 J/cm^2$ has also been recommended by the British Photodermatology Group.

The dermatologist undertaking photopatch testing generally does not know the MED of his patients, which is usually not of absolute importance. However, exposure to $5 J/cm^2$ of UVA can give a very severe sunburn-type reaction on the exposed skin of very light-sensitive individuals and if such sensitivity seems possible, the UVA MED can be determined beforehand by irradiating defined small areas of the skin of the back in sequence with increasing doses of UVA from the same light source as that to be used for the photopatch testing.

In the series reported by Cronin (1984) the photoallergic contact reactions to musk ambrette were elicited by 1 J/cm² of the UVA, while the previously mentioned photoallergic contact reaction to 2-ethoxy-p-methoxycinnamate (English *et al.*, 1987) in an Asian was elicited by 2 J/cm² of UVA. Further, the threshold dose of UVA to produce a photoallergic contact reaction to isopropyl dibenzoylmethane was also 2 J/cm² as determined by incremental exposure from 0.5 to 5 (Murphy *et al.*, 1990b). Finally, Wennersten *et al.* (1986) commented that many of the reactions obtained to phenothiazines during photopatch testing in their clinics with 5 J/cm² UVA may have been phototoxic at that dose rather than photoallergic, while there is also some evidence that irradiation with more than 5 J/cm² may not increase the rate of detection of true photoallergic responses in any case.

Recommended UVA dose

Although there still needs to be a thorough evaluation of the optimum UVA exposure dose to elicit photoallergic patch test responses reliably in sensitized individuals, it seems appropriate to suggest that 5 J/cm² is normally suitable. However, 0.5 MED dose should be given when the degree of photosensitivity is exquisite.

Source of UVA

Any artificial source of light with a broad spectral UVA output is suitable for photopatch testing, small units such as those used for hand and foot PUVA being an example. If significant UVB is present in the output, however, this needs to be filtered.

The energy output of the light source chosen must be measured initially and monitored at intervals to detect any fluctuation. The Waldmann Lichttechnik UV meter may serve, for example, as a standard monitoring device, although other such devices may also be used. At St John's Institute of Dermatology, the light source is a bank of Philips TL-44D

25/09 fluorescent tubes, while the Philips TLK 40W/09N fluorescent tube is also free from UVB contamination.

ALLERGEN APPLICATION AND READINGS: RECOMMENDED METHODS

Normally, individuals investigated by photopatch testing should also be patch tested with a standard general series of contact allergens, with a series of allergens which may cause contact reactions on the face and with any skin care products being used, if appropriate. Patch testing to such allergens may be undertaken at the same time as the photopatch testing. Substances for photopatch testing, the so-called photo or light series, are applied in duplicate as parallel series on either side of the back. Additional substances, where relevant, for such testing may include drugs such as thiazide diuretics (White, 1983), benzydamine (Frosch and Weickel, 1989) and occupational contactants such as thiourea, used as an antioxidant in photocopy paper (Dooms-Goossens *et al.*, 1987).

After two days, the sites are examined for reactions, which are then recorded in the usual fashion. The light series which is not for irradiation is then masked with opaque material and the second irradiated with UVA and covered with opaque material; in temperate climates, however, it may not be necessary in practical terms to re-cover the allergens for this second two-day period. After a further two days, the opaque covers are removed and any reactions again recorded.

Some variations on this scheme are used. For example, the sites for irradiation may be occluded with the allergen for one day only while the readings may also be undertaken at a different time (Hölzle *et al.*, 1987) and there is no evidence that this decreased time of occlusion affects detection of any photoallergens. It does, however, permit readings one day after irradiation, which may show early photoreactions, and a three-day postirradiation reading, at which time any photoallergic reactions may conceivably be more obvious. In addition, to produce positive photopatch test reactions to methylcoumarin, the substance must be applied shortly before irradiation.

PHOTOSCARIFICATION TEST

If penetration of photopatch test substances through the stratum corneum is likely to be poor, then increased penetration may be obtained by first scarifying or tape-stripping the skin (Hölzle *et al.*, 1987).

INTERPRETATION OF RESULTS

No reaction at an unirradiated site with a reaction at the equivalent irradiated site signifies a photoallergic response, while equal reactions at both sites are interpreted as contact allergy alone. Reactions at both sites but with the irradiated site showing a significantly greater reaction suggests that contact and photocontact allergy to the same substance co-exist. A marginal reaction or a marginally greater reaction at the exposed site may perhaps be a phototoxic response.

Although positive photoallergic contact reactions are usually quite definite, it may sometimes be necessary, as with ordinary patch testing, to differentiate between toxic and allergic reactions. One method is to undertake the test again with a serial dilution series of the suspected photoallergen while also varying the irradiation dose, a technique called photopatch test mapping (Takashima *et al.*, 1991). A positive response at a very low concentration or irradiation dose then points to photoallergy rather than phototoxicity.

REFERENCES

Bruze, M., Gruvberger, B. and Thune, P. (1988) Contact and photocontact allergy to glyceryl para-aminobenzoate. *Photodermatology*, **5**, 162–5.

Cirne De Castro, J.L., Pereira, M.A., Prates Nunes, F. and Pereira dos Santos, A. (1986) Successful treatment of a musk ambrette sensitive persistent light reactor with azathioprine. *Photodermatology*, **3**, 241–2.

Cronin, E. (1984) Photosensitivity to musk ambrette. *Contact Dermatitis*, **11**, 88–92.

De Groot, A.C., Weyland, J.W. and Nater J.P. (1994) *Unwanted Effects of Cosmetics and Drugs Used in Dermatology*, 3rd edn, Elsevier, Amsterdam, pp. 136–54.

DeLeo, V.A. and Harber, L.C. (1986) Contact photodermatitis, in *Contact Dermatitis*, (ed. A.A. Fisher), Lea and Febiger, Philadelphia, p. 465.

Dooms-Goossens, A., Chrispels, M.T., De Veylden, H. *et al.* (1987) Contact and photocontact sensitivity problems associated with thiourea and its derivatives: a review of the literature and case reports. *British Journal of Dermatology*, **116**, 573–9.

Ducombs, G., Benezra, C., Talaga, P. *et al.* (1990) Patch testing with the "sesquiterpene lactone mix": a marker for contact allergy to Compositae and other sesquiterpene lactone-containing plants. *Contact Dermatitis*, in press.

English, J.S.C. and White, I.R. (1986) Allergic contact dermatitis from isopropl dibenzoylmethane. *Contact Dermatitis*, **15**, 94.

English, J.S.C., White, I.R. and Cronin, E. (1987) Sensitivity to sunscreens. *Contact Dermatitis*, **17**, 159–62.

English J.S.C., Norris, P., White, I. and Cronin, E. (1989) Variability in the clinical patterns of Compositae dermatitis. *British Journal of Dermatology*, **121** (suppl 34), 27.

Frain-Bell, W. and Johnson, B.E. (1979) Contact sensitivity to chrysanthemum and the photosensitivity dermatitis and actinic reticuloid syndrome. *British Journal of Dermatology*, **101**, 491–501.

Frosch, P.J. and Weickel, R. (1989) Photokontaktallergie durch Benzydamin (Tantum). *Hautarzt*, **40**, 771–3.

Hjorth, N., Roed-Petersen J. and Thomson K. (1976) Airborne contact dermatitis from Compositae oleoresins stimulates photodermatitis. *British Journal of Dermatology*, **95**, 613–20.

Hölzle, E., Plewig, G. and Lehmann, P. (1987) Photodermatoses – diagnostic procedures and their interpretation. *Photodermatology*, **4**, 109–14.

Ibbotson, S.H., Farr, P.M., Beck, M. *et al.* (1997) Photopatch testing: methods and indications. *British Journal of Dermatology*,

Jansén, C.J., Wennersten, G., Rystedt, I., Thune, P. and Brodthagen, H. (1982) The Scandinavian standard photopatch test procedure. *Contact Dermatitis*, **8**, 155–8.

Larsen, W. (1978) *Photoallergy to Musk Ambrette Found in Aftershave Lotion.* Presented at the American Academy of Dermatology Meeting, San Francisco.

LeRoy, D. and Dompmartin, A. (1989) Connubial photosensitivity to musk ambrette. *Photodermatology*, **6**, 137–9.

Lindberg, L., Larkö, O. and Roupe, G. (1986) Successful PUVA treatment for musk ambrette induced persistent light reaction. *Photodermatology*, **3**, 111–12.

Murphy, G.M. and White, I.R. (1987) Photoallergic contact dermatitis to 2-ethoxy-p-methoxycinnamate. *Contact Dermatitis*, **16**, 296.

Murphy, G.M., White, I.R. and Hawk, J.L.M. (1990a) Allergic airborne contact dermatitis to Compositae with photosensitivity – chronic actinic dermatitis in evolution. *Photodermatology*, **7**, 38–9.

Murphy, G.M., White, I.R. and Cronin, E. (1990b) Immediate and delayed photocontact dermatitis to isopropyl dibenzoylmethane. *Contact Dermatitis*, **22**, 129–31.

Norris, P.G. and Hawk, J.L.M. (1990) Chronic actinic dermatitis: a unifying concept. *Archives of Dermatology* **126**, 376–8.

Norris, P., Hawk, J.L.M. and White, I.R. (1988) Photoallergic contact dermatitis from Fentichlor. *Contact Dermatitis*, **18**, 318–20.

Schauder, S. and Ippen, H. (1986) Photoallergic and allergic contact dermatitis from dibenzoylmethanes. *Photodermatology*, **3**, 140–7.

Schauder, S. and Ippen, H. (1988) Lichtschutzfilterhaltige Präparate in der Bundesrepublik Deutschland 1988. *Zeitschrift für Hautkrankheiten*, **63**, 707–63.

Takashima, A., Yamatoto, K., Kimura, S., Takakuwa, Y. and Mizuno, N. (1991) Allergic contact and photocontact dermatitis due to psoralens in patients with psoriasis treated with topical PUVA. *British Journal of Dermatology*, **124**, 37–42.

Thune, P. (1984) Contact and photocontact allergy to sunscreens. *Photodermatology*, **1**, 5–9.

Thune, P., Jansen, C., Wennersten, G. *et al.* (1988) The Scandinavian multicenter photopatch study (1980-85) – final report. *Photobiology*, **5**, 261–9.

Wennersten, G., Thune, P., Jansen, C.T. and Brodthagen, H. (1986) Photocontact dermatitis: current status with emphasis on allergic contact photosensitivity (CPS) occurrence, allergens, and practical phototesting. *Seminars in Dermatology*, **5**, 277–89.

White, I.R. (1983) A positive photopatch test with hydrochlorothiazide. *Contact Dermatitis*, **9**, 237.

Wilkinson, D.S. (1962) Patch test reactions to certain halogenated salicylanilides. *British Journal of Dermatology*, **74**, 302–6.

Wrangsjö, K., Ros A.M. and Wahlberg J.E. (1990) Contact allergy to Compositae plants in patients with summer exacerbating dermatitis. *Contact Dermatitis*, **22**, 148–54.

APPENDIX C
BASIC GUIDELINES ON THE ESTABLISHMENT OF A UVB/PUVA TREATMENT CENTRE

Charles R. Taylor and Bernhard Ortel

This appendix provides a brief summary of practical information relating to the creation of a phototherapy and photochemotherapy treatment centre. Discussed sequentially are the three basic requirements of every centre, namely space, equipment and staff.

SPACE

LOCATION

To be successful, a UVB/PUVA treatment facility should be centrally located so as to draw upon considerable numbers of patients, affiliation with a university hospital usually guaranteeing such referrals. Within the hospital itself, the unit should be located near both inpatient and outpatient units. Further, because of the importance of patient privacy and the risk of inadvertent additional ultraviolet exposure, it could be argued that the centre might be more safely situated in an area of the building with few or no windows, although the need for adequate ventilation dictates proximity to a proper system of heat evacuation. Access to a 220-volt power supply is also necessary for most phototherapy units.

ACCESSIBILITY

The centre should be readily accessible to public transport and since the demand for treatments is highest at the beginning and end of the standard work day, a centre only open from 9 am to 5 pm is less useful for most patients than one providing a service both before and after work hours and at weekends. Handicapped access is also an important issue so if the centre is not on the ground floor, access by means of a lift is essential.

DESIGN

Waiting area

Ideally, the treatment centre should contain a patient waiting area immediately adjacent to the treatment room itself. As patients may not arrive on time, and treatment units may not be immediately available for use, this space should be comfortable with adequate incandescent lighting, regularly updated magazines, waste receptacles and coat hooks. Piped-in soft music may also be considered to soothe those who are anxious, angry or impatient. This waiting area should be easily monitored visually from the treatment room, for example, through a counter window through which patient and technician can communicate. Educational signs may also serve a critical role in the waiting area, for example, reminding patients to inform their physicians or nurses of any new medications commenced since their last treatment or reinforcing the need for adequate eye protection.

Storage

Storage space will be needed for the supplies required by the unit such as theatre gowns, goggles, towels, emollients, spare bulbs, pillow cases (useful for head cover) and total sunblock or plasters (for nipple or mole protection). Because the main hospital charts may not be available as often as needed, separate records for the phototherapy treatments should also usually be kept on site. If necessary, a copy of the treatment record can be periodically forwarded to the main hospital records.

Treatment area

One of the first decisions to be made concerns the number of units the centre must purchase. As a rough guideline, each treatment unit can handle approximately one patient every 15 minutes and an estimate of patient numbers to be handled must therefore be made early.

Most stand-up light treatment boxes need space of about 3×2.7 m to allow for the unit itself (about 1.7×1.7 m) and an adjacent area for the patient to change (about 1.3×1 m) which should be equipped with a small stool for the patient to sit on, hooks for clothing, a mirror, paper towels and a wastebasket. A hand and foot unit requires approximately 1.7×1.3 m while a lie-down unit needs an area of about 3.3×2.3 m. This last unit, which takes up a lot of space, is nevertheless useful for patients who cannot stand for the treatment duration, but may be cost effective only in a large, busy referral centre. Each treatment unit needs its own separate, self-contained space.

In order to shield the operator and provide privacy for each patient, drapes must be suspended from the ceiling to the floor between each unit; however, to ensure sufficient circulation of air throughout the treatment centre, space should be left at the top and bottom of each curtain, always provided that the patient is afforded complete privacy and that those outside the unit are protected from stray radiation. Alternatively, fixed walls and doors may be used, again leaving enough overhead and floor clearance for air circulation, but hinged changing room doors take up more space than folding doors or curtains.

Finally, the floors should be made of easy-to-clean, non slippery tiles or wood. If the floor colour is too dark, small accumulations of psoriatic scale are easily visible and our unit therefore has a tan floor tile that hides fallen scales fairly well while allowing for easy cleaning.

Special requirements

If bath PUVA and soaks are to be provided, additional allowance must be made for the necessary plumbing. In addition, patients certainly appreciate showering facilities to remove the oils used for UVB therapy or the perspiration which ensues during any long phototherapy treatment in hot weather.

EQUIPMENT

LIGHT SOURCES

There are many products available for use in a light treatment centre and while there have been few published direct comparisons, most such equipment has very similar features regarding safety and operation. Consequently, choice of equipment will depend primarily on the exact perceived need and available budget. With a knowledge of the centre's anticipated patient volume, one then needs to decide how many and what type of sources should be available. Choices include units that produce broad-band UVB, narrow-band UVB, broad-band UVA and combination UVB/UVA. The latter is mostly useful for atopic dermatitis while the broad-band UVA sources (for PUVA) have the widest established applicability to date.

The essential part of any treatment system is the type of lamp inside, namely a fluorescent or metal halide source. Most units employ the former, in which the intensity may be enhanced by increased tube length and the addition of internal reflectors. Such lamps are typically available in two, four and six foot long units which can be mounted in banks or cabinets designed specifically for phototesting or therapy. The number of bulbs in a unit is also important, fewer meaning longer treatment times.

So-called standard UVB fluorescent bulbs have an emission spectrum from about 270 to 390 nm with a peak near 313, about 60% of the emission thus being UVB while the remainder is predominantly UVA. There is, however, some visible emission and a very small amount of UVC.

Through an alteration of the phosphor-filtering system, the Philips Lighting Company has now also developed a narrow-band fluorescent UVB lamp emitting almost exclusively at 310–313 nm. Although such lamps require a higher UV dosage, there is evidence that they are most effective and safer with less tendency to produce erythema than traditional broadband UVB bulbs and they have thus recently become favoured recently for several indications. Narrow-band UVB bulbs are currently slightly longer than the standard fluorescent bulbs used in full-body stand-up units in the United States and thus require a special unit in which to mount them; however, for European standards, such bulbs can be used interchangeably in existing treatment units.

UVA bulbs emit largely from 320 to 400 nm with about 5% of their output in UVB and less in the visible, most marketed lamps for PUVA having similar emission spectra such that the small differences that exist are probably not important in clinical practice. While many cabinets can accommodate either UVB or UVA bulbs, it is impractical to change the bulb type on a regular basis.

Some units are instead equipped with metal halide lamps, which provide an emission spectrum from 250 nm through to the visible spectrum. Filters are then utilized to restrict this emission to the UVB/UVA (> 295 nm) or UVA (> 315 nm). Because such lamps have a high irradiance, treatment times are shorter; however, their cost is slightly greater than that of fluorescent bulbs and they require manual changing of the filters for UVB/UVA to UVA treatment and vice versa.

Many treatment units come as a small cabinet with a door, while others consist of stand-up panels, sometimes hinged and on wheels to form an easily opened shell. Some patients find completely enclosed units claustrophobic and prefer them to be open at the top. Further, because of the heat generated by such units, those that are open at the top or air conditioned are most appreciated by patients. Lie-down units resemble a single bed with a hinged canopy top; bulbs are present in the bed portion and sometimes in the cover. Hand and foot units resemble a small player organ with receptacles for both hands and both feet, each having bulbs above and below, while most units for phototesting are mobile panels of usually fluorescent bulbs. Generally, in each case there is a small computer that regulates the function of the light unit, and ease of operation is usually the main criterion for choosing among the various unit types.

SAFETY ISSUES

To protect the patient from accidental laceration due to bulb breakage, many units have Teflon sleeves over the bulbs, which are already enclosed behind a wire mesh. For additional safety, stand-up units should also have a rail for patients to hold on to, a UV-opaque window through which the operator can observe the patient and a dual time alarm system in case one timer malfunctions.

Eye protection is critical for patients undergoing therapy and a routine question for the operator to ask of each patient before operating the start button is whether the patient has goggles on. Large wraparound goggles offer the best protection but result in untanned periorbital rings if the face receives treatment; thus patients receiving facial exposure usually prefer small, tightly fitting goggles.

STAFF

TRAINING

All supervising physicians, nurses and other operators must receive careful instruction in the various treatment protocols. Nurses make ideal staff for delivering phototherapy because they are already well versed in the skills of patient communication and excellent at motivating patients to comply with the many safety and efficacy-oriented details. All staff should be trained in basic life support measures.

JOB SPECIFICS

Patients

Prior to the commencement of phototherapy, patients should sign an appropriate consent form, receive printed information and instructions concerning their therapy, receive protective goggles, have a negative circulating antinuclear factor titre recorded on file and, in the case of PUVA therapy, have baseline and yearly eye examinations. Those who administer the therapy should also ensure that all patients are seen regularly by a supervising doctor.

Equipment

To measure the irradiance of a phototherapy source, a device known as a **radiometer** is used. Typically, these are so-called vacuum diodes because they are cheaper and more durable than the other types. Such a device consists of a probe or sensor, placed within the irradiation field, and an electronic meter, which reports the irradiance in mW/cm^2. Either automatic radiometry by means of a probe built into the unit or regular but intermittent radiometry with a portable radiometer and separate probes for the different spectral bands is essential. When the latter technique is used, measurements should be taken daily when the bulbs are new and weekly once the readings have stabilized. Measurement conditions also need to be standardized, particularly with the probe being kept at a fixed distance from the bulbs. Thus, provided the technician is appropriately protected from UV light exposure, he or she can stand in the unit with the probe held successively toward each of the four sides of the lamp unit, an average reading then being taken. Automatic radiometry, on the other hand, has the disadvantage that the sensor may become dirty from dust or perspiration, thus underestimating the true exposure. In addition, patients may either inadvertently or intentionally block the probe, thus resulting in overexposure. Therefore, besides the periodic changing of the bulbs, ultraviolet radiation systems also need regular cleaning to remove the dust and psoriatic scale which rapidly accumulate within the unit.

Documentation

A dated log of the dosimetry measurements for each of the treatment units should be maintained, in which periodic changes of the bulbs and repairs should also be recorded. Meticulous record keeping regarding patient treatments is also essential and a flow sheet recording the treatment number and individual and cumulative regional doses (face, trunk, extremities) in both time and mJ/cm^2 or J/cm^2 is essential. In addition, a space for noting additional comments, such as whether the patient complained of itching or burning or had recently started a new medication, is also useful. Failure to attend for a regularly scheduled treatment should also be duly entered in the flow sheet, while the technician who administered any treatment should place his or her initials beside the treatment entry. Some centres may instead install a computer base for the ongoing recording of treatment numbers and cumulative doses per course. Such a system can serve as a database for studies and case records.

APPENDIX D
TESTING FOR THE CUTANEOUS PORPHYRIAS

George H. Elder

Confirmation or exclusion of the diagnosis of cutaneous porphyria is usually straightforward in a patient who presents with skin lesions suggestive of the disease, provided the required investigations are appropriately selected, correctly carried out and expertly interpreted. Whether these investigations are undertaken locally or at a specialist centre will depend on the degree of expertise required. Thus, the investigations for latent porphyria in asymptomatic relatives are often complex procedures and in this case are best referred.

This appendix focuses on three problems: the differentiation of a cutaneous porphyria from other similar disorders, the precise identification of that type of porphyria and the screening of relatives, where necessary, for latent porphyria. It thus emphasizes the need for careful selection of the appropriate tests in each case. The methods available for such testing have been reviewed (Bonkovsky and Barnard, 1997; Elder *et al.*. 1990; Kushner, 1991). The diagnostic criteria for the main types of cutaneous porphyria are shown in Table D.1, while full details of the patterns of haem precursor overproduction in these disorders and their uncommon variants are provided in Chapter 13.

SAMPLE SELECTION AND STABILITY

The selection of samples is determined by a patient's clinical presentation (Table D.2).

When the distinction between suspected erythropoietic protoporphyria (EPP) or a bullous porphyria is uncertain, urine should be collected in addition to ethylenediamine tetra-acetic acid (EDTA) anticoagulated blood. Cutaneous porphyria during childhood is unusual and always requires full investigation. The choice of samples for family screening depends on the type of porphyria under investigation; family studies should therefore not be undertaken until the diagnosis has been unequivocally established in the proband.

Porphyrins are reasonably stable in solution provided they are protected from light and oxidants. Porphobilogen (PBG) is less stable, however, and may polymerize rapidly to form uroporphyrin and various brownish-red pyrrolic pigments. Thus, fresh random samples of urine are more suitable than 24-hour collections for porphyria investigation: collection over 24 hours delays analysis and the expression of analyte concentration per mole of creatinine is preferable to that over time. Urine should be analysed for PBG and porphyrins, and faecal samples for porphyrins, as soon as practicable after collection, although concentrations are unlikely to change sufficiently over 48 hours to produce an incorrect diagnosis, particularly if the sample is kept in the dark at 4°C. However, very dilute urine samples with creatinine concentrations of less than 4 mmol/l are

Table D.1   Overproduction of haem precursors: minimum criteria for laboratory diagnosis of cutaneous porphyrias

Disorder	Plasma[1]	Erythrocytes	Urine	Faeces
Congenital erythropoietic porphyria (CEP)	615–620		Uroporphyrin I Coproporphyrin I	Coproporphyrin I
Porphyria cutanea tarda (PCT)	615–620		Uroporphyrins I and III Heptacarboxylic porphyrin	Isocoproporphyrin Heptacarboxylic porphyrin
Hereditary coproporphyria (HCP)	615–620		Coproporphyrin III Porphobilinogen[2]	Coproporphyrin III
Variegate porphyria (VP)	624–626		Coproporphyrin III Porphobilinogen[2]	Coproporphyrin III Protoporphyrin IX
Erythropoietic protoporphryia (EPP)	626–634	Protoporphyrin IX (not zinc chelate)		

See Chapter 13 for other abnormalities of overproduction of haem precursors in these conditions
[1] Porphyrin fluorescence emission maxima (nm)
[2] Usually normal in the absence of symptoms of acute porphyria

Table D.2   Samples required for diagnosis of the cutaneous porphyrias

Clinical presentation	Sample
1. Suspected bullous porphyria	
Adults	Fresh, random urine; EDTA blood **or** faeces[1]
Patients with chronic renal failure	EDTA blood; faeces
Children	Fresh, random urine; faeces; EDTA blood
2. Suspected erythropoietic protoporphyria	EDTA blood

EDTA: ethylenediamine tetra-acetic acid-anticoagulated.
EDTA blood is convenient for the analysis of plasma and erythrocyte porphyrins.
[1] Faecal samples are essential if plasma fluorescence analysis is not available and will be required in addition to EDTA blood if initial plasma and urinary investigations suggest porphyria but exclude porphyria cutanea tarda and variegate porphyria. Sample requirements for the methods cited in the text are 5 ml EDTA blood, 20 ml urine and 5–10 g (wet weight) faeces

unsuitable for analysis. Urine and faecal samples are stable for weeks at -20°C, while EDTA-anticoagulated blood samples kept in the dark show no loss of protoporphyrin for up to eight days at room temperature or for eight weeks at 8°C or lower (Chisholm and Brown, 1975). Thus, EDTA blood, urine and faecal samples can safely be sent to specialist laboratories at ambient temperature without additional preservatives provided they arrive within 24–48 hours of collection.

RECOMMENDED METHODS

The detection and measurement of porphyrins are based on their spectroscopic and solubility properties, the compounds having characteristic electronic absorption spectra with a strongly absorbing, so-called Soret peak at around 400 nm. Thus, irradiation at about this wavelength excites an intense red fluorescence at around 600 nm, the precise wavelengths of maximum absorption and emission for each porphyrin depending on the nature of the side chains, but such differences are not usually sufficient to allow accurate differentiation of the individual porphyrins in a mixture by spectroscopy alone. Current methods for the separation of individual porphyrins which depend on differences in their solubility that are determined mainly by the nature of their side chains. Solvent partition methods have been widely used for the fractionation of porphyrin mixtures; however, these fractions are rarely pure and the methods have therefore been largely replaced by chromatographic techniques, particularly thin-layer chromatography (TLC) and high-pressure liquid chromatography (HPLC).

PORPHYRINS IN PLASMA

Fluorescence emission spectroscopy is a specific and sensitive qualitative method for the detection of increased porphyrin concentrations in plasma (Long *et al.*, 1993; Poh-Fitzpatrick, 1980). With this technique, plasma is diluted 1:10 with phosphate-buffered saline and scanned between 550 nm and 650 nm at an excitation wavelength of 405 nm in a spectrofluorometer that should be fitted with a red-sensitive photomultiplier. The presence of porphyrin is then shown by an emission peak between 615 and 634 nm, depending on the type of porphyrin present (Fig. D.1). Ideally, the spectrofluorometer should be sufficiently sensitive to give a full-scale deflection when calibrated with 10 nmol/l of coproporphyrin in 1.5 M HCl, while it is also important first to establish criteria for a normal scan by running sufficient samples of normal plasma (Long *et al.*, 1993). Occasional samples show background levels because of the presence of interfering compounds. If doubt persists quantitative measurement of the total plasma porphyrin (Seubert *et al.*, 1985) may help, except in variegate porphyria (VP) where the porphyrin is bound to protein and thus difficult to quantify.

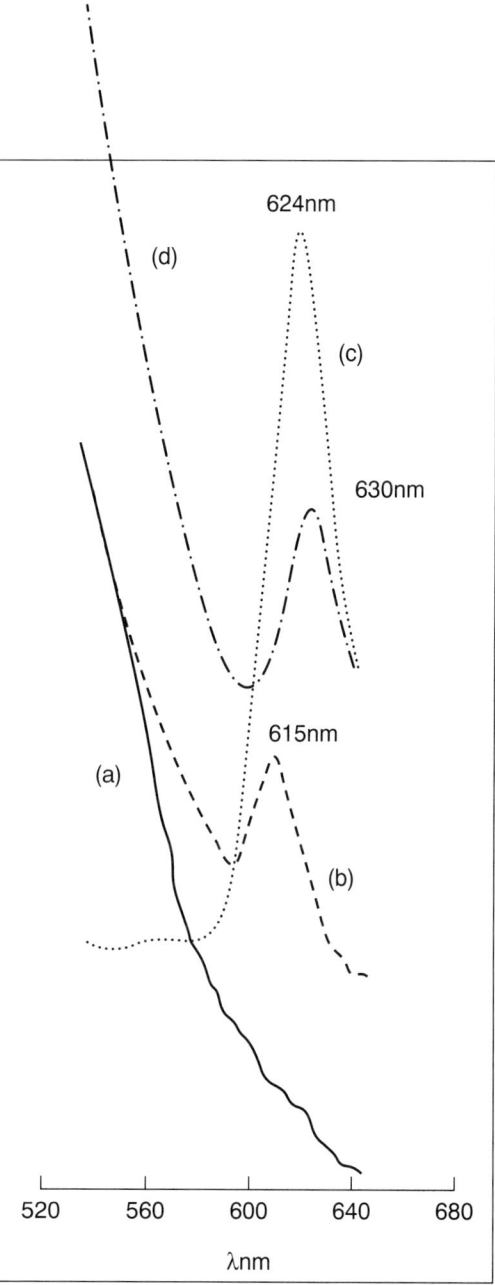

Figure D.1 Fluorescence emission spectra of plasma diluted ten-fold with phosphate-buffered saline. Plasma from normal subject (a) and from patients with porphyria cutanea tarda (b), variegate porphyria (c) and erythropoietic protoporphyria (d). Excitation was at 405 nm.

PORPHYRINS IN URINE

Qualitative screening tests for increased urinary porphyrin based on the examination of urine for red fluorescence by means of an ultraviolet lamp fitted with a Wood's filter, either directly or after concentration of the porphyrins by solvent extraction, are insensitive and should be replaced by quantitative spectrophotometric (Deacon, 1988; Jones and Sweeney, 1979) or fluorometric methods (Poulos and Lockwood, 1980; Westerlund et al., 1988). Thus, direct spectrophotometry of acidified urine with measurement of the Soret peak (Deacon, 1988, Elder et al., 1990) is a simple method sufficiently sensitive to detect porphyrin concentrations within the normal range. If suitable equipment is available, spectrofluorometry of acidified urine (Poulos and Lockwood, 1980) or derivative spectroscopy (Jones and Sweeney, 1979) are almost as simple and more accurate. The urinary acidification converts any porphyrinogens in the urine to porphyrins.

The measurement of urinary porphyrins after their separation is then necessary for differentiation of the cutaneous porphyrias (see Table D.1). However, solvent partition methods are cumbersome and do not provide sufficient separation and should therefore be replaced by TLC (Elder et al., 1990; Henderson, 1989) or HPLC, preferably the latter because it provides easier quantification, separates porphyrin isomers more easily and often requires less sample preparation. In particular, the ammonium acetate-organic modifier reverse-phase HPLC systems introduced by Lim and co-workers (Lim and Peters, 1984; Rossi and Curnow, 1986) are robust and provide complete separation of all the porphyrins of clinical importance, including the type I and III isomers.

PORPHYRIN PRECURSORS IN URINE

Measurement of the haem precursors PBG and aminolaevulinic acid (ALA) may be required for differentiation of the bullous porphyrias (see Table D.1) and since diagnostically significant increases in excretion may be below the limit of detection of the screening tests for PBG, their quantitative measurement is essential. Commercial kits based on the ion-exchange chromatographic methods of Mauzerall and Granick (1956) are available for both compounds.

PORPHYRINS IN FAECES

Qualitative screening tests for the assessment of increased faecal porphyrin concentrations based on solvent extraction techniques have been criticized as insensitive and difficult to interpret (Deacon, 1988). They should thus be replaced by a simple, quantitative test such as that described by Lockwood et al. (1985) for the measurement of total ether-soluble porphyrins. However, if the porphyrin concentration is to be expressed per unit dry weight, as recommended, the drying procedure needs to be carefully standardized. Fractionation of porphyrins may then be accomplished by TLC or HPLC. TLC requires prior methyl esterification of porphyrins and, as for urine, HPLC is the more convenient method. If the solvent system described above for urine is used, the porphyrin acid extract for the Lockwood procedure can be injected into the HPLC system without the need for further purification.

PORPHYRINS IN WHOLE BLOOD

A reliable, simple and rapid method for the detection of increased erythrocyte porphyrin concentrations is essential if EPP is not to be missed. Several quantitative, fluorometric micromethods fulfil these criteria (Chisholm and Brown, 1975; Piomelli, 1977). Qualitative methods based on solvent extraction followed by visual inspection for porphyrin fluorescence are likely to give false-negative results and should be discarded. Fluorescence microscopy of erythrocytes (Rimington and

Cripps, 1965), another diagnostic technique, is reliable only in expert centres and needs to be supported by quantification.

Quantitative fluorometric micromethods include an acid extraction stage which dissociates zinc from zinc-protoporphyrin. Thus, they measure the total porphyrin concentration and do not distinguish between the two forms of protoporphyrin, zinc-protoporphyrin and zinc-free protoporphyrin, that occur in erythrocytes. The two forms can be separated by HPLC (Rossi and Curnow, 1986) or the distinction made as satisfactorily and more easily by fluorescence emission spectroscopy of a neutral, ethanol extract of whole blood (Garden *et al.*, 1977) (Fig. D.2). This simple method therefore makes a very reliable screening test for EPP, which is excluded if zinc-protoporphyrin is the major component.

INTERPRETATION

ACUTE PHOTOSENSITIVITY

EPP is an uncommon cause of acute photosensitivity that may at times be difficult to distinguish clinically from commoner causes without laboratory investigation. The essential first investigation is measurement of the patient's erythrocyte porphyrin concentration (see Table D.1), a normal concentration excluding EPP, while if the concentration is increased, demonstration that most of the porphyrin is free protoporphyrin confirms the diagnosis. No further tests are required as other causes of raised protoporphyrin concentration, such as iron deficiency, increase zinc-protoporphyrin; on the other hand, iron deficiency may occasionally coincide with photosensitivity and misdiagnosis is avoided if the two forms of protoporphyrin are thus distinguished. A normal plasma fluorescence scan also provides strong evidence against EPP but in practice, erythrocyte porphyrin measurement is a more useful first test because, unlike plasma, the same sample can then be used to confirm the diagnosis.

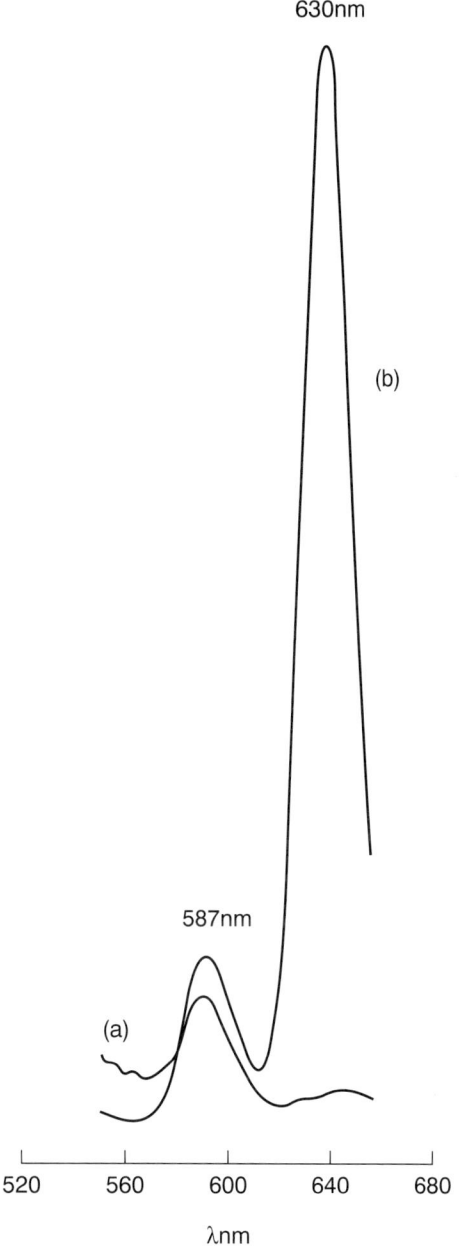

Figure D.2 Fluorescence emission spectra of ethanol extracts of whole blood from a normal subject (a) and patient with erythropoietic protoporphyria (b).

THE BULLOUS PORPHYRIAS

Most patients in this group have porphyria cutanea tarda (PCT), although its distinctive skin lesions and those of other bullous porphyrias (see Table D.1) are the same. The main problem is its differentiation from drug- or sunbed-induced pseudoporphyria and chronic renal failure, especially when treated by long-term haemodialysis, all of which have similar skin lesions.

Urine and either plasma or faecal samples should be obtained for the initial investigation, unless the patient has renal failure, which makes faecal analysis essential (see Table D.2). Plasma is otherwise more convenient than faeces, which are unlikely to be required unless the urine and plasma analyses exclude PCT. On the other hand, the diagnosis of PCT cannot be made unequivocally by either urinary porphyrin measurements or plasma fluorescence scanning alone; thus, some patients with VP have a urinary porphyrin pattern resembling that of PCT (see Chapter 13), while plasma scanning does not distinguish PCT from hereditary coproporphyria (HCP), congenital erythropoietic porphyria (CEP) or hepatoerythropoietic porphyria (HEP).

In a patient with active skin lesions, the demonstration of increased plasma and urinary porphyrin concentrations together provides very strong evidence for porphyria, the position of the plasma porphyrin fluorescence emission peak differentiating VP from the other bullous porphyrias (see Fig. D.1). Thus, a peak at 624–626 nm establishes VP, while peaks in the 615–620 nm region suggest PCT but do not distinguish it from the much less common conditions HCP, HEP and CEP, including its adult-onset form. Subsequent fractionation of the urinary porphyrins to show predominantly uroporphyrin and heptacarboxylic porphyrin, together with a plasma porphyrin fluorescent emission peak at 615–620 nm, however, confirms PCT in an adult (see Table D.1); in children, on the other

hand, measurement of erythrocyte uroporphyrinogen decarboxylase is necessary to distinguish PCT from HEP (see Chapter 13). Thereafter, further analysis of individual porphyrins in faeces, and of porphyrin precursors in the urine, is unlikely to change a diagnosis of PCT, VP or HEP based on this sequence of investigation. However, measurements of individual porphyrins and their isomers in faeces are essential to differentiate HCP from CEP (see Table D.1), if prior fractionation of the urinary porphyrins has not revealed a pattern typical of PCT in a patient with a plasma fluorescence emission peak at 615–620 nm.

Urinary total porphyrin concentrations may occasionally be normal in VP if skin lesions are healing or mild, but the plasma fluorescence scan is always diagnostic (Long *et al.*, 1993). In PCT, however, the reverse may occur as skin lesions heal; thus, urinary total porphyrin excretion may remain abnormal even when the raised plasma porphyrin concentration has settled. As remission progresses, the total urinary porphyrin levels then return to normal before the relative concentrations of the individual porphyrins. Thus, it may still be possible to make a diagnosis of PCT in a patient who has not been investigated until the skin lesions have healed, provided the urinary porphyrins are fractionated.

The usefulness of plasma porphyrin fluorescence scanning for the diagnosis of the bullous porphyrias has been emphasized above. If the method is not available, however, analysis of both urine and faeces is essential (see Table D.1) because if faecal analysis is omitted, VP and other bullous porphyrias may be mistaken for PCT.

The diagnosis of PCT in a patient with chronic renal failure may be difficult (see Table D.2), plasma uroporphyrin concentrations being increased in renal failure alone and sometimes overlapping the usually higher levels found when PCT is also present (Poh-Fitzpatrick *et al.*, 1982; Seubert *et al.*,

1985). In addition, urine is often unavailable and analysis of the faecal porphyrins is thus necessary to reveal the typical pattern of PCT (see Tables D.1 and D.2).

ABNORMAL PORPHYRIN EXCRETION NOT CAUSED BY PORPHYRIA

Abnormalities of porphyrin metabolism not caused by porphyria do not usually coincide with skin lesions but may occasionally cause diagnostic confusion. The commonest of these abnormalities is coproporphyrinuria secondary to alcoholism, cholestasis, drug intake and various other miscellaneous disorders (Bonkovsky and Barnard, 1998; Elder *et al.*, 1990). However, faecal porphyrin excretion is normal in these conditions, excluding all the bullous porphyrias, as is the plasma porphyrin fluorescence scan, unless cholestasis is severe. An increased concentration of faecal protoporphyrin and other dicarboxylic porphyrin without urinary, plasma or erythrocyte abnormalities is also occasionally found during the investigation of suspected cutaneous porphyria, the usual cause being minor gastrointestinal haemor-

rhage, including that caused by those non-steroidal anti-inflammatory agents that may also cause pseudoporphyria, with the subsequent conversion of haem to dicarboxylic porphyrins by gut bacteria. Tests for occult blood may, however, be negative, particularly if the bleeding occurs high in the gut. A high meat diet and certain dietary oddities, for example, the excessive consumption of brewers' yeast (Lim *et al.*, 1984), may have the same effect.

SCREENING OF FAMILIES FOR LATENT CUTANEOUS PORPHYRIA

Once the decision has been made to screen a family for latent porphyria (see Chapter 13), the next step is to establish unequivocally the diagnosis in the proband, since this then determines the choice of investigation. Such latent porphyria can be detected by metabolite measurements, enzyme assay or DNA analysis.

Metabolite measurements are useful initially, being fairly simple technically, but they have important limitations (Table D.3), their sensitivity being low and their values

Table D.3   Metabolic methods for detection of latent cutaneous porphyrias

Disorder	Metabolites	Limitation
Porphyria cutanea tarda (type II)	Uroporphyrin and heptacarboxylic porphyrin in urine; isocoproporphyrin in faeces	Low sensitivity
Hereditary coproporphyria	Coproporphyrin isomer III/I ratio in faeces[1]	Sensitivity high in adults; sensitivity in children not established
Variegate porphyria	Fluorescence emission spectroscopy of plasma[2]	Normal before puberty. Over the age of 15 years, sensitivity is 86% and the specificity 100%
	Faecal porphyrin analysis[2]	Normal before puberty. Over the age of 15 years, sensitivity is 36%
Erythropoietic protoporphyria	Erythrocyte free protoporphyrin	Low sensitivity

[1] Blake *et al.*, 1992
[2] Long *et al.*, 1993

Table D.4 Enzyme methods for detection of latent cutaneous porphyrias

Disorder	Enzyme measurement	Sample
Porphyria cutanea tarda (type II)	Uroporphyrinogen decarboxylase	Erythrocytes
Hereditary coproporphyria	Coproporphyrinogen oxidase	Lymphocytes (L, EBV-L); fibroblasts
Variegate porphyria	Protoporphyrinogen oxidase	Lymphocytes (L, EBV-L); fibroblasts
Erythropoietic protoporphyria	Ferrochelatase	Lymphocytes (L, EBV-L); fibroblasts

L, peripheral blood lymphocytes; L, EBV-L, Epstein–Barr virus-transformed lymphoblastoid cells

being normal before puberty in VP and HCP. Enzyme measurements, on the other hand, have the advantage that they are abnormal at all ages and, in theory, should distinguish clearly between affected and unaffected individuals; however, in practice there is overlap between the normal and abnormal ranges with most methods. Nevertheless, they are useful when metabolite measurements are normal and DNA methods not available (Kappas, *et al.*, 1995; Nordmann and Deybach, 1990). Table D.4 lists the enzyme methods and sample requirements for detection of the latent cutaneous porphyrias. DNA methods designed to detect a specific mutation are likely to become the investigations of choice for the detection of latent porphyria during the next few years. However, mutational analysis in all the inherited porphyrias is complicated by their extensive allelic heterogeneity, which in most countries makes it necessary to identify the causative mutation in each family. Nevertheless, DNA methods for the diagnosis of latent acute intermittent porphyria have now been established and validated (Puy *et al.*, 1997) and similar approaches are steadily becoming available for the inherited cutaneous porphyrias (Kirsch *et al.*, 1998; Elder, 1998).

REFERENCES

Blake, D., McManus, J., Cronin, V. *et al.* (1992) Fecal coproporphyrin isomers in hereditary coproporphyria. *Clinical Chemistry*, **38**, 96-100.

Bonkovsky, H. and Barnard, G. (1998) Diagnosis of porphyric syndromes. *Seminars in Liver Disease*, **18**, 57–66.

Chisholm, J.J. and Brown, D.H. (1975) Microscale photofluorometric determination of 'free erythrocyte porphyrin' (protoporphyrin IX). *Clinical Chemistry*, **21**, 1669–82.

Deacon, A.C. (1988) Performance of screening tests for porphyria. *Annals of Clinical Biochemistry*, **25**, 392–7.

Elder, G.H., Smith, S.G. and Smyth, S.J. (1990) Laboratory investigation of the porphyrias. *Annals of Clinical Biochemistry*, **27**, 395–412.

Elder, G.H. (1998) Genetic defects in the porphyrias. *Clinics in Dermatology*, **16**, 225–34.

Garden, J.S., Mitchell, D.G. and Jackson, K.W. (1977) Improved ethanol extraction procedure for determining zinc protoporphyrin in whole blood. *Clinical Chemistry*, **23**, 1585–9.

Henderson, M.J. (1989) Thin-layer chromatography of faecal porphyrins for the diagnosis of porphyria. *Clinical Chemistry*, **35**, 1043–4.

Jones, K.G. and Sweeney, G.D. (1979) Quantitation of urinary porphyrins by use of second derivative spectroscopy. *Clinical Chemistry*, **25**, 71–4.

Kappas, A., Sassa, S., Galbraigh, R.A. *et al.* (1995) The porphyrias, in *The Metabolic and Molecular Basis of Inherited Disease*, 7th edn, (eds C.R. Scriver, A.L. Beaudet, W.S. Sly *et al.*), McGraw-Hill, New York, pp. 2103–59.

Kirsch, R.E., Meissner, P.N. and Hijt, R.J. (1998) Variegate porphyria. *Seminars in Liver Disease*, **18**, 33–42.

Kushner, J.P. (1991) Laboratory diagnosis of the porphyrias. *New England Journal of Medicine*, **324**, 1432–4.

Lim, C.K. and Peters, T.J. (1984) Urine and faecal porphyrin profiles by reversed-phase high-performance liquid chromatography in the porphyrias. *Clinical Chemistry Acta*, **139**, 55–63.

Lim, C.K., Rideout, J.M. and Peters, T.J. (1984) Pseudoporphyria associated with consumption of brewer's yeast. *British Medical Journal*, **288**, 1640.

Lockwood, W.H., Poulos, V., Rossi, E. *et al.* (1985) Rapid procedure for fecal porphyrin assay. *Clinical Chemistry*, **31**, 1163–7.

Long, C., Smyth, S.J., Woolf, J. *et al.* (1993) Detection of latent variegate porphyria by fluorescence emission spectroscopy of plasma. *British Journal of Dermatology*, **129**, 9–13.

Mauzerall, D. and Granick, S. (1956) The occurrence and determination of δ-amino-levulinic acid and porphobilinogen in urine. *Journal of Biological Chemistry*, **219**, 435–6.

Nordmann, Y. and Deybach, J-C. (1990) Human hereditary porphyrias, in *Biosynthesis of Heme and Chlorophylls*, (ed. H.A. Dailey), McGraw-Hill, New York, pp. 491–542.

Piomelli, S. (1977) Free erythrocyte porphyrin in the detection of undue absorption of lead and of iron deficiency. *Clinical Chemistry*, **23**, 264–9.

Poh-Fitzpatrick, M.B. (1980) A plasma porphyrin fluorescence marker for variegate porphyria. *Archives of Dermatology*, **116**, 543–7.

Poh-Fitzpatrick, M.B., Sosin, A.E. and Bemis, J.(1982) Porphyrin levels in plasma and erythrocytes of chronic haemolysis patients.*Journal of the American Academy of Dermatology*, **7**, 100–4.

Poulos, V. and Lockwood, W.H. (1980) Direct spectrofluorometric determination of porphyrin in diluted urine. *International Journal of Biochemistry*, **12**, 1051–2.

Puy, H., Deybach, J.C., Lamoril, J. *et al.* (1997) Molecular epidemiology and diagnosis of PBG deaminase gene defects in acute intermittent porphyria. *American Journal of Human Genetics*, **60**, 1373–83.

Rimington, C. and Cripps, D.J. (1965) Biochemical and fluorescence-microscopy screening tests for erythropoietic protoporphyria. *Lancet*, **i**, 624–46.

Rossi, E. and Curnow, D.H. (1986) Porphyrins, in *Hplc of Small Molecules: A Practical Approach*, (ed. C.K. Lim), IRL Press, Oxford, pp. 261–303.

Seubert, S., Seubert, A., Rumpf, K.W. *et al.* (1985) A porphyria cutanea tarda-like distribution pattern of porphyrins in plasma, hemodialysate, hemofiltrate, and urine of patients on chronic haemodialysis. *Journal of Investigative Dermatology*, **85**, 107–9.

Westerlund, J., Pudek, M. and Schreiber, W.E. (1988) A rapid and accurate spectro-fluorometric method for quantification and screening of urinary porphyrins. *Clinical Chemistry*, **34**, 345–51.

INDEX

All entries which appear in *italic* refer to tables and entries in **bold** refer to illustrations.

24